T0226725

Upper Gastrointestinal Bleeding Management

Editor

JOHN R. SALTZMAN

GASTROINTESTINAL ENDOSCOPY CLINICS OF NORTH AMERICA

www.giendo.theclinics.com

Consulting Editor
CHARLES J. LIGHTDALE

July 2015 • Volume 25 • Number 3

ELSEVIER

1600 John F. Kennedy Boulevard • Suite 1800 • Philadelphia, Pennsylvania, 19103-2899

http://www.theclinics.com

GASTROINTESTINAL ENDOSCOPY CLINICS OF NORTH AMERICA Volume 25, Number 3
July 2015 ISSN 1052-5157, ISBN-13: 978-0-323-39098-9

Editor: Kerry Holland
Developmental Editor: Donald Mumford

Gastrointestinal Endoscopy Clinics of North America (ISSN 1052-5157) is published quarterly by Elsevier Inc., 360 Park Avenue South, New York, NY 10010-1710. Months of issue are January, April, July, and October. Business and Editorial Offices: 1600 John F. Kennedy Blvd., Suite 1800, Philadelphia, PA, 19103-2899. Periodicals postage paid at New York, NY and additional mailing offices. Subscription prices are $335.00 per year for US individuals, $486.00 per year for US institutions, $175.00 per year for US students and residents, $370.00 per year for Canadian individuals, $576.00 per year for Canadian institutions, $465.00 per year for international individuals, $576.00 per year for international institutions, and $245.00 per year for Canadian and foreign students/residents. To receive student/resident rate, orders must be accompanied by name of affiliated institution, date of term, and the *signature* of program/residency coordinator on institution letterhead. Orders will be billed at individual rate until proof of status is received. Foreign air speed delivery is included in all *Clinics* subscription prices. All prices are subject to change without notice. **POSTMASTER:** Send address change to *Gastrointestinal Endoscopy Clinics of North America*, Elsevier Health Sciences Division, Subscription Customer Service, 3251 Riverport Lane, Maryland Heights, MO 63043. **Customer Service: 1-800-654-2452 (US). From outside the United States, call 1-314-447-8871. Fax: 1-314-447-8029. E-mail: JournalsCustomerService-usa@elsevier.com (for print support) or JournalsOnlineSupport-usa@elsevier.com (for online support).**

Reprints. For copies of 100 or more, of articles in this publication, please contact the Commercial Reprints Department, Elsevier Inc., 360 Park Avenue South, New York, NY 10010-1710. Tel. 212-633-3874; Fax: 212-633-3820; E-mail: reprints@elsevier.com.

Gastrointestinal Endoscopy Clinics of North America is covered in *Excerpta Medica, MEDLINE/PubMed (Index Medicus), and MEDLINE/MEDLARS.*

Contributors

CONSULTING EDITOR

CHARLES J. LIGHTDALE, MD
Professor of Medicine, Division of Digestive and Liver Diseases, Columbia University Medical Center, New York, New York

EDITOR

JOHN R. SALTZMAN, MD, FACP, FACG, FASGE, AGAF
Director of Endoscopy, Brigham and Women's Hospital; Associate Professor of Medicine, Harvard Medical School, Gastroenterology Division, Boston, Massachusetts

AUTHORS

NEENA S. ABRAHAM, MD, MSCE, FACG, FASGE, AGAF
Professor of Medicine, Division of Gastroenterology and Hepatology, Department of Medicine, Mayo Clinic, Scottsdale, Arizona; Division of Health Care Policy and Research, Department of Health Services Research; Associate Director, Robert D. and Patricia E. Kern Center for the Science of Health Care Delivery, Mayo Clinic, Rochester, Minnesota

MEER AKBAR ALI, MD
Digestive Health Institute, Division of Gastroenterology and Liver Disease, University Hospitals Case Medical Center, Cleveland, Ohio

MARC BARDOU, MD, PhD
Gastroenterology Department and Centre d'Investigations Clinique, CHU de Dijon, Dijon, France

ALAN N. BARKUN, MD, MSc
Division of Gastroenterology, McGill University Health Center; Epidemiology and Biostatistics and Occupational Health, McGill University, Montreal, Quebec, Canada

ABDUL Q. BHUTTA, MD
Lecturer, Department of Internal Medicine, Yale University School of Medicine; Hospitalist, Section of Hospital Medicine, Yale-New Haven Hospital, New Haven, Connecticut

ANDREW S. BROCK, MD
Assistant Professor of Medicine; Director, Small Bowel Endoscopy, Department of Internal Medicine, Medical University of South Carolina, Charleston, South Carolina

CRISTINA BUCCI, MD, PhD
Gastroenterology Unit, University of Salerno, Salerno, Italy

DANIEL BUJANDA, MD
Department of Internal Medicine, University of Texas Southwestern Medical School, Dallas, Texas

YEN-I CHEN, MD
Division of Gastroenterology, McGill University Health Center, McGill University, Montreal, Quebec, Canada

BYRON CRYER, MD
Professor of Medicine, Department of Internal Medicine, University of Texas Southwestern Medical School; Medical Service, Gastroenterology Section, Dallas VA Medical Center, Dallas, Texas

NARAYAN DHAREL, MBBS, PhD
Senior GI Fellow, Division of Gastroenterology, Department of Internal Medicine, Virginia Commonwealth University School of Medicine, Richmond, Virginia

KYLE J. FORTINSKY, MD
Department of Medicine, Toronto General Hospital, University of Toronto, Toronto, Ontario, Canada

LARISSA L. FUJII-LAU, MD
Instructor of Medicine, Division of Gastroenterology and Hepatology, Washington University, St Louis, Missouri

GUADALUPE GARCIA-TSAO, MD
Professor of Medicine, Section of Digestive Diseases, Yale University School of Medicine, New Haven, Connecticut; Chief, Section of Digestive Diseases, VA-CT Healthcare System, West Haven, Connecticut

GREGORY G. GINSBERG, MD, FASGE, AGAF
Director, Endoscopic Service, Professor of Medicine, Professor of Surgery, Division of Gastroenterology, Department of Medicine, University of Pennsylvania Perelman School of Medicine, Philadelphia, Pennsylvania

IAN M. GRALNEK, MD, MSHS, FASGE
Associate Professor of Medicine, Rappaport Faculty of Medicine, Technion-Israel Institute of Technology; Chief, The Institute of Gastroenterology and Liver Diseases, Ha'Emek Medical Center, Afula, Israel

ASHWANI KAPOOR, MBBS
Senior Therapeutic Endoscopy Fellow, Division of Gastroenterology, Department of Internal Medicine, Virginia Commonwealth University School of Medicine, Richmond, Virginia

IYAD KHAMAYSI, MD
Lecturer; Rappaport Faculty of Medicine, Technion-Israel Institute of Technology; Director of the Interventional Endoscopy Unit, Interventional Endoscopy Unit, Department of Gastroenterology, Rambam Health Care Campus, Haifa, Israel

MICHAEL J. LEVY, MD
Professor of Medicine, Division of Gastroenterology and Hepatology, Mayo Clinic, Rochester, Minnesota

RICCARDO MARMO, MD
Endoscopy Unit, Division of Gastroenterology, L.Curto Hospital, Polla-Salerno, Italy

KEYUR PARIKH, MD
Digestive Health Institute, Division of Gastroenterology and Liver Disease, University Hospitals Case Medical Center, Cleveland, Ohio

MICHAEL W. RAJALA, MD, PhD
Instructor of Medicine, Division of Gastroenterology, Department of Medicine, University of Pennsylvania Perelman School of Medicine, Philadelphia, Pennsylvania

DON C. ROCKEY, MD
Professor of Medicine, Chairman, Department of Internal Medicine, Medical University of South Carolina, Charleston, South Carolina

GIANLUCA ROTONDANO, MD, FASGE, FACG
Division of Gastroenterology, Maresca Hospital, Torre del Greco, Italy

JOHN R. SALTZMAN, MD, FACP, FACG, FASGE, AGAF
Director of Endoscopy, Brigham and Women's Hospital; Associate Professor of Medicine, Harvard Medical School, Gastroenterology Division, Boston, Massachusetts

ARUN J. SANYAL, MBBS, MD
Professor of Medicine, Physiology and Molecular Pathology, Division of Gastroenterology, Department of Internal Medicine, Virginia Commonwealth University School of Medicine, Richmond, Virginia

TRACEY G. SIMON, MD
Department of Medicine, Brigham and Women's Hospital, Boston, Massachusetts

JOSEPH J.Y. SUNG, MD, PhD, FRCP
State Key Laboratory of Digestive Disease, Faculty of Medicine, Institute of Digestive Disease; Department of Medicine and Therapeutics, Faculty of Medicine, The Chinese University of Hong Kong, Hong Kong, China

THOMAS TIELLEMAN, MD
Department of Internal Medicine, University of Texas Southwestern Medical School, Dallas, Texas

ANNE C. TRAVIS, MD
Division of Gastroenterology, Hepatology and Endoscopy, Department of Medicine, Brigham and Women's Hospital, Harvard Medical School, Boston, Massachusetts

RICHARD C.K. WONG, MD
Digestive Health Institute, Division of Gastroenterology and Liver Disease, University Hospitals Case Medical Center, Cleveland, Ohio

SUNNY H. WONG, MBChB, DPhil, MRCP
State Key Laboratory of Digestive Disease, Faculty of Medicine, Institute of Digestive Disease; Department of Medicine and Therapeutics, Faculty of Medicine; Li Ka Shing Institute of Health Sciences, Faculty of Medicine, The Chinese University of Hong Kong, Hong Kong, China

LOUIS M. WONG KEE SONG, MD
Associate Professor of Medicine, Division of Gastroenterology and Hepatology, Mayo Clinic, Rochester, Minnesota

Contents

> Although the incidence of nonvariceal upper gastrointestinal bleeding (UGIB) has been decreasing worldwide, nonvariceal UGIB continues to be a significant problem. Even with the advent of advanced endoscopic procedures and potent medications to suppress acid production, UGIB carries significant morbidity and mortality. Some of the most common risk factors for nonvariceal UGIB include *Helicobacter pylori* infection, nonsteroidal antiinflammatory drugs (NSAIDs), aspirin, selective serotonin reuptake inhibitors, and other antiplatelet and anticoagulant medications. In patients with cardiovascular disease and kidney disease, UGIB tends to be more severe and has greater morbidity. Many of the newer NSAIDs have been removed from the market.

> Acute nonvariceal upper gastrointestinal bleeding remains an important cause of hospital admission with an associated mortality of 2-14%. Initial patient evaluation includes rapid hemodynamic assessment, large-bore intravenous catheter insertion and volume resuscitation. A hemoglobin transfusion threshold of 7 g/dL is recommended, and packed red blood cell transfusion may be necessary to restore intravascular volume and improve tissue perfusion. Patients should be risk stratified into low- and high-risk categories, using validated prognostic scoring systems such as the Glasgow-Blatchford, AIMS65 or Rockall scores. Effective early management of acute, nonvariceal upper gastrointestinal hemorrhage is critical for improving patient outcomes.

> Upper gastrointestinal (UGI) endoscopy is the cornerstone of diagnosis and management of patients presenting with acute UGI bleeding. Once hemodynamically resuscitated, early endoscopy (performed within 24 hours of

patient presentation) ensures accurate identification of the bleeding source, facilitates risk stratification based on endoscopic stigmata, and allows endotherapy to be delivered where indicated. Moreover, the preendoscopy use of a prokinetic agent (eg, IV erythromycin), especially in patients with a suspected high probability of having blood or clots in the stomach before undergoing endoscopy, may result in improved endoscopic visualization, a higher diagnostic yield, and less need for repeat endoscopy.

Antithrombotic drugs (anticoagulants, aspirin, and other antiplatelet agents) are used to treat cardiovascular disease and to prevent secondary thromboembolic events. These drugs are independently associated with an increased risk of gastrointestinal bleeding (GIB), and, when prescribed in combination, further increase the risk of adverse bleeding events. Clinical evidence to inform the choice of endoscopic hemostatic procedure, safe temporary drug cessation, and use of reversal agents is reviewed to optimize management following clinically significant GIB.

Nonvariceal upper gastrointestinal bleeding (UGIB) is a major cause of morbidity and mortality worldwide. Mortality from UGIB has remained 5-10% over the past decade. This article presents current evidence-based recommendations for the medical management of UGIB. Preendoscopic management includes initial resuscitation, risk stratification, appropriate use of blood products, and consideration of nasogastric tube insertion, erythromycin, and proton pump inhibitor therapy. The use of postendoscopic intravenous proton pump inhibitors is strongly recommended for certain patient populations. Postendoscopic management also includes the diagnosis and treatment of Helicobacter pylori, appropriate use of proton pump inhibitors and iron replacement therapy.

Acute variceal hemorrhage (AVH) is a lethal complication of portal hypertension and should be suspected in every patient with liver cirrhosis who presents with upper gastrointestinal bleed. AVH-related mortality has decreased in the last few decades from 40% to 15%–20% due to advances in the general and specific management of variceal hemorrhage. This review summarizes current management of AVH and prevention of recurrent hemorrhage with a focus on pharmacologic therapy.

Gastroesophageal variceal hemorrhage is a medical emergency with high morbidity and mortality. Endoscopic therapy is the mainstay of management of bleeding varices. It requires attention to technique and the appropriate choice of therapy for a given patient at a given point in time. Subjects must be monitored continuously after initiation of therapy for control of bleeding, and second-line definitive therapies must be introduced quickly if endoscopic and pharmacologic treatment fails.

Upper gastrointestinal bleeding remains one of the most common challenges faced by gastroenterologists and endoscopists in daily clinical practice. Endoscopic management of nonvariceal bleeding has been shown to improve clinical outcomes, with significant reduction of recurrent bleeding, need for surgery, and mortality. Early upper gastrointestinal endoscopy is recommended in all patients presenting with upper gastrointestinal bleeding within 24 hours of presentation, although appropriate resuscitation, stabilization of hemodynamic parameters, and optimization of comorbidity before endoscopy are essential.

One of the most important advances in gastroenterology has been the use of endoscopic hemostasis techniques to control nonvariceal upper gastrointestinal bleeding, particularly when high-risk stigmata are present. Several options are available, including injection therapy, sprays/topical agents, electrocautery, and mechanical methods. The method chosen depends on the nature of the lesion and experience of the endoscopist. This article reviews the available mechanical hemostatic modalities.

Topical hemostatic agents and powders are an emerging modality in the endoscopic management of upper and lower gastrointestinal bleeding. This systematic review demonstrates the effectiveness and safety of these agents with special emphasis on TC-325 and Ankaferd Blood Stopper. The unique noncontact/nontraumatic application, ability to cover large areas of bleed, and ease of use make these hemostatic agents an attractive option in certain clinical situations, such as massive bleeding with poor visualization, salvage therapy, and diffuse bleeding from luminal malignancies.

Endoscopic treatment of gastrointestinal (GI) bleeding is considered the first line of therapy. Although standard techniques, such as epinephrine injection, through-the-scope hemoclips, bipolar coagulation, argon plasma coagulation, and band ligation are routinely used, some GI bleeds are refractory to these therapies. Newer technologies have emerged to assist with the treatment of GI bleeding. This article highlights endoscopic and endoscopic ultrasound-guided therapies that may be used by experienced endoscopists for the primary control of GI bleeding or for cases refractory to standard hemostatic techniques.

Peptic ulcer bleeding is a common emergency. Management of ulcer bleeding requires prompt risk stratification, initiation of pharmacotherapy, and timely evaluation for endoscopy. Although endoscopy can achieve primary hemostasis in more than 90% of peptic ulcer bleeding, rebleeding may occur in up to 15% of patients after therapeutic endoscopy and is associated with heightened mortality. Early identification of high-risk patients for rebleeding is important. Depending on bleeding severity and center availability, patients with rebleeding may be managed by second endoscopy, transarterial angiographic embolization, or surgery. This article reviews the current management of peptic ulcers with an emphasis on rebleeding.

Upper gastrointestinal (GI) bleeding is an important clinical condition managed routinely by endoscopists. Diagnostic and therapeutic options vary immensely based on the source of bleeding and it is important for the gastroenterologist to be cognizant of both common and uncommon etiologies. The focus of this article is to highlight and discuss unusual sources of upper GI bleeding, with a particular emphasis on both the clinical and endoscopic features to help diagnose and treat these atypical causes of bleeding.

Videos of hemostasis obtained following injection of epinephrine followed by bipolar diatheramy and then hemoclip placement; treatment of a variceal bleed by placement of 2 hemoclips; and the proper technique for guillotining off an adherent clot from an ulcer in the lesser curvature of the stomach accompany this article

Effective endoscopic therapy for upper gastrointestinal (GI) bleeding has been shown to reduce rebleeding, need for surgery, and mortality. Effective endoscopic management of acute upper GI bleeding can be challenging and worrying. This article provides advice that is complementary to the in-depth reviews that accompany it in this issue. Topics include initial management, resuscitation, when and where to scope, benefits and limitations of devices, device selection based on lesion characteristics, improving visualization to localize the lesion, and tips on how to reduce the endoscopist's trepidation about managing these cases.

GASTROINTESTINAL ENDOSCOPY CLINICS OF NORTH AMERICA

ISSUE OF RELATED INTEREST

Gastroenterology Clinics of North America, December 2014, (Vol 43, No. 4)
Upper Gastrointestinal Bleeding
Ian Gralnek, MD, *Editor*

THE CLINICS ARE AVAILABLE ONLINE!
Access your subscription at:
www.theclinics.com

Foreword

Upper Gastrointestinal Bleeding: New Management for an Evolving Emergency

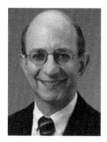

Charles J. Lightdale, MD
Consulting Editor

Just about every clinical gastroenterologist must be ready to effectively manage upper gastrointestinal bleeding. During the past 5 years, it has become clear that many methods and skills used in the past no longer apply. The patients who present with hematemesis and melena tend to be older and sicker, frequently taking anticoagulants, antiplatelet agents, antidepressants, aspirin, or nonsteroidal anti-inflammatory drugs. How to assess these emergent patients, how to resuscitate and stabilize them, and when to perform upper gastrointestinal endoscopy are critical issues. Understanding the application of the newest methods to identify and stop the bleeding is central to successful management. Working in concert with emergency room and intensive care physicians, interventional radiologists, anesthesiologists, and skilled nurses also requires a collegial team approach and up-to-date knowledge. Bleeding from the upper gastrointestinal tract is the most common and one of the most demanding emergencies for gastroenterologists. It is of the utmost importance to be as prepared and ready as possible.

This issue of *Gastrointestinal Endoscopy Clinics of North America* is devoted exclusively to advances and improvements in the management of upper gastrointestinal bleeding. I am extremely grateful to the editor of this issue, Dr John R. Saltzman, Director of Endoscopy at Brigham and Women's Hospital, Boston, Massachusetts. Dr Saltzman has been a leader and innovator in gastrointestinal endoscopy and his high-impact scholarship continues in this issue, which should have a significant influence on the management of gastrointestinal bleeding. He has taken a comprehensive approach here, finding an extraordinary group of author-experts to cover every key aspect. Readers of this issue should feel comfortable and confident that they are current in their knowledge and approach in dealing with this emergency. All practicing

Gastrointest Endoscopy Clin N Am 25 (2015) xiii–xiv
http://dx.doi.org/10.1016/j.giec.2015.05.001
1052-5157/15/$ – see front matter © 2015 Published by Elsevier Inc.

giendo.theclinics.com

gastroenterologists—trainees to senior attending physicians—should read this issue from cover to cover. I consider it to be essential reading.

Charles J. Lightdale, MD
Department of Medicine
Columbia University Medical Center
161 Fort Washington Avenue
New York, NY 10032, USA

E-mail address:
CJL18@columbia.edu

Preface

Advances and Improvements in the Management of Upper Gastrointestinal Bleeding

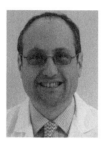

John R. Saltzman, MD, FACP, FACG, FASGE, AGAF
Editor

Upper gastrointestinal bleeding is the primary gastrointestinal emergency leading to hospitalization and urgent endoscopy in the United States. Compared with prior decades, patients with upper gastrointestinal bleeding are older, are more likely to have complex medical problems, and are more likely to be receiving anticoagulant and antithrombotic agents. However, while the patients we treat are now more complicated, there have also been many significant advancements in the medical and endoscopic therapies for upper gastrointestinal bleeding, and there are strong data showing that mortality from upper gastrointestinal bleeding is decreasing. Given this rapidly evolving field, it is crucial that physicians caring for patients with upper gastrointestinal bleeding be aware of the many recent changes in patient management. I am honored to be the guest editor of this issue of *Gastrointestinal Endoscopy Clinics of North America* dedicated to upper gastrointestinal bleeding at this time of rapid progression in the field. The authors of the articles in this issue are international experts who are recognized thought-leaders in upper gastrointestinal bleeding.

The last several years have seen significant changes in the initial management of patients with upper gastrointestinal bleeding, with more restrictive transfusion thresholds, increased use of risk stratification scores, and discontinuation of routine nasogastric tubes. In addition, there are new data and recommendations on the optimal timing of endoscopy. Concurrent with the evolution of endoscopic management, medical therapies have been developed with recent changes in proton pump inhibitor administration recommendations as well as the use of prokinetics to improve endoscopic visualization. Many modifications in endoscopic therapy have been developed, including the use of endoscopic ultrasound-guided angiotherapy, topical sprays (eg, hemostatic nanopowders), and over-the-scope clips. The medical and endoscopic management of esophageal and gastric variceal bleeding is also changing, including

Gastrointest Endoscopy Clin N Am 25 (2015) xv–xvi
http://dx.doi.org/10.1016/j.giec.2015.04.001
1052-5157/15/$ – see front matter © 2015 Published by Elsevier Inc.

the use of injected glues. This issue discusses all of these important areas as well as management of rebleeding and of unusual causes of upper gastrointestinal bleeding. I highly recommend reading "Tips and Tricks on How to Optimally Manage Patients with Upper Gastrointestinal Bleeding," which provides practical insights on improving management, as well as the "Zen of Endoscopy."

To provide optimal care to our patients, it is critical that practicing gastroenterologists be familiar with the many recent advances in management of upper gastrointestinal bleeding. This issue of *Gastrointestinal Endoscopy Clinics of North America* provides a comprehensive overview of the management of patients with upper gastrointestinal bleeding by experts who provide state-of-the-art updates as well as practical clinical pearls. I am deeply indebted to all of the contributors and hope that you find this issue helpful in your practice.

John R. Saltzman, MD, FACP, FACG, FASGE, AGAF
Brigham and Women's Hospital
Harvard Medical School
Gastroenterology Division
75 Francis Street
Boston, MA 02115, USA

E-mail address:
jsaltzman@partners.org

Epidemiology and Risk Factors for Upper Gastrointestinal Bleeding

 CrossMark

Thomas Tielleman, MD[a], Daniel Bujanda, MD[a],
Byron Cryer, MD[a,b],*

KEYWORDS

- Epidemiology • NSAIDs • Aspirin • Clopidogrel • *Helicobacter pylori* • Mortality
- Risk factors • Incidence

KEY POINTS

- Incidence of nonvariceal upper gastrointestinal bleeding (UGIB) has been decreasing worldwide. However, nonvariceal UGIB continues to be a significant problem.
- The most common risk factors for nonvariceal UGIB include *Helicobacter pylori* infection, nonsteroidal antiinflammatory medications (NSAIDs), aspirin, selective serotonin reuptake inhibitors, and other antiplatelet and anticoagulant medications.
- More recently observed important risks for UGIB are cardiovascular disease, heart failure, left ventricular assist devices, and renal failure.
- Despite the introduction of cyclooxygenase-2 inhibitors, which were introduced to decrease UGIB, bleeding from NSAIDs continues to be a problem.
- Introduction of newer antiplatelet agents and newer oral anticoagulants has contributed to the persisting incidence of UGIB.

INTRODUCTION

Upper gastrointestinal bleeding (UGIB) is defined as hemorrhage that involves the mouth to the duodenum proximal to the ligament of Treitz. Common causes of UGIB include peptic ulcer disease (PUD) and ulcers of the esophagus, erosions of the upper gastrointestinal (GI) tract, variceal bleeding, gastroesophageal reflux disease, Mallory-Weiss tears, vascular lesions, malignancy, and other less common

Disclosures: B. Cryer discloses has consulting relationships with Iroko Pharmaceuticals; McNeil Consumer Healthcare; Ritter Pharma, Inc; Sanofi-Aventis Pharmaceuticals; Sandoz Pharmaceuticals; Sucampo, Inc; and Takeda Pharmaceuticals.
[a] Department of Internal Medicine, University of Texas Southwestern Medical School, Dallas, TX 75390, USA; [b] Medical Service, Gastroenterology Section 111B1, Dallas VA Medical Center, 4500 S Lancaster Road, Dallas, TX 75216, USA
* Corresponding author. Medical Service, Gastroenterology Section (111B1), Dallas VA Medical Center, 4500 S Lancaster Road, Dallas, TX 75216.
E-mail address: byron.cryer@utsouthwestern.edu

causes. Between 40% and 50% of patients who have UGIB present with hematemesis and 90% to 98% with either melena or hematochezia.[1] The disease is commonly divided into 2 types: nonvariceal and variceal, and the primary focuses of this article are the epidemiology and risk factors of nonvariceal bleeding. Even with the use of advanced endoscopic procedures and potent medications to suppress acid production, UGIB still carries significant morbidity and mortality. Although studies have reported a decreased incidence in UGIB in the United States (96–82 per 100,000)[2,3] it still accounts for nearly 300,000 hospitalizations per year, with a mortality of approximately 5%.[3,4] PUD still accounts for most nonvariceal bleeding (37%)[5] and is higher among elderly men, those who use aspirin and nonsteroidal antiinflammatory drugs (NSAIDs), and in areas with high *Helicobacter pylori* prevalence.[3,4] In the United States in 2004, there were about 700,000 ambulatory care visits with peptic ulcer as the first-listed diagnosis, with a total cost of approximately $1.4 billion.[5]

RISK FACTORS

The most common risk factors for nonvariceal UGIB include *H pylori* infection, NSAIDs/aspirin, and other antiplatelet and anticoagulant medication use.[4,6] *H pylori* infection and NSAID use are both independent and synergistic risk factors for peptic ulcer–related bleeding.[7] Studies from the 1980s and 1990s show that *H pylori* was present in more than 90% of patients with duodenal ulcers and approximately 70% of patients with gastric ulcers.[8,9] However, more recent Western studies have suggested that there is a changing cause of PUD, with the overall PUD incidence decreasing and the proportion of *H pylori*–negative PUD increasing.[3,10,11] A Dutch study of the incidence of duodenal and gastric ulcers in a district hospital found that the incidence of duodenal ulcer disease has been decreasing with a decline in the prevalence of *H pylori*.[11] A review of 73 worldwide published studies from 1999 to 2008 evaluating patients with duodenal ulcers showed that 88% of patients were infected with *H pylori*, with a decrease to 77% infected when including the studies from 2003 to 2008.[12] There has been an overall decline in the prevalence of *H pylori*–positive PUD and an increase in non-NSAID, non–*H pylori* PUD. According to a prospective multicenter study involving 32 hospitals in France, 40% of PUD was related to *H pylori* infection alone, 18.7% to gastrotoxic drugs alone (NSAIDs, aspirin, and/or cyclooxygenase [COX]-2 inhibitors), 19.8% had *H pylori* infection in the setting of gastrotoxic drugs, and 21.6% had neither *H pylori* infection nor gastrotoxic drug use.[13] Therefore, although *H pylori* and gastrotoxic drugs make up approximately 80% of PUD and PUD-related bleeding, there is a significant subsection of idiopathic ulcers as well.

There has been a well-established correlation between NSAID use and the increased risk of UGIB. The prevalence of PUD in patients with regular NSAID use is approximately 15% to 30%.[14] In addition to NSAID use independently increasing the risk of GI adverse effects, there are multiple other risk factors that have been associated with nonvariceal UGIB that are potentiated in the presence of NSAID use (**Fig. 1**).[15–17]

COX-2 inhibitors were first introduced in the hope that they would provide the analgesic and antiinflammatory benefits of nonselective NSAIDs without the adverse GI side effects. There is evidence that there is a reduced risk of upper GI complications and ulcers compared with those associated with nonselective NSAIDs.[18–20] However, overall, there is still an increased risk of upper GI complications and symptomatic gastroduodenal ulcers with COX-2 selective inhibitors compared with no use at all.[21,22]

Recently, a 2014 case series analysis of 7 population-based health care databases for 114,835 patients with UGIB analyzed various drug combinations with NSAIDs, low-dose aspirin, and COX-2 inhibitors. Monotherapy with nonselective NSAIDs was

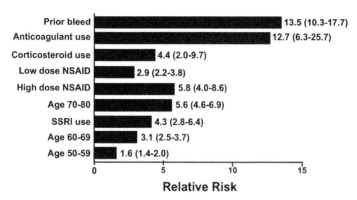

Fig. 1. Risk factors for serious GI adverse events with NSAIDs; relative risks and 95% confidence intervals. SSRI, selective serotonin reuptake inhibitor. (*Data from* Refs.[15–17])

shown to increase the relative risk of UGIB by a factor of 4.3, compared with monotherapy with COX-2 inhibitors (relative risk of 2.9) and monotherapy with low-dose aspirin (relative risk of 3.1).[22] Combination therapy also increases risk of UGIB, with the greatest increase seen with the combination of NSAIDs with corticosteroids (**Table 1**). Other studies have also shown an increased risk for the combination of NSAIDs and aspirin,[23–25] whereas other suggested risk factors from studies include alcohol consumption, history of prior peptic ulcers,[6] and smoking.[26]

There is growing evidence that use of selective serotonin reuptake inhibitors (SSRIs) is associated with an increased risk of UGIB, and that this risk is further increased by the concurrent use of NSAIDs and SSRIs. Previous reviews of a small number of studies have reported a substantial risk of UGIB with SSRIs. However, more recent studies have produced variable results. A meta-analysis of 4 observational studies showed an odds ratio (OR) of 2.36 (95% confidence interval [CI], 1.44, 3.85) for use of SSRI-associated UGIB.[27] A more recent 2014 systematic review of 19 case-control studies showed a significant risk with an OR of 1.66 (95% CI, 1.44, 1.92).[17] Moreover, the combination of SSRIs and NSAIDs further increases UGIB risk to an OR of 4.25 (95% CI, 2.82, 6.42) (see **Fig. 1**).[17] Because serotonin induces platelet aggregation, it has been postulated that SSRIs increase UGIB risk by decreasing platelet-generated serotonin, resulting in impaired platelet aggregation and hemostasis.[27–29] It has also been hypothesized that, because SSRIs increase gastric acid secretion, they may alternatively increase risks of peptic ulcers and UGIB from ulcers of the upper GI tract.[30,31]

In patients with ulcers in whom tests for *H pylori* are negative and the history is also negative for NSAID or SSRI usage, important considerations are whether the tests for *H pylori* may be falsely negative because of concurrent use of proton pump inhibitors (PPIs); whether the patient might be taking an NSAID product that is unfamiliar to the patient (such as an over-the-counter NSAID); whether the patient might be taking an NSAID product that is part of a combination medication (such as combination analgesics or combination cough and cold medications); or whether the patient might have a gastric acid hypersecretory condition, such as Zollinger-Ellison syndrome.

PREVALENCE/INCIDENCE

The overall reported incidence rates for acute UGIB vary from 48 to 160 cases per 100,000 population per year, with higher incidences reported among men and the elderly.[4] The most common cause of acute UGIB continues to be PUD, with reported incidences as high as 67% of all acute UGIB (**Table 2**).[4,32,33]

Table 1
Relative risk of diagnosed UGIB during exposure to specific drug groups (with corresponding 95% confidence intervals [CIs]) in monotherapy and in combination with other drugs

Drug Groups[a]	Monotherapy		Combination with: nsNSAIDs		COX-2 Inhibitors		Low-dose Aspirin	
	N	IRR (95% CI)	N	IRR (95% CI)	N	IRR (95% CI)	N	IRR (95% CI)
No drug[a]	69,664	1.00 (reference)	NA		NA		NA	
nsNSAIDs	3327	4.27 (4.11–4.44)	NA		NA		416	6.77 (6.09–7.53)
COX-2 inhibitors	635	2.90 (2.67–3.15)	NA		NA		131	7.49 (6.22–9.02)
Low-dose aspirin	4733	3.05 (2.94–3.17)	416	6.77 (6.09–7.53)	131	7.49 (6.22–9.02)	NA	
Corticosteroids	1378	4.07 (3.83–4.32)	244	12.82 (11.17–14.72)	40	5.95 (4.25–8.33)	190	8.37 (7.14–9.81)
SSRIs	1793	2.06 (1.94–2.18)	210	6.95 (5.97–8.08)	65	5.82 (4.45–7.62)	401	4.60 (4.09–5.17)
GPAs	5279	1.61 (1.56–1.66)	678	3.90 (3.59–4.24)	95	2.37 (1.92–2.93)	607	2.54 (2.32–2.78)
Aldosterone antagonists	1211	3.27 (3.06–3.50)	76	11.00 (8.63–14.03)	10	4.02 (2.07–7.81)	131	5.01 (4.13–6.08)
Ca channel blockers	3546	1.57 (1.51–1.63)	363	4.45 (3.98–4.98)	77	3.11 (2.46–3.93)	1123	3.07 (2.86–3.29)
Anticoagulants	1760	3.01 (2.85–3.19)	143	8.69 (7.30–10.35)	21	5.01 (3.21–7.82)	168	6.94 (5.86–8.22)
Antiplatelets (excluding aspirin)	994	1.74 (1.61–1.87)	87	6.50 (5.19–8.15)	9	1.73 (0.87–3.44)	246	5.49 (4.71–6.41)
Nitrates	2572	2.55 (2.43–2.68)	172	5.82 (4.97–6.82)	49	5.09 (3.79–6.82)	859	3.79 (3.51–4.10)

Note: n refers to the number of UGIB events during exposure to specific drug groups (the total number does not add up to 114,835 because of diagnoses of UGIB in the "other drug" category).

Abbreviations: GPA, gastroprotective agent; IRR, incidence rate ratio; NA, not applicable; nsNSAID, nonselective nonsteroidal antiinflammatory drug; SSRI, selective serotonin reuptake inhibitor.

[a] No use of the predefined drugs of interest.

From Masclee GM, Valkhoff VE, Coloma PM, et al. Risk of upper gastrointestinal bleeding from different drug combinations. Gastroenterology 2014;147(4):787; with permission.

Table 2
Incidences of various causes of acute UGIB

Cause	Incidence (%)
PUD	20–67
Erosive disease	4–31
Bleeding varices	4–20
Esophagitis	3–12
Mallory-Weiss tears	4–12
Malignancy	2–8
Vascular lesions	2–8
Esophageal ulcers	2–6
Idiopathic/unknown cause	3–19

Data from Refs.[4,32,33]

The overall incidence of acute UGIB, particularly PUD, decreased toward the end of the twentieth century and has now stabilized in the twenty-first century.[3,34] In the United States, the incidence rates for hospital discharges that carried the diagnosis of PUD decreased from 1400 per 100,000 in 1979 to approximately 700 per 100,000 in 2004 (**Fig. 2**).[5] In addition, a 2012 article in the *American Journal of Gastroenterology* by Laine and colleagues[35] indicated that there were 36 million inpatient visits for PUD across approximately 620 US hospitals from 2001 to 2009. Although alarming, these data revealed decreases in overall UGIB from 78.4 to 60.6 per 100,000 over that 8-year time frame. Furthermore, there was a decrease in peptic ulcer bleeding from 48.7 to 32.1 per 100,000 as well (**Fig. 3**). Corroborating these earlier data are UGIB rates from a more recent 2014 longitudinal study of UGIB hospitalizations in the United States that used the Nationwide Inpatient Sample and indicated

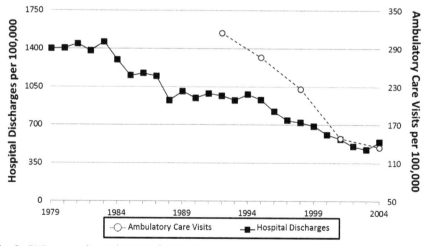

Fig. 2. PUD: age-adjusted rates of ambulatory care visits and hospital discharges with all listed diagnoses in the United States between 1979 and 2004. (*Data from* Everhart JE, Ruhl CE. Burden of Digestive Diseases in the United States Part I: Overall and Upper Gastrointestinal Diseases. Gastroenterology 2009;136:385.)

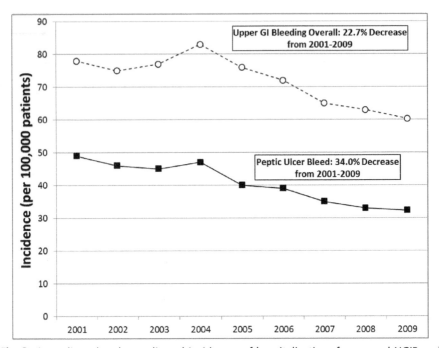

Fig. 3. Age-adjusted and sex-adjusted incidences of hospitalizations for general UGIB and for peptic ulcer bleeding. (*Adapted from* Laine L, Yang H, Chang SC, et al. Trends for incidence of hospitalization and death due to GI complications in the United States from 2001 to 2009. Am J Gastroenterol 2012;107(8):1192; with permission.)

that nonvariceal UGIB incidence declined from 108 to 78 cases per 100,000 persons from 1994 to 2009, respectively (**Table 3**).[3]

WORLDWIDE/REGIONAL INCIDENCE

Worldwide incidences of UGIB from geographic locations around the globe are shown in **Table 3**.[3,24,36–39] The variability in incidence rates is mainly caused by the variance of methodology used in diagnosing UGIB. However, despite this limitation, the information corroborates decreasing incidence of UGIB all over the world. It has been suggested that the decreases in PUD and UGIB are caused by an overall decrease in

Table 3		
Changes in incidence rates in all UGIB or UGIB caused by PUD in different regions of the world		
Location	**Decrease in Incidence in UGIB**	**Reference**
United States	108 per 100,000 in 1994 to 78 per 100,000 in 2009	3
Spain	54.6 per 100,000 in 1996 to 25.8 per 100,000 in 2005	24
Veneto region (Italy)	64.4 per 100,000 in 2001 to 35.9 per 100,000 in 2010	36
Netherlands	61.7 per 100,000 in 1993 per 1994 to 47.7 per 100,000 in 2000	38
New Zealand	53.6 per 100,000 in 2001–2005 to 45.8 per 100,000 in 2006–2010	39
Sweden	63.9 per 100,000 in 1987 to 35.3 per 100,000 in 2005	37

H pylori prevalence in addition to an increased use of acid-suppressing medications.[36,40,41] Although UGIB and peptic ulcer bleeding are decreasing in the general population overall, rates of hospitalization because of ulcer complications are increasing in elderly populations.[42] This paradoxic observation is thought to be caused by longer life expectancy in Western countries leading to increased occurrences of cardiovascular and rheumatic diseases that are associated with an increased use of aspirin and NSAIDs among the elderly population.[43]

Studies from other parts of the world also show this trend in decreasing PUD. A study from Sweden reported a 44% decrease in peptic ulcer bleeding from 1987 to 2005 and a study from Spain reported a 52% decrease from 1996 to 2005.[24,37]

MORTALITY

Despite advances in diagnosis and treatment of UGIB, it is still a condition that carries a high morbidity and mortality. The overall mortality from all UGIB is approximately 5%.[4] Age and comorbidities portend a worse prognosis and there are several calculators that can predict UGIB mortality, the Rockall scoring system being one of the most validated systems.[44] In a study that analyzed UGIB in the National Hospital Discharge Survey over 3 decades from 1979 to 2009, mortality risk from UGIB from gastric causes decreased by 55.8% (5.2% in the first decade to 2.3% in the third). UGIB caused by gastric ulcers and gastritis showed the greatest decrease and the most pronounced decrease was seen on hospital day 1, especially in patients with heart and renal failure.[45] In 2 large studies of mortality related to UGIB over time in the United States there was a reduction in mortality (**Fig. 4**),[3] a phenomenon that was consistent across various age groups (**Fig. 5**).[35] Although not well defined, decreases in *H pylori* and prevention strategies with NSAIDs have led to decreases in the incidence of UGIB.[42] However, decreases in mortality are more likely caused by advances in medical management with PPIs combined with more effective

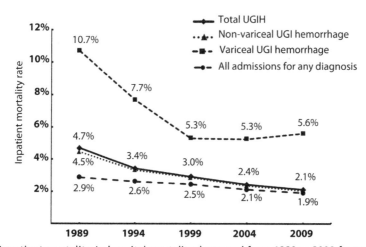

Fig. 4. Inpatient mortality. In-hospital mortality decreased from 1989 to 2009 for total, nonvariceal, and variceal GI hemorrhage. The rate of decline of in-hospital mortality was faster than that of all patients admitted to a hospital for any reason. UGI, upper GI; UGIH, upper GI hemorrhage. (*From* Abougergi MS, Travis AC, Saltzman JR. The in-hospital mortality rate for upper GI hemorrhage has decreased over 2 decades in the United States: a nationwide analysis. Gastrointest Endosc 2014. http://dx.doi.org/10.1016/j.gie.2014.09.027; with permission.)

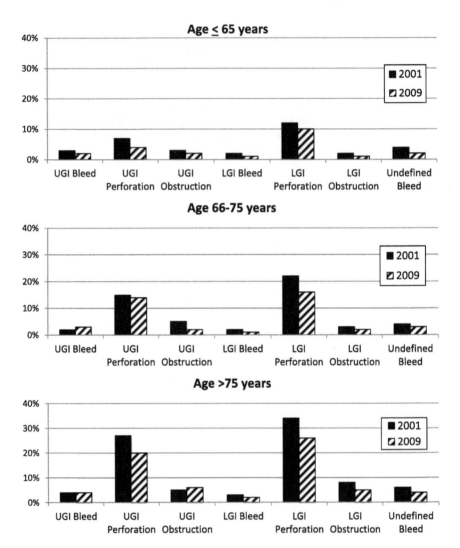

Fig. 5. Case fatality rates (%) for GI complications in different age groups. LGI, lower GI. (*Adapted from* Laine L, Yang H, Chang SC, et al. Trends for incidence of hospitalization and death due to GI complications in the United States from 2001 to 2009. Am J Gastroenterol 2012;107(8):1193; with permission.)

endoscopic therapies and shorter time to endoscopy. Supporting this premise are data indicating that, in the United States, rates of endoscopy, early endoscopy, and endoscopic therapy have increased substantially over the past 20 years.[3] Furthermore, improved care in emergency departments, improved geriatric care, and improvements in critical care medicine are also thought to have contributed to the decreasing mortality of UGIB.[45] Geographically, the mortality from UGIB in different parts of the world is variable (3%–11%) and difficult to assess, mainly because of differences in methodologies in diagnosis and populations studied. More uniform standards in reporting are needed for data on UGIB to be useful for comparison.

CLINICAL CORRELATION

Although the overall incidence of acute UGIB is decreasing, the overall occurrence of acute UGIB remains high. Certain clinical scenarios can increase the potential for the development of acute UGIB, especially clinical situations related to cardiovascular disease and renal failure.

Impact of Concomitant Cardiovascular Disease

Cardiovascular disease is a significant and leading cause of death in the United States. Percutaneous coronary intervention is a mainstay in coronary artery disease and continues to evolve with regard to prevention of stent rethrombosis with the development of dual antiplatelet therapies and drug-eluting stents. A population-based case-control study in Denmark from 2000 to 2004 found that the use of combined antithrombotic regimens increased by 425% in the 4-year study period.[46] However, the increased antiplatelet activity associated with antithrombotic medications also leads to an increased risk of acute UGIB. Foley and colleagues[47] reviewed multiple published studies evaluating the risks of GI bleeding related to percutaneous coronary intervention and antiplatelet therapies, including novel antiplatelet therapies such as clopidogrel (**Table 4**).

A 2012 study from a 1200-bed tertiary care center in Israel followed all patients admitted to the coronary care unit who were admitted with acute coronary syndrome (ACS) over an 11-year period (totaling 7240 patients from October 1996 to November 2007) and analyzed the number of those patients who developed UGIB during their hospital stay.[48] UGIB was developed by 0.9% of patients and the combination of unfractionated heparin with glycoprotein IIb/IIIa inhibitors was strongly associated with UGIB (OR, 2.87; 95% CI, 1.66–4.97). These patients also had a significantly higher mortality than patients with ACS who did not develop UGIB (33% vs 5%; $P<.001$).[48]

Table 4
Comparison of GI bleeding incidence in clinical studies evaluating antiplatelet regimens

Study	%	%	Number of Patients	Odds Ratio (95% CI)
Meta-analysis: aspirin (50–162.5 mg/d) vs placebo	2.3	1.5	49,917	1.59 (1.4–1.81)
Meta-analysis: aspirin (162.5–1500 mg/d vs placebo	3	1.4	16,060	1.96 (1.51–2.43)
CAPRIE aspirin 325 mg vs clopidogrel: severe GI hemorrhage	0.71	0.49	19,185	1.45 (1.00–2.09)
MATCH aspirin (75 mg) and clopidogrel 75 mg vs clopidogrel 75 mg: all life-threatening bleeds including GI	1.4	0.6	7578	2.46 (1.48–4.10)
MATCH aspirin (75 mg) vs clopidogrel: all major bleeds including GI	1.12	0.29	7578	3.87 (1.99–7.53)
CURE aspirin (75–325 mg) + clopidogrel vs aspirin (75–325 mg): life-threatening GI bleeds	1.3	0.7	12,562	1.79 (1.25–2.56)

Abbreviations: CAPRIE, clopidogrel versus aspirin in patients at risk of ischaemic events; CURE, clopidogrel in unstable angina to prevent recurrent events; MATCH, aspirin and clopidogrel compared with clopidogrel alone after recent ischaemic stroke or transient ischaemic attack in high-risk patients.
$P<.05$ for all studies listed.
Data from Refs.[47,52–55]

Another cardiovascular disease with associated increased risks of UGIB is advanced heart failure, specifically in patients who are placed on left ventricular assist devices (LVADs). There have been multiple case reports and case series that have described frequent GI bleeding in association with the use of LVADs. A 2013 article by Islam and colleagues[49] reviewed 10 case reports and 22 case series covering 1543 patients with LVADs, and 20.5% of these patients developed GI bleeding. These lesions were often related to arteriovenous malformations and were found throughout the GI tract, but seemed to be more frequent in the upper GI tract. Furthermore, the use of anticoagulation did not seem to predispose patients to an increased number of GI bleeding episodes.

Impact of Concomitant Renal Failure

Impaired kidney function is also associated with increased risk of UGIB.[50] Chronic kidney disease and end-stage renal disease (ESRD) are growing problems, with more than 600,000 patients in the United States requiring maintenance dialysis or kidney transplantation.[50] A 2011 study in Taiwan assessed a cohort of patients with prior history of peptic ulcer bleeding and divided them into 6447 patients with ESRD and 25,788 matched controls. Over a 10-year period, there was a significantly increased incidence of peptic ulcer rebleeding in patients with ESRD compared with controls (**Fig. 6**).[51] The effects of uremia in impairing platelet function is thought to mechanistically underlie the observation of increased UGIB in renal failure. Furthermore, although the overall trend in acute UGIB has decreased,[3,5,35] a 2012 study assessing close to 1 million patients from the US renal data revealed that rates of nonvariceal UGIB in patients undergoing dialysis had not decreased in the previous 10 years.[50] However, this study did show improvements in 30-day mortality over that time span, with decreases of 2.3% to 2.8% per year, suggesting improvements in medical care. However, the burden of acute UGIB in the setting of ESRD remains considerable.

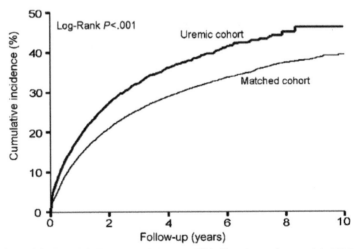

Fig. 6. Cumulative incidences of peptic ulcer rebleeding in patients with ESRD (uremic) compared with controls matched by age, gender, and gastroprotective agent use over a 10-year period. There is a significant increase in incidence of peptic ulcer rebleeding in patients with kidney disease compared with those without. (*From* Wu CY, Wu MS, Kuo KN, et al. Long-term peptic ulcer rebleeding risk estimation in patients undergoing haemodialysis: a 10-year nationwide cohort study. Gut 2011;60(8):1040; with permission.)

SUMMARY/DISCUSSION

Although UGIB has declined in incidence worldwide, it continues to be a major public health concern. Major risk factors for UGIB, such as NSAIDs and *H pylori*, from a worldwide perspective continue to be major contributors to this persisting problem. Although *H pylori* prevalence has declined in the United States, this infection continues to have a considerable presence worldwide. During the past 2 decades, approaches to improving the GI safety of NSAIDs were developed and were mainly directed toward discovery of COX-2–selective NSAIDs, agents that were expected to minimize the risk of GI injury. However, the results from multiple clinical studies have shown that treatment with COX-2 inhibitors may increase the risk for cardiovascular complications and has consequently resulted in limited use of these agents in clinical practice. More recently observed important risks for UGIB are use of SSRIs, cardiovascular disease, heart failure, LVADs, and renal failure. Complicating the current clinical problem of UGIB is that introduction of new antiplatelet agents and new oral anticoagulants has contributed to the persistence of UGIB. Despite the advent of advanced endoscopic procedures and potent medications to suppress acid production, UGIB still carries significant morbidity and mortality. Thus, UGIB continues to be an important concern and management problem for gastroenterologists.

REFERENCES

1. Fallah MA, Prakash C, Edmundowicz S. Acute gastrointestinal bleeding. Med Clin North Am 2000;84(5):1183–208.
2. Zhao Y, Encinosa W. Hospitalizations for gastrointestinal bleeding in 1998 and 2006: statistical brief #65. Healthcare Cost and Utilization Project (HCUP) statistical briefs. Rockville (MD): Agency for Health Care Policy and Research (US); 2006.
3. Abougergi MS, Travis AC, Saltzman JR. The in-hospital mortality rate for upper GI hemorrhage has decreased over 2 decades in the United States: a nationwide analysis. Gastrointest Endosc 2014. http://dx.doi.org/10.1016/j.gie.2014.09.027.
4. Rotondano G. Epidemiology and diagnosis of acute nonvariceal upper gastrointestinal bleeding. Gastroenterol Clin North Am 2014;43(4):643–63.
5. Everhart JE, Ruhl CE. Burden of Digestive Diseases in the United States Part I: Overall and Upper Gastrointestinal Diseases. Gastroenterology 2009;136: 376–86.
6. Nagata N, Niikura R, Sekine K, et al. Risk of peptic ulcer bleeding associated with *Helicobacter pylori* infection, nonsteroidal anti-inflammatory drugs, low-dose aspirin, and antihypertensive drugs: a case-control study. J Gastroenterol Hepatol 2015;30(2):292–8.
7. Papatheodoridis GV, Sougioultzis S, Archimandritis AJ. Effects of *Helicobacter pylori* and nonsteroidal anti-inflammatory drugs on peptic ulcer disease: a systematic review. Clin Gastroenterol Hepatol 2006;4(2):130–42.
8. Kuipers EJ, Thijs JC, Festen HP. The prevalence of *Helicobacter pylori* in peptic ulcer disease. Aliment Pharmacol Ther 1995;9(Suppl 2):59–69.
9. Marshall BJ. Helicobacter pylori. Am J Gastroenterol 1994;89(Suppl 8): S116–28.
10. Musumba C, Jorgensen A, Sutton L, et al. The relative contribution of NSAIDs and *Helicobacter pylori* to the aetiology of endoscopically-diagnosed peptic ulcer disease: observations from a tertiary referral hospital in the UK between 2005 and 2010. Aliment Pharmacol Ther 2012;36(1):48–56.

11. Groenen MJ, Kuipers EJ, Hansen BE, et al. Incidence of duodenal ulcers and gastric ulcers in a Western population: back to where it started. Can J Gastroenterol 2009;23(9):604–8.

12. Gisbert JP, Calvet X. Review article: *Helicobacter pylori*-negative duodenal ulcer disease. Aliment Pharmacol Ther 2009;30(8):791–815.

13. Charpignon C, Lesgourgues B, Pariente A, et al. Peptic ulcer disease: one in five is related to neither *Helicobacter pylori* nor aspirin/NSAID intake. Aliment Pharmacol Ther 2013;38(8):946–54.

14. Laine L. Approaches to nonsteroidal anti-inflammatory drug use in the high-risk patient. Gastroenterology 2001;120(3):594–606.

15. Piper JM, Ray WA, Daugherty JR, et al. Corticosteroid use and peptic ulcer disease: role of nonsteroidal anti-inflammatory drugs. Ann Intern Med 1991;114(9):735–40.

16. Garcia Rodriguez LA, Jick H. Risk of upper gastrointestinal bleeding and perforation associated with individual non-steroidal anti-inflammatory drugs. Lancet 1994;343(8900):769–72.

17. Anglin R, Yuan Y, Moayyedi P, et al. Risk of upper gastrointestinal bleeding with selective serotonin reuptake inhibitors with or without concurrent nonsteroidal anti-inflammatory use: a systematic review and meta-analysis. Am J Gastroenterol 2014;109(6):811–9.

18. Bombardier C, Laine L, Reicin A, et al. Comparison of upper gastrointestinal toxicity of rofecoxib and naproxen in patients with rheumatoid arthritis. VIGOR Study Group. N Engl J Med 2000;343(21):1520–8.

19. Schnitzer TJ, Burmester GR, Mysler E, et al. Comparison of lumiracoxib with naproxen and ibuprofen in the Therapeutic Arthritis Research and Gastrointestinal Event Trial (TARGET), reduction in ulcer complications: randomised controlled trial. Lancet 2004;364(9435):665–74.

20. Masclee GM, Valkhoff VE, van Soest EM, et al. Cyclo-oxygenase-2 inhibitors or nonselective NSAIDs plus gastroprotective agents: what to prescribe in daily clinical practice? Aliment Pharmacol Ther 2013;38(2):178–89.

21. Garcia Rodriguez LA, Hernandez-Diaz S. The risk of upper gastrointestinal complications associated with nonsteroidal anti-inflammatory drugs, glucocorticoids, acetaminophen, and combinations of these agents. Arthritis Res 2001;3(2):98–101.

22. Masclee GM, Valkhoff VE, Coloma PM, et al. Risk of upper gastrointestinal bleeding from different drug combinations. Gastroenterology 2014;147(4):784–92.

23. Sorensen HT, Mellemkjaer L, Blot WJ, et al. Risk of upper gastrointestinal bleeding associated with use of low-dose aspirin. Am J Gastroenterol 2000;95(9):2218–24.

24. Lanas A, Perez-Aisa MA, Feu F, et al. A nationwide study of mortality associated with hospital admission due to severe gastrointestinal events and those associated with nonsteroidal antiinflammatory drug use. Am J Gastroenterol 2005;100(8):1685–93.

25. Weil J, Colin-Jones D, Langman M, et al. Prophylactic aspirin and risk of peptic ulcer bleeding. BMJ 1995;310(6983):827–30.

26. Kurata JH, Nogawa AN. Meta-analysis of risk factors for peptic ulcer. Nonsteroidal antiinflammatory drugs, *Helicobacter pylori*, and smoking. J Clin Gastroenterol 1997;24(1):2–17.

27. Serebruany VL. Selective serotonin reuptake inhibitors and increased bleeding risk: are we missing something? Am J Med 2006;119(2):113–6.

28. Halperin D, Reber G. Influence of antidepressants on hemostasis. Dialogues Clin Neurosci 2007;9(1):47–59.

29. Li N, Wallen NH, Ladjevardi M, et al. Effects of serotonin on platelet activation in whole blood. Blood Coagul Fibrinolysis 1997;8(8):517–23.
30. Andrade C, Sandarsh S, Chethan KB, et al. Serotonin reuptake inhibitor antidepressants and abnormal bleeding: a review for clinicians and a reconsideration of mechanisms. J Clin Psychiatry 2010;71(12):1565–75.
31. Abdel Salam OM. Fluoxetine and sertraline stimulate gastric acid secretion via a vagal pathway in anaesthetised rats. Pharm Res 2004;50(3):309–16.
32. Hreinsson JP, Kalaitzakis E, Gudmundsson S, et al. Upper gastrointestinal bleeding: incidence, etiology and outcomes in a population-based setting. Scand J Gastroenterol 2013;48(4):439–47.
33. Khamaysi I, Gralnek IM. Acute upper gastrointestinal bleeding (UGIB) - initial evaluation and management. Best Pract Res Clin Gastroenterol 2013;27(5):633–8.
34. Quan S, Frolkis A, Milne K, et al. Upper-gastrointestinal bleeding secondary to peptic ulcer disease: incidence and outcomes. World J Gastroenterol 2014; 20(46):17568–77.
35. Laine L, Yang H, Chang SC, et al. Trends for incidence of hospitalization and death due to GI complications in the United States from 2001 to 2009. Am J Gastroenterol 2012;107(8):1190–5.
36. Cavallaro LG, Monica F, Germana B, et al. Time trends and outcome of gastrointestinal bleeding in the Veneto region: a retrospective population based study from 2001 to 2010. Dig Liver Dis 2014;46(4):313–7.
37. Ahsberg K, Ye W, Lu Y, et al. Hospitalisation of and mortality from bleeding peptic ulcer in Sweden: a nationwide time-trend analysis. Aliment Pharmacol Ther 2011; 33(5):578–84.
38. van Leerdam ME, Vreeburg EM, Rauws EA, et al. Acute upper GI bleeding: did anything change? Time trend analysis of incidence and outcome of acute upper GI bleeding between 1993/1994 and 2000. Am J Gastroenterol 2003;98(7):1494–9.
39. Irwin J, Ferguson R, Weilert F, et al. Incidence of upper gastrointestinal haemorrhage in Maori and New Zealand European ethnic groups, 2001-2010. Intern Med J 2014;44(8):735–41.
40. Lewis JD, Bilker WB, Brensinger C, et al. Hospitalization and mortality rates from peptic ulcer disease and GI bleeding in the 1990s: relationship to sales of nonsteroidal anti-inflammatory drugs and acid suppression medications. Am J Gastroenterol 2002;97(10):2540–9.
41. Perez-Aisa MA, Del Pino D, Siles M, et al. Clinical trends in ulcer diagnosis in a population with high prevalence of Helicobacter pylori infection. Aliment Pharmacol Ther 2005;21(1):65–72.
42. Lanas A, Garcia-Rodriguez LA, Polo-Tomas M, et al. The changing face of hospitalisation due to gastrointestinal bleeding and perforation. Aliment Pharmacol Ther 2011;33(5):585–91.
43. Higham J, Kang JY, Majeed A. Recent trends in admissions and mortality due to peptic ulcer in England: increasing frequency of haemorrhage among older subjects. Gut 2002;50(4):460–4.
44. Wang CY, Qin J, Wang J, et al. Rockall score in predicting outcomes of elderly patients with acute upper gastrointestinal bleeding. World J Gastroenterol 2013;19(22):3466–72.
45. Taefi A, Cho WK, Nouraie M. Decreasing trend of upper gastrointestinal bleeding mortality risk over three decades. Dig Dis Sci 2013;58(10):2940–8.
46. Hallas J, Dall M, Andries A, et al. Use of single and combined antithrombotic therapy and risk of serious upper gastrointestinal bleeding: population based case-control study. BMJ 2006;333(7571):726.

47. Foley P, Foley S, Kinnaird T, et al. Clinical review: gastrointestinal bleeding after percutaneous coronary intervention: a deadly combination. QJM 2008;101(6): 425–33.
48. Shalev A, Zahger D, Novack V, et al. Incidence, predictors and outcome of upper gastrointestinal bleeding in patients with acute coronary syndromes. Int J Cardiol 2012;157(3):386–90.
49. Islam S, Cevik C, Madonna R, et al. Left ventricular assist devices and gastrointestinal bleeding: a narrative review of case reports and case series. Clin Cardiol 2013;36(4):190–200.
50. Yang JY, Lee TC, Montez-Rath ME, et al. Trends in acute nonvariceal upper gastrointestinal bleeding in dialysis patients. J Am Soc Nephrol 2012;23(3): 495–506.
51. Wu CY, Wu MS, Kuo KN, et al. Long-term peptic ulcer rebleeding risk estimation in patients undergoing haemodialysis: a 10-year nationwide cohort study. Gut 2011;60(8):1038–42.
52. Derry S, Loke YK. Risk of gastrointestinal haemorrhage with long term use of aspirin: meta-analysis. BMJ 2000;321(7270):1183–7.
53. Harker LA, Boissel JP, Pilgrim AJ, et al. Comparative safety and tolerability of clopidogrel and aspirin: results from CAPRIE. CAPRIE Steering Committee and Investigators. Clopidogrel Versus Aspirin in Patients at Risk of Ischaemic Events. Drug Saf 1999;21(4):325–35.
54. Diener HC, Bogousslavsky J, Brass LM, et al. Aspirin and clopidogrel compared with clopidogrel alone after recent ischaemic stroke or transient ischaemic attack in high-risk patients (MATCH): randomised, double-blind, placebo-controlled trial. Lancet 2004;364(9431):331–7.
55. Mehta SR, Yusuf S. The Clopidogrel in Unstable angina to prevent Recurrent Events (CURE) trial programme; rationale, design and baseline characteristics including a meta-analysis of the effects of thienopyridines in vascular disease. Eur Heart J 2000;21(24):2033–41.

Initial Assessment and Resuscitation in Nonvariceal Upper Gastrointestinal Bleeding

Tracey G. Simon, MD[a], Anne C. Travis, MD[b],
John R. Saltzman, MD[b],*

KEYWORDS

- Gastrointestinal bleeding • Nonvariceal hemorrhage • Risk stratification • AIMS65
- Glasgow-Blatchford score

KEY POINTS

- In-hospital mortality ranges from 2% to 14% in patients with upper gastrointestinal bleeding and is most often related to multiorgan failure or advanced metastatic disease.
- Initial rapid evaluation includes a thorough history and assessment of vital signs including orthostatics and blood tests. Effective intravenous access and volume infusion is critical.
- Early evaluation and stratification for mortality and rebleeding risk should be performed using validated prognostic scoring systems, such as the Glasgow-Blatchford, AIMS65, or Rockall score.
- Blood transfusions should target a restrictive transfusion threshold in most patients, as restrictive strategies have been associated with improved patient outcomes.

INTRODUCTION

Acute nonvariceal upper gastrointestinal bleeding (UGIB) remains a common and potentially life-threatening medical condition requiring a prompt, accurate assessment and timely medical and endoscopic management. It has a reported annual incidence of 50 to 150 cases per 100,000 adults and results in considerable patient morbidity as well as utilization of hospital resources.[1–3] Despite improvements in medical therapy with proton pump inhibitors and endoscopic interventions, there is a 2% to 14% mortality rate, with some reports noting up to 27% mortality rates in elderly patients or in those with significant comorbid conditions.[4–6] The most recent reports have found that current

[a] Department of Medicine, Brigham and Women's Hospital, 75 Francis Street, Boston, MA 02215, USA; [b] Division of Gastroenterology, Hepatology and Endoscopy, Department of Medicine, Brigham and Women's Hospital, Harvard Medical School, 75 Francis Street, Boston, MA 02115, USA
* Corresponding author.
E-mail address: jsaltzman@partners.org

Gastrointest Endoscopy Clin N Am 25 (2015) 429–442
http://dx.doi.org/10.1016/j.giec.2015.02.006
1052-5157/15/$ – see front matter

in-hospital mortality in the United States is about 2%.[6] Death among patients admitted with acute nonvariceal UGIB is less often a direct result of the bleeding event. Rather, cardiopulmonary collapse, sepsis, and/or metastatic cancer account for most in-hospital mortality.[7] This finding was demonstrated in a prospective cohort study of patients admitted to a Hong Kong hospital with acute nonvariceal UGIB; of the patients who died, 80% died of non–bleeding-related causes.[8] In addition to appropriate management of the acute bleed, patients with UGIB also require global, supportive management.

The principal components of early management in acute, nonvariceal UGIB include resuscitation, risk stratification, acid suppression, and endoscopy for diagnosis and appropriate intervention. Accurate patient evaluation and assessment of risk is of critical importance, both to improve patient outcomes and minimize health care costs.

DEFINITIONS

An acute GI bleeding event should be clearly characterized with respect to the suspected source of bleeding, bleeding rate, and estimated volume of blood loss. UGIB is defined as bleeding proximal to the ligament of Treitz and may manifest as hematemesis or passage of blood from the rectum (**Table 1**). Hematemesis can contain either fresh blood or clots, consistent with a more acute and active bleed. Specks of dark, granular blood, often described as *coffee grounds* suggest a less active bleed. Blood from the rectum that originates proximal to the ligament of Treitz may appear as black, tarry-appearing stool with a distinct odor, called *melena*. Notably, a middle (small bowel) GI bleed or a slow colonic bleed might also manifest as melena. Finally, maroon-colored stool and/or bright red blood per the rectum may be seen in a brisk upper GI hemorrhage.

The most common cause of nonvariceal UGIB is peptic ulcer disease, which accounts for 31% to 67% of cases.[2,9] This cause is followed by erosive upper GI disease (7%–31%), including esophagitis (3%–12%), malignancy (2%–8%), and Mallory-Weiss tears (4%–8%).[10–12] In 2% to 8% of patients, uncommon causes, including hemobilia, angiodysplasia, aortoenteric fistula, Dieulafoy lesion, or gastric antral vascular ectasia, are found.

HISTORY AND PHYSICAL EXAMINATION

A thorough history detailing symptoms and past medical history may provide insight into the cause of the bleeding (see **Table 1**). Symptoms of acute UGIB may include epigastric pain, dyspepsia, lightheadedness, dizziness, and/or syncope.[5,13]

Table 1
Clinical manifestations of UGIB

	Sources of GI Bleeding					
	Esophagus	Stomach	Duodenum	Small Intestine[a]	Right Colon	Left Colon
Hematemesis	X	X	X	—	—	—
Coffee-ground emesis	X	X	X	—	—	—
Melena	X	X	X	X	X	—
Guaiac-positive stool	X	X	X	X	X	X
BRBPR	(If severe)	(If severe)	(If severe)	(If severe)	X	X

Abbreviation: BRBPR, bright red blood per rectum.
[a] Small bowel distal to the ligament of Treitz.

Symptoms such as dizziness or syncope may be the result of anemia or volume deple-tion. Patients should be asked about a history of prior abdominal pain, bleeding, his-tory of coagulopathy (both inherent and/or related to anticoagulants and antiplatelet agents), nonsteroidal antiinflammatory drug/aspirin use, medications associated with pill esophagitis, *Helicobacter pylori* infection, and smoking status, which is a risk factor for malignancy. The patients' history may also suggest the source of bleeding if there is evidence of liver disease, alcohol abuse, presence of abdominal aortic aneurysm or a prior aortic graft, or known GI malignancy.

Vital signs are of critical importance in the evaluation of patients with acute upper GI hemorrhage. Patients should be assessed for orthostatic hypotension and the pres-ence of shock.[14] Isolated resting tachycardia is a notable finding, as it is the first sign of volume loss and can be seen with mild to moderate hypovolemia.[15]

LABORATORY EVALUATION

Routine laboratory studies should include a complete blood count (CBC), basic meta-bolic panel, coagulation panel, liver tests including albumin, type, and screen. Hemo-globin or hematocrit should be checked every 2 to 12 hours, depending on the severity of the bleed (generally every 6 hours initially with acute GI bleeding). In the acute setting, hemoglobin and hematocrit may initially be normal, as both plasma and red blood cells are lost in equal proportions in whole blood. It is only with time and resus-citation that equilibration occurs and these lab values start to fall, revealing the true degree of blood loss. On the CBC, note should be made of both the mean corpuscular volume (MCV) and the red blood cell distribution width (RDW), as a low MCV and elevated RDW suggest the presence of iron deficiency anemia and a chronic bleed or an acute-on-chronic GI bleed. In addition, a low platelet count may suggest the presence of portal hypertension.

The blood urea nitrogen (BUN)-to-creatinine ratio can be a helpful clinical tool for sug-gesting the location of the bleeding source. In an acute UGIB, the BUN increases as a result of blood degradation and subsequent reabsorption in the small intestine; a BUN-to-creatinine ratio greater than 36 has been shown to be 90% sensitive for UGIB.[16]

Fluid Resuscitation

The first step in the management of patients with UGIB is to provide adequate fluid resuscitation. Patients should receive nothing by mouth, and a bolus of crystalloid fluid (normal saline or Lactated Ringer solution) should be rapidly infused to maintain blood pressure and correct hypovolemia while patients are being typed and cross-matched for blood products.

Early and adequate intravenous (IV) access for volume resuscitation is of critical importance, and the practitioner is often faced with a decision about what type of percutaneous IV catheter to use. Most patients should have 2 large-bore (18-gauge or larger) peripheral IV catheters placed. Factors that influence the speed of fluid resuscitation include catheter length and diameter, the use of pressure with infused fluids, and the type and temperature of infusate. Studies have shown that large-bore peripheral IV catheters demonstrate an 18% to 164% increase in flow rate compared with the same gauge catheters used in central veins because of the shorter length of peripheral catheters.[17,18] Unless the use of a central vein permits the inser-tion of a catheter larger in diameter and shorter in length than could be placed periph-erally, a large-bore peripheral IV catheter may permit more rapid fluid administration.[19] Additionally, it is important to note that piggybacking blood into an existing IV line, rather than infusing blood directly into a separate catheter, can significantly decrease flow rates (340 mL/min vs 20 mL/min).[17] It is important for practitioners to select IV catheters carefully in order to optimize resuscitation in patients with acute UGIB. A comparison of various venous catheters is shown in **Table 2**.

NASOGASTRIC LAVAGE

Nasogastric lavage (NGL) has traditionally been part of the initial assessment of patients with UGIB. However, studies have failed to show a clear benefit of NGL on clinical outcomes; nasogastric tube insertion has been rated the most painful of commonly performed emergency department procedures.[20] Although no large randomized controlled trial of NGL exists, the largest retrospective study of 632 patients admitted with upper GI bleeding found no improvement in 30-day mortality or length of hospital stay, and no significant difference in transfusion requirements or need for surgery after NGL.[21] Although it has been argued that NGL could improve visualization at the time of endoscopy, a multicenter randomized trial demonstrated that IV erythromycin is equivalent to NGL in terms of endoscopic visualization.[22] As a result, current clinical guidelines do not recommend routine NGL in the management of patients with UGIB.[13–15]

Video Capsule Endoscopy

In an attempt to improve risk stratification and identify moderate- and high-risk patients, recent attention has focused on real-time bedside video capsule endoscopy (VCE) for the rapid identification of patients likely to have stigmata of high-risk bleeding at the time of endoscopy. The feasibility of bedside VCE performed in the emergency department in the triage of acute UGIB has been described.[23] Several studies have reported that rapid VCE accurately predicts those patients most likely to have high-risk endoscopic stigmata of bleeding, with high degrees of sensitivity and specificity.[24,25] VCE has several advantages: it can be easily and rapidly performed in an emergency triage setting; it does not require sedation; it poses minimal risk to patients; it permits accurate assessment of patients' need for urgent endoscopy; it does not interfere with subsequent upper endoscopy. Moreover, VCE offers an opportunity to more accurately predict which patients may be at the highest risk of recurrent bleeding, need for endoscopic intervention, or death. However, thus far there are no randomized trials of VCE compared with using validated risk prognostic scores in patients with UGIB. In addition, the cost-effectiveness of this approach has not been formally analyzed, which is important because the cost of VCE is significant.

Table 2 Comparison of flow rates through various intravenous (IV) catheters	
Type and Diameter of Venous Catheter	**Maximum Flow Rate**
20-gauge	60 mL/min
18-gauge	105 mL/min
16-gauge	220 mL/min
Triple lumen catheter	
Medial (blue)/proximal (white) lumen (18-gauge)	26 mL/min
Distal (brown) lumen (16-gauge)	52 mL/min
Cordis: 8.5 French (100 mm)	126 mL/min 333 mL/min under pressure[a]
Intraosseous line	80 mL/min 150 mL/min under pressure[a]

[a] Pressure defined as pressure bag inflated to 300 mm Hg.

RISK STRATIFICATION

The 2010 international consensus and the 2012 guidelines from the American College of Gastroenterology (ACG) recommend that patients with acute UGIB undergo endoscopy within 24 hours of presentation unless they are identified as low risk for rebleeding, need for intervention (including blood transfusion, endoscopic intervention or surgery), or death.[26–28] To determine which low-risk patients may be suitable for safe early discharge and outpatient management, a growing body of literature has focused on the validation of prognostic scoring systems. In addition, these scores can predict which patients are at high risk for poor outcomes. These scores use a combination of clinical, laboratory, and, in some cases, endoscopic parameters to direct appropriate patient intervention and care.

Pre-Endoscopic Risk Scores

The Glasgow Blatchford Risk Score (GBRS), the AIMS65 score, and the clinical Rockall score are among the best-studied pre-endoscopic risk scores. The GBRS was developed to predict the need for hospital-based intervention (blood transfusion, endoscopic therapy, or surgery) among patients with UGIB; this score assigns points to measures of systolic blood pressure, BUN, hemoglobin, and other variables, such as pulse, melena, syncope, hepatic disease, and cardiac failure. Scores range from 0 to 23, with higher scores indicating a higher risk. Patients with a GBRS of 0 have a less than 1% likelihood of requiring endoscopic intervention and, therefore, may safely be discharged before undergoing endoscopy.[29–35] However, 90% of patients have a GBRS greater than 0 and, therefore, would require inpatient management.[36] A more recent study used a higher GBRS cutoff, and found that a cutoff of 1 or less was 99.2% sensitive and 39.8% for identifying low-risk patients and, if used, would decrease the number of patients admitted for UGIB by half.[37]

The AIMS65 score is an easily calculated bedside score used to predict mortality in patients with acute UGIB. Developed from a retrospective cohort of 29,222 patients admitted to the hospital with acute UGIB, there were 5 admission factors independently associated with increased in-patient mortality.[38,39] These factors include

- Albumin less than 3.0 g/dL
- International normalized ratio (INR) greater than 1.5
- Altered mental status
- Systolic blood pressure of 90 mm Hg or less
- Age older than 65 years

The AIMS65 score was validated in a cohort of 32,504 patients and has recently been shown to predict mortality more accurately than the GBRS.[39,40]

The clinical Rockall score, a modified version of the full Rockall score (see later discussion), is used for pre-endoscopic prognostication.[41] In a retrospective analysis of 341 patients admitted with acute UGIB, a clinical Rockall score greater than 3 was associated with a significantly increased rate of rebleeding and surgery as well as increased overall mortality.[42] However, in studies comparing the clinical Rockall score with the GBRS, the GBRS has been found to be superior for predicting mortality and the need for clinical intervention.[36,43,44]

Pre-endoscopic scoring systems are effective for the identification of those lowest-risk patients who may be safe for early discharge and outpatient follow-up. However, they are limited in their ability to accurately distinguish high- from moderate-risk patients. Recent studies have reported that both the GBRS and the clinical Rockall scores are not useful predictors of adverse clinical outcomes in patients outside of the very lowest risk category (ie, GBRS of 0).[45] A summary of the AIMS65, GBRS, and clinical Rockall scores can be found in **Table 3**.

Postendoscopic Prognostic Scores

The American Baylor score, among the first UGIB scores derived in 1993, incorporates 5 clinical and endoscopic variables to predict rebleeding after endoscopic therapy for nonvariceal UGIB.[46] The Cedars-Sinai Predictive Index incorporates endoscopic findings, hemodynamics, comorbidities, and time from onset of symptoms in order to predict patient outcomes and length of stay.[47]

The most widely used postendoscopic scoring system is the Rockall score, which was developed from a large, prospective UK hospital audit, and incorporates variables, including age, hemodynamics, comorbidity, endoscopic diagnosis, and endoscopic findings, to assess the risk of death among patients with acute UGIB.[41] Among those with a Rockall score of 1 or less, the rate of rebleeding was found to be 3.8% and mortality was 0%.

Table 3
Components of the AIMS65, Glasgow-Blatchford, and clinical Rockall risk scores

AIMS65 Score		Glasgow-Blatchford Risk Score		Clinical Rockall Score	
Risk Factor	Points	Risk Factor	Points	Risk Factor	Points
Albumin <3.0 g/dL	1	BUN, mg/dL		SBP <100 mm Hg	2
INR >1.5	1	≥18.2 to <22.4	2	Pulse >100 bpm	1
Altered mental status	1	≥22.4 to <28.0	3	**Age**	
SBP ≤90 mm Hg	1	≥28.0 to <70.0	4	<60 y	0
Age >65 y	1	≥70.0	6	60–79 y	1
		Hemoglobin, men g/dL		>80 y	2
		≥12.0 to <13.0	1	**Comorbidities**	
		≥10.0 to <12.0	3	None	0
		<10.0	6	Any	2
		Hemoglobin, women g/dL		Renal or liver failure or advanced malignancy	3
		≥10.0 to <12.0	1		
		<10.0	6		
		SBP, mm Hg			
		100–109	1		
		90–99	2		
		<90	3		
		Other parameters			
		Heart rate ≥100 bpm	1		
		Melena	1		
		Syncope	2		
		Liver disease	2		
		Heart failure	2		
Maximum score	5	*Maximum score*	23	*Maximum score*	7

Abbreviations: bpm, beats per minute; SBP, systolic blood pressure.

The Baylor, Cedars-Sinai, and Rockall scores have all been shown to predict mortality more accurately than they predict rebleeding.[48] However, the Rockall score has also been shown to be superior to both the Baylor and Cedars-Sinai scores in identifying low-risk patients who may be candidates for outpatient management.[48] In a recent prospective trial designed to compare the accuracy of the GBRS with the Rockall, Baylor, and Cedars-Sinai scoring systems, the GBRS more accurately identified those patients with UGIB most likely to require inpatient management and those who could safely be discharged with close outpatient care.[49]

In 2010, the Italian Progetto Nazionale Emorragi Digestiva (PNED) score was derived to predict the mortality of patients presenting with nonvariceal UGIB.[50] The 10-variable calculation results in a score total ranging from 0 to 24 points. It was developed using both new and previously identified predictive factors for mortality and incorporated both clinical and endoscopic data. The PNED score is the first score to use failure of endoscopic hemostasis as one of the weighted variables in its calculation. The study found that the PNED score was accurate at predicting mortality (area under the receiver operating characteristic curve [AUROC] 0.81, 95% confidence interval [CI] 0.72–0.90). A score of less than 2 was associated with 0% mortality; a score of 5 to 8 was associated with 10% mortality; a score of 9 or greater had a 32% mortality rate. The PNED score was superior to the Rockall score for predicting 30-day mortality; however, the PNED score requires additional validation.

In 2009, the Chinese University of Hong Kong (CUHK) Prediction Score was developed with mortality as the primary outcome variable.[51] The score focuses on patients with UGIB from peptic ulcers and does not include other sources of hemorrhage. Consecutive patients with endoscopic stigmata of active bleeding, visible vessels, or adherent clots were recruited; risk factors for mortality were identified in the derivation cohort using multiple stepwise logistic regression. A prediction model was then developed and included factors such as age, comorbid illnesses, hypovolemic shock, in-hospital bleeding, rebleeding, and need for surgery. When applied to a validation cohort, the model had good predictive ability for mortality (AUROC 0.73).

Other scores, including the Forrest Score and the Spanish Almela score, have been created but have not yet been externally validated in prospective, international patient populations.[50] A comparison of major risk-stratification scores in acute UGIB is shown in **Table 4**.

APPROACH TO BLOOD TRANSFUSION

The purpose of packed red blood cell transfusion is to restore oxygen delivery and maintain adequate regional and global tissue perfusion. Currently, international consensus and the ACG's practice guidelines recommend a threshold for initiation of blood transfusions of hemoglobin less than or equal to 7 g/dL among patients with acute nonvariceal UGIB and less than or equal to 8 g/dL in patients with variceal bleeding.[26]

The decision to initiate blood transfusions must be individualized, and the optimal transfusion strategy remains a subject of controversy. Transfusion is clearly indicated in any patient with acute UGIB and evidence of hypovolemia, shock, significant ongoing hemorrhage, or tissue hypoxia (ie, cardiac ischemia). In such patients, a more liberal approach to blood transfusions (ie, targeting hemoglobin greater than 9–10 g/dL) is appropriate. Other comorbidities, including recent cardiac surgery or certain hematologic malignancies, may require a more liberal transfusion approach.[26,52]

In critically ill patients, a liberal approach to blood transfusion has been associated with adverse clinical outcomes and increased mortality, compared with a more restrictive strategy.[53–55] A 2008 meta-analysis of observational studies compiled from the

Table 4
Characteristics of UGIB scores

Score	Author (Reference), Year	Before or After Endoscopy	Outcome	Population	Patients	Results
Glasgow-Blatchford	Blatchford et al,[29] 2000	Before	Need for intervention	United Kingdom	1748	AUROC = 0.92
AIMS65	Saltzman et al,[39] 2011	Before	Mortality	United States	29,222	AUROC = 0.80
Rockall	Rockall et al,[41] 1996	After (clinical score before endoscopy)	Mortality	United Kingdom	4185	N/A, rates per score group reported
Italian PNED	Marmo et al,[50] 2010	After	Mortality	Italy	1360	AUROC = 0.81
CUHK	Chiu et al,[51] 2009	After	Mortality	China	3220	AUROC = 0.84

Abbreviations: N/A, not applicable.

surgical, trauma, and intensive care settings found that when compared with not transfusing, blood transfusion was associated with a higher risk of death and adverse events, including nosocomial infection, multiorgan dysfunction, and acute respiratory distress syndrome.[56] The harm associated with liberal transfusion strategies may be related to increased splanchnic and portal pressures,[57,58] exacerbation of coagulopathies,[59] and immunologic factors.[60]

Although previous guidelines recommended transfusion thresholds of 9 to 10 g/dL, mounting evidence has demonstrated the safety and efficacy of the more restrictive approach, with a target hemoglobin of 7 to 8 g/dL. In 3 recent randomized trials of critically ill patients admitted to the intensive care unit, patients who received transfusions targeting hemoglobin greater than 7 g/dL had no increase in morbidity or mortality rates and no increase in hospital length of stay.[61] However, the generalizability of these trials is limited, as patients with UGIB were largely excluded from analysis.

The most direct evidence favoring a restrictive approach to blood transfusions in acute UGIB comes from a randomized trial published in 2013.[62] In this trial, 921 consecutive adults with acute UGIB were randomly assigned to receive blood transfusions if their hemoglobin value was less than 9 g/dL (liberal transfusion arm) or to receive transfusions only for a hemoglobin value less than 7 g/dL (restrictive transfusion arm). Patients with exsanguinating hemorrhage were excluded. Those in the restrictive transfusion arm had lower overall mortality rates compared with the liberal transfusion arm (5% vs 9%; adjusted hazard ratio 0.55, 95% CI 0.33–0.92; $P = .02$), as well as lower overall rates of further bleeding (10% vs 16%; $P = .01$). In a recent meta-analysis of 4 randomized trials comparing outcomes in patients with acute UGIB assigned to restrictive versus liberal transfusion strategies, mortality was significantly reduced in patients in the restrictive transfusion arms (odds ratio [OR] 0.52, 95% CI 0.31–0.87; $P = .01$); this group also had a significantly shorter hospital length of stay (standard mean difference −0.17, 95% CI −0.30 to −0.04; $P = .009$).[63]

MANAGEMENT OF COAGULOPATHY

Among patients presenting with acute UGIB, research has suggested a relationship between an elevated INR (>1.5) and increased mortality.[64,65] However, a mild to moderate INR elevation does not seem to affect the effectiveness of hemostasis during endoscopic intervention or overall mortality. This was first shown in a retrospective cohort study of 52 anticoagulated patients presenting with acute UGIB, who were compared with 50 matched controls not previously on anticoagulation.[66] If needed, patients received fresh frozen plasma to decrease their INR to between 1.5 and 2.5 before endoscopy. Both the rates of hemostasis and overall mortality were similar among anticoagulated and nonanticoagulated patients (91% vs 92%, and 0% vs 4%, respectively).

A moderately elevated INR at the time of endoscopy has not been shown to impact outcomes, such as initial control of bleeding or rate of rebleeding.[67] A 2007 retrospective analysis of 233 patients with acute nonvariceal UGIB evaluated the impact of an elevated INR at the time of endoscopy on patient outcomes.[68] Patients were divided into 2 groups according to an INR cutoff level of 1.3. Fifty-six percent had an INR less than or equal to 1.3, and 44% had an INR greater than 1.3 (95% of those subjects had an INR between 1.3 and 2.7). The two groups did not vary in terms of rebleeding rate, transfusion requirement, need for surgery, length of stay, or mortality rate. In a Canadian multicenter study of 1869 patients, 462 patients (24.7%) had an elevated INR at the time of presentation (mean INR 1.5 ± 1.7), including an INR greater than 2.5 in 7.6%. In this study, the INR did not add to the prediction of rebleeding; however, similar to the AIMS65 study, an INR greater than 1.5 did predict mortality (OR 1.96, 95% CI 1.13–3.41).[65]

These studies suggest that endoscopic therapy can be safely performed in patients who are mildly to moderately anticoagulated, and the most recent consensus recommendations state that correction of a moderate coagulopathy (INR up to 2.5) should not delay endoscopy.[26]

PLATELET TRANSFUSION THRESHOLDS

Uncertainty exists regarding optimal platelet values and target thresholds for platelet transfusion among patients with acute, nonvariceal UGIB. In a systematic review of 18 studies (including 4 randomized controlled trials and 6 cohort studies), it was concluded that there is insufficient evidence for determining the proper target platelet level in this patient population.[69] However, based on expert opinions and consensus statements, they proposed a platelet transfusion threshold of 50×10^9/L (or 100×10^9/L if altered platelet function is suspected) among patients with acute UGIB.

SUMMARY

Acute nonvariceal UGIB remains an important cause of hospital admission and is associated with significant mortality. Rapid and effective patient assessment and appropriate intravascular volume resuscitation are critical components of early management. Patients should then be risk-stratified according to hemodynamic status, ongoing bleeding, comorbidities, age, and laboratory test results. Both pre-endoscopic and postendoscopic risk stratification scores assist in patient triage and may improve patient outcomes and decrease health care spending through standardization of care.

REFERENCES

1. Vreeburg EM, Snel P, de Bruijne JW, et al. Acute upper gastrointestinal bleeding in the Amsterdam area: incidence, diagnosis, and clinical outcome. Am J Gastroenterol 1997;92:236–43.
2. van Leerdam ME, Vreeburg EM, Rauws EA, et al. Acute upper GI bleeding: did anything change? Time trend analysis of incidence and outcome of acute upper GI bleeding between 1993/1994 and 2000. Am J Gastroenterol 2003;98:1494–9.
3. Targownik LE, Nabalamba A. Trends in management and outcomes of acute nonvariceal upper gastrointestinal bleeding: 1993–2003. Clin Gastroenterol Hepatol 2006;4:1459–66.
4. Weng SC, Shu KH, Tarng DC, et al. In-hospital mortality risk estimation in patients with acute nonvariceal upper gastrointestinal bleeding undergoing hemodialysis: a retrospective cohort study. Ren Fail 2013;35:243–8.
5. Laine L, Peterson WL. Bleeding peptic ulcer. N Engl J Med 1994;331:717–27.
6. Abougergi MS, Travis AC, Saltzman JR. Impact of day of admission on mortality and other outcomes in upper GI hemorrhage: a nationwide analysis. Gastrointest Endosc 2014;80:228–35.
7. Sostres C, Lanas A. Epidemiology and demographics of upper gastrointestinal bleeding: prevalence, incidence, and mortality. Gastrointest Endosc Clin N Am 2011;21:567–81.
8. Sung JJ, Tsoi KK, Ma TK, et al. Causes of mortality in patients with peptic ulcer bleeding: a prospective cohort study of 10,428 cases. Am J Gastroenterol 2010;105:84–9.

9. van Leerdam ME. Epidemiology of acute upper gastrointestinal bleeding. Best Pract Res Clin Gastroenterol 2008;22:209–24.

10. Loperfido S, Baldo V, Piovesana E, et al. Changing trends in acute upper-GI bleeding: a population-based study. Gastrointest Endosc 2009;70:212–24.

11. Hearnshaw SA, Logan RF, Lowe D, et al. Acute upper gastrointestinal bleeding in the UK: patient characteristics, diagnoses and outcomes in the 2007 UK audit. Gut 2011;60:1327–35.

12. Nahon S, Hagege H, Latrive JP, et al. Epidemiological and prognostic factors involved in upper gastrointestinal bleeding: results of a French prospective multi-center study. Endoscopy 2012;44:998–1008.

13. Rivkin K, Lyakhovetskiy A. Treatment of nonvariceal upper gastrointestinal bleeding. Am J Health Syst Pharm 2005;62:1159–70.

14. Lanier JB, Mote MB, Clay EC. Evaluation and management of orthostatic hypotension. Am Fam Physician 2011;84:527–36.

15. Cappell MS, Friedel D. Initial management of acute upper gastrointestinal bleeding: from initial evaluation up to gastrointestinal endoscopy. Med Clin North Am 2008;92:491–509, xi.

16. Ernst AA, Haynes ML, Nick TG, et al. Usefulness of the blood urea nitrogen/creatinine ratio in gastrointestinal bleeding. Am J Emerg Med 1999;17:70–2.

17. Dutky PA, Stevens SL, Maull KI. Factors affecting rapid fluid resuscitation with large-bore introducer catheters. J Trauma 1989;29:856–60.

18. Hodge D 3rd, Fleisher G. Pediatric catheter flow rates. Am J Emerg Med 1985;3:403–7.

19. Macnab A, Christenson J, Findlay J, et al. A new system for sternal intraosseous infusion in adults. Prehosp Emerg Care 2000;4:173–7.

20. Singer AJ, Richman PB, Kowalska A, et al. Comparison of patient and practitioner assessments of pain from commonly performed emergency department procedures. Ann Emerg Med 1999;33:652–8.

21. Huang ES, Karsan S, Kanwal F, et al. Impact of nasogastric lavage on outcomes in acute GI bleeding. Gastrointest Endosc 2011;74:971–80.

22. Pateron D, Vicaut E, Debuc E, et al. Erythromycin infusion or gastric lavage for upper gastrointestinal bleeding: a multicenter randomized controlled trial. Ann Emerg Med 2011;57:582–9.

23. Gralnek IM, Ching JY, Maza I, et al. Capsule endoscopy in acute upper gastrointestinal hemorrhage: a prospective cohort study. Endoscopy 2013;45:12–9.

24. Gutkin E, Shalomov A, Hussain SA, et al. Pillcam ESO ((R)) is more accurate than clinical scoring systems in risk stratifying emergency room patients with acute upper gastrointestinal bleeding. Therap Adv Gastroenterol 2013;6:193–8.

25. Rubin M, Hussain SA, Shalomov A, et al. Live view video capsule endoscopy enables risk stratification of patients with acute upper GI bleeding in the emergency room: a pilot study. Dig Dis Sci 2011;56:786–91.

26. Barkun AN, Bardou M, Kuipers EJ, et al. International consensus recommendations on the management of patients with nonvariceal upper gastrointestinal bleeding. Ann Intern Med 2010;152:101–13.

27. Barkun A, Bardou M, Marshall JK, et al, Nonvariceal Upper GIBCCG. Consensus recommendations for managing patients with nonvariceal upper gastrointestinal bleeding. Ann Intern Med 2003;139:843–57.

28. Sung JJ, Chan FK, Chen M, et al. Asia-Pacific Working Group consensus on nonvariceal upper gastrointestinal bleeding. Gut 2011;60:1170–7.

29. Blatchford O, Murray WR, Blatchford M. A risk score to predict need for treatment for upper-gastrointestinal haemorrhage. Lancet 2000;356:1318–21.

30. Cebollero-Santamaria F, Smith J, Gioe S, et al. Selective outpatient management of upper gastrointestinal bleeding in the elderly: results from the SOME Bleeding Study. Ochsner J 1999;1:195–201.

31. Romagnuolo J, Barkun AN, Enns R, et al. Simple clinical predictors may obviate urgent endoscopy in selected patients with nonvariceal upper gastrointestinal tract bleeding. Arch Intern Med 2007;167:265–70.

32. de Groot NL, Bosman JH, Siersema PD, et al. Prediction scores in gastrointestinal bleeding: a systematic review and quantitative appraisal. Endoscopy 2012;44:731–9.

33. Almela P, Benages A, Peiro S, et al. A risk score system for identification of patients with upper-GI bleeding suitable for outpatient management. Gastrointest Endosc 2004;59:772–81.

34. Cipolletta L, Bianco MA, Rotondano G, et al. Outpatient management for low-risk nonvariceal upper GI bleeding: a randomized controlled trial. Gastrointest Endosc 2002;55:1–5.

35. Masaoka T, Suzuki H, Hori S, et al. Blatchford scoring system is a useful scoring system for detecting patients with upper gastrointestinal bleeding who do not need endoscopic intervention. J Gastroenterol Hepatol 2007;22:1404–8.

36. Stanley AJ, Ashley D, Dalton HR, et al. Outpatient management of patients with low-risk upper-gastrointestinal haemorrhage: multicentre validation and prospective evaluation. Lancet 2009;373:42–7.

37. Laursen SB, Dalton HR, Murray IA, et al. Performance of new thresholds of the Glasgow Blatchford score in managing patients with upper gastrointestinal bleeding. Clin Gastroenterol Hepatol 2015;13:115–21.e2.

38. Liang PS, Saltzman JR. A national survey on the initial management of upper gastrointestinal bleeding. J Clin Gastroenterol 2014;48(10):e93–8.

39. Saltzman JR, Tabak YP, Hyett BH, et al. A simple risk score accurately predicts in-hospital mortality, length of stay, and cost in acute upper GI bleeding. Gastrointest Endosc 2011;74:1215–24.

40. Nakamura S, Matsumoto T, Sugimori H, et al. Emergency endoscopy for acute gastrointestinal bleeding: prognostic value of endoscopic hemostasis and the AIMS65 score in Japanese patients. Dig Endosc 2014;26:369–76.

41. Rockall TA, Logan RF, Devlin HB, et al. Risk assessment after acute upper gastrointestinal haemorrhage. Gut 1996;38:316–21.

42. Wang CY, Qin J, Wang J, et al. Rockall score in predicting outcomes of elderly patients with acute upper gastrointestinal bleeding. World J Gastroenterol 2013;19:3466–72.

43. Stanley AJ, Dalton HR, Blatchford O, et al. Multicentre comparison of the Glasgow Blatchford and Rockall scores in the prediction of clinical end-points after upper gastrointestinal haemorrhage. Aliment Pharmacol Ther 2011;34:470–5.

44. Pang SH, Ching JY, Lau JY, et al. Comparing the Blatchford and pre-endoscopic Rockall score in predicting the need for endoscopic therapy in patients with upper GI hemorrhage. Gastrointest Endosc 2010;71:1134–40.

45. Chandra S, Hess EP, Agarwal D, et al. External validation of the Glasgow-Blatchford bleeding score and the Rockall score in the US setting. Am J Emerg Med 2012;30:673–9.

46. Saeed ZA, Winchester CB, Michaletz PA, et al. A scoring system to predict rebleeding after endoscopic therapy of nonvariceal upper gastrointestinal hemorrhage, with a comparison of heat probe and ethanol injection. Am J Gastroenterol 1993;88:1842–9.

47. Hay JA, Maldonado L, Weingarten SR, et al. Prospective evaluation of a clinical guideline recommending hospital length of stay in upper gastrointestinal tract hemorrhage. JAMA 1997;278:2151–6.
48. Camellini L, Merighi A, Pagnini C, et al. Comparison of three different risk scoring systems in non-variceal upper gastrointestinal bleeding. Dig Liver Dis 2004;36:271–7.
49. Laursen SB, Hansen JM, Schaffalitzky de Muckadell OB. The Glasgow Blatchford score is the most accurate assessment of patients with upper gastrointestinal hemorrhage. Clin Gastroenterol Hepatol 2012;10:1130–5.e1.
50. Marmo R, Koch M, Cipolletta L, et al. Predicting mortality in non-variceal upper gastrointestinal bleeders: validation of the Italian PNED score and prospective comparison with the Rockall score. Am J Gastroenterol 2010;105:1284–91.
51. Chiu PW, Ng EK, Cheung FK, et al. Predicting mortality in patients with bleeding peptic ulcers after therapeutic endoscopy. Clin Gastroenterol Hepatol 2009;7:311–6 [quiz: 253].
52. Laine L, Jensen DM. Management of patients with ulcer bleeding. Am J Gastroenterol 2012;107:345–60 [quiz: 361].
53. Robinson WP 3rd, Ahn J, Stiffler A, et al. Blood transfusion is an independent predictor of increased mortality in nonoperatively managed blunt hepatic and splenic injuries. J Trauma 2005;58:437–44 [discussion: 444–5].
54. Malone DL, Dunne J, Tracy JK, et al. Blood transfusion, independent of shock severity, is associated with worse outcome in trauma. J Trauma 2003;54:898–905 [discussion: 905–7].
55. Hebert PC, Wells G, Blajchman MA, et al. A multicenter, randomized, controlled clinical trial of transfusion requirements in critical care. Transfusion requirements in critical care investigators, Canadian Critical Care Trials Group. N Engl J Med 1999;340:409–17.
56. Marik PE, Corwin HL. Efficacy of red blood cell transfusion in the critically ill: a systematic review of the literature. Crit Care Med 2008;36:2667–74.
57. Kravetz D, Sikuler E, Groszmann RJ. Splanchnic and systemic hemodynamics in portal hypertensive rats during hemorrhage and blood volume restitution. Gastroenterology 1986;90:1232–40.
58. Castaneda B, Morales J, Lionetti R, et al. Effects of blood volume restitution following a portal hypertensive-related bleeding in anesthetized cirrhotic rats. Hepatology 2001;33:821–5.
59. Halland M, Young M, Fitzgerald MN, et al. Characteristics and outcomes of upper gastrointestinal hemorrhage in a tertiary referral hospital. Dig Dis Sci 2010;55:3430–5.
60. Vamvakas EC, Blajchman MA. Transfusion-related immunomodulation (TRIM): an update. Blood Rev 2007;21:327–48.
61. Carson JL, Terrin ML, Noveck H, et al. Liberal or restrictive transfusion in high-risk patients after hip surgery. N Engl J Med 2011;365:2453–62.
62. Villanueva C, Colomo A, Bosch A. Transfusion for acute upper gastrointestinal bleeding. N Engl J Med 2013;368:1362–3.
63. Wang J, Bao YX, Bai M, et al. Restrictive vs liberal transfusion for upper gastrointestinal bleeding: a meta-analysis of randomized controlled trials. World J Gastroenterol 2013;19:6919–27.
64. Baker RI, Coughlin PB, Gallus AS, et al. Warfarin reversal: consensus guidelines, on behalf of the Australasian Society of Thrombosis and Haemostasis. Med J Aust 2004;181:492–7.
65. Shingina A, Barkun AN, Razzaghi A, et al. Systematic review: the presenting international normalised ratio (INR) as a predictor of outcome in patients with

upper nonvariceal gastrointestinal bleeding. Aliment Pharmacol Ther 2011;33: 1010–8.

66. Choudari CP, Rajgopal C, Palmer KR. Acute gastrointestinal haemorrhage in anti-coagulated patients: diagnoses and response to endoscopic treatment. Gut 1994;35:464–6.

67. Barkun A, Sabbah S, Enns R, et al. The Canadian Registry on Nonvariceal Upper Gastrointestinal Bleeding and Endoscopy (RUGBE): endoscopic hemostasis and proton pump inhibition are associated with improved outcomes in a real-life setting. Am J Gastroenterol 2004;99:1238–46.

68. Wolf AT, Wasan SK, Saltzman JR. Impact of anticoagulation on rebleeding following endoscopic therapy for nonvariceal upper gastrointestinal hemorrhage. Am J Gastroenterol 2007;102:290–6.

69. Razzaghi A, Barkun AN. Platelet transfusion threshold in patients with upper gastrointestinal bleeding: a systematic review. J Clin Gastroenterol 2012;46: 482–6.

Nonvariceal Upper Gastrointestinal Bleeding

Timing of Endoscopy and Ways to Improve Endoscopic Visualization

Iyad Khamaysi, MD[a,b], Ian M. Gralnek, MD, MSHS, FASGE[a,c],*

KEYWORDS

- Upper gastrointestinal bleeding • Endoscopy • Prokinetic agent
- Peptic ulcer bleeding

KEY POINTS

- The first priority in the management of upper gastrointestinal bleeding (UGIB) is correcting fluid losses and restoring hemodynamic stability.
- After hemodynamic stabilization, patients should undergo "early" upper endoscopy, now routinely defined as performance within 24 hours of patient presentation.
- The availability GI endoscopists proficient in endoscopic hemostasis and support staff with technical expertise enables performance of endoscopy on a 24/7 basis and is recommended.
- Routine use of a prokinetic in all UGIB patients is not recommended.
- Use of a prokinetic in patients with a suspected high probability of having blood or clots in the stomach may improve endoscopic visualization and diagnostic yield.

INTRODUCTION

Acute upper gastrointestinal bleeding (UGIB) refers to gross GI blood loss originating proximal to the ligament of Treitz that usually manifests as fresh blood hematemesis, "coffee ground" emesis, and/or melena with or without hemodynamic compromise.[1–5] Hematochezia may be the presenting sign in patients with extremely brisk UGIB, yet this clinical presentation is uncommon.[6] Traditional negative patient

Neither Prof I.M. Gralnek nor Dr I. Khamaysi have any commercial or financial conflict of interests to declare for this article.
[a] Rappaport Faculty of Medicine, Technion-Israel Institute of Technology, Israel; [b] Interventional Endoscopy Unit, Department of Gastroenterology, Rambam Health Care Campus, Haifa, Israel; [c] The Institute of Gastroenterology and Liver Diseases, Ha'Emek Medical Center, Afula, Israel
* Corresponding author. Rappaport Faculty of Medicine, Technion-Israel Institute of Technology, Institute of Gastroenterology and Liver Diseases, Ha'Emek Medical Center, Afula, Israel.
E-mail address: ian_gr@clalit.org.il

outcomes include rebleeding and mortality, with patient mortality commonly associated with decompensation of preexisting comorbid medical conditions precipitated by the acute bleeding event.[1–3,7]

In most clinical settings, the great majority (80%–90%) of episodes of acute UGIB are secondary to nonvariceal causes, the foremost being peptic ulcer bleeding. Upper endoscopy is the most accurate and practical method for diagnosing the source of acute UGIB. Subsequently, appropriate endoscopic therapy significantly reduces mortality, rebleeding, requirement for transfusion, hospital stay, and health care costs. Even in the absence of specific endoscopic hemostasis therapy, the prognostic information obtained from upper endoscopy can significantly reduce the use of health care resources.[1–4]

TIMING OF ENDOSCOPY

The first priority in UGIB patient management is correcting fluid losses and restoring hemodynamic stability. Volume resuscitation should be initiated with crystalloid intravenous (IV) fluids with the use of large-bore IV catheters (eg, 2 peripheral catheters of 16–18 gauge or a central catheter if peripheral venous access is not attainable). To maintain adequate oxygen-carrying capacity, especially in older patients with coexisting cardiopulmonary comorbidities, the use of supplemental oxygen and transfusion of plasma expanders (eg, packed red blood cells) should be considered. When indicated, correction of coagulopathy should be undertaken but should not delay performance of upper endoscopy.[1–3] This can be achieved using fresh frozen plasma and in selected cases (if the platelet count is <50,000) transfusion of platelets.

Blood transfusions should be considered in patients with a hemoglobin level below 70 g/L. Early transfusions (given within 12 hours of patient presentation) have been shown to be associated with higher rates of rebleeding and a higher 30-day mortality.[8] Villanueva and colleagues recently reported on 921 patients with UGIB randomly assigned to either a restrictive (transfuse at a hemoglobin level of ≤70 g/L) or liberal (transfuse at a hemoglobin level of ≤90 g/L) transfusion strategy. Those who received the restrictive blood transfusion strategy had significantly lower mortality at 45 days (95% vs 91%; hazard ratio [HR], 0.55; 95% CI, 0.33–0.92), less rebleeding (10% vs 16%; HR, 0.68; 95% CI, 0.47–0.98), and fewer overall adverse events.[9] However, in the subset of nonvariceal UGIB patients, significantly improved outcomes were limited to a reduced need for surgery and only statistical trends suggesting less rebleeding and improved survival. These blood transfusion thresholds may not necessarily apply to patients with significant medical comorbidities (ie, acute coronary syndrome, symptomatic peripheral ischemia, stroke, or transient ischemic attack). Such patients may benefit from a more liberal transfusion policy in an attempt to avoid disease exacerbations induced by significant GI blood loss.

After hemodynamic stabilization, patients should undergo "early" upper endoscopy (now routinely defined as performance within 24 hours of patient presentation).[1–3] Some high-risk patients, such as those with acute coronary syndrome or a suspected bowel perforation, may benefit from deferring endoscopy until their clinical situation is more fully evaluated and stabilized. Low-risk patients, identified using a pre-endoscopy risk stratification score (eg, Glasgow-Blatchford) can be considered for outpatient management.[9] Very early or emergent upper endoscopy, performed within 2 to 12 hours of patient presentation, has not been shown to confer any additional benefit or alter patient outcomes compared with 'early' endoscopy.[10] In patients who require endoscopic hemostasis therapy, early upper endoscopy results in improved patient outcome. Cooper and colleagues[11] reported that early endoscopy significantly reduced rebleeding and surgery in patients who required endoscopic hemostasis. It has also been shown that, compared with patients who undergo routine endoscopy, early endoscopy is safe and reduces the hospital duration of stay for all patients, regardless of need for endotherapy.[12–15] Early endoscopy (performed within 24 hours of patient presentation) is performed, therefore, because of its potential to improve clinical outcomes in the subset of patients who require endoscopic hemostasis and overall reduces hospital length of stay and health care costs.

Studies of urgent endoscopy[16,17] (ie, endoscopy performed within only a few hours of patient presentation) have not shown any differences in patient outcomes compared with routine timed performance of endoscopy. Several randomized, controlled trials and retrospective cohort studies have examined "very early endoscopy" at less than 2 to 3, less than 6, less than 8, or less than 12 hours compared with endoscopy performed at less than 24 to 48 hours.[16] Very early endoscopy yielded higher rates of finding high-risk endoscopic stigmata of bleeding, and thus, higher rates of endoscopic hemostasis, but without demonstrable improved outcomes of rebleeding, need for surgery, or duration of hospitalization.[13,17] In higher risk patients, 1 study randomizing patients to upper endoscopy fewer than 12 hours versus longer than 12 hours from patient presentation, detected a significantly reduced need for blood transfusions and shorter hospitalization (4 vs 14.5 days) in the subgroup of patients with coffee grounds or bloody nasogastric aspirate.[18] Moreover, an observational study demonstrated that longer time to endoscopy predicted all-cause, "in hospital" mortality in patients with a Blatchford score of 12 or higher.[19] The American College of Gastroenterology's recent guidelines on peptic ulcer bleeding suggest that upper endoscopy performed within 12 hours of patient presentation may be considered in high-risk patients. Similarly, the United Kingdom UGIB toolkit produced by the Academy of Royal Medical Colleges recommends upper endoscopy within 6 to 12 hours in "urgent-risk" patients, a practice that is currently not supported by high-quality evidence for nonvariceal UGIB,[2] although appropriate in the context of suspected variceal bleeding where upper endoscopy within 12 hours is recommended.

Data from bleeding registries show that a significant proportion of UGIB patients have a delay of greater than 24 hours before undergoing upper endoscopy.[20,21] Reasons behind such delays are likely multifactorial; however, several reports from administrative databases report a "weekend effect," whereby UGIB patients presenting on weekends are less likely to undergo early endoscopy and have higher mortality, which may or may not be owing to the delay in receiving endoscopy.[20–22] Nevertheless, endoscopy within 24 hours of patient presentation should be targeted as a standalone quality indicator when managing patients with acute UGIB.[23] The availability both of on-call GI endoscopists proficient in endoscopic hemostasis and on-call support staff with technical expertise in the usage of endoscopic devices enables performance of endoscopy on a 24/7 basis and is recommended.

IMPROVING VISUALIZATION

Upper GI endoscopy in the bleeding patient should be carried out in an adequately equipped setting by qualified endoscopists and support staff. Ideally, a therapeutic upper endoscope with a large single channel (eg, ≥3.3 mm so as to allow the use of 10-F size devices) should be used. Upper GI endoscopes with a 6-mm "jumbo" channel or double-channel are available and may occasionally be advantageous to use. All devices for endoscopic hemostasis (injection needles and solutions, multi-polar/bipolar contact thermal probes, mechanical devices such as through the scope hemoclips and larger size over-the-scope clips, band-ligating devices, and topical hemostatic powders) should all be available for use. The assistance of an anesthesiologist is required in patients with severe ongoing hematemesis or an inability to control their airway such that endotracheal intubation should be considered in such selected cases to prevent aspiration.

In patients with acute UGIB, the quality of the endoscopic examination can be adversely affected by poor visibility owing to obscuring blood, clots, and fluids in the gastric lumen and duodenum. It is reported that, in 3% to 19% of UGIB cases, no obvious cause is identified.[20,24,25] This may in part be related to the presence of bloody debris impairing endoscopic visualization. In addition to the use of water jet irrigation and adequate suction through the working channel of the endoscope, the patient may also need to be rolled over into various positions to move fluids/clots and thereby improve endoscopic visualization, especially of the gastric fundus. In cases of large fundal blood clots, one may also consider inserting a large-bore nasogastric or orogastric tube to clear the stomach and repeat the endoscopic examination shortly thereafter.

The use of IV prokinetic agents should also be considered during the pre-endoscopy patient management phase. A recent metaanalysis of 3 randomized, controlled trials using erythromycin and 2 abstracts using metoclopramide and including a total of 162 patients evaluated the effectiveness of prokinetic agents before index endoscopy in patients presenting with acute UGIB.[26] This metaanalysis demonstrated that an IV prokinetic administered up to 2 hours before endoscopy in patients with acute UGIB improved endoscopic visualization and decreased significantly the need for repeat endoscopy to determine the site and cause of bleeding (odds ratio [OR], 0.55; 95% CI, 0.32–0.94). However, there was no improvement in other clinical outcomes, including hospital length of stay, blood transfusion requirements, or need for surgery, and this observed treatment effect was not preserved when analyzing metoclopramide alone. Two more recent metaanalyses solely evaluating erythromycin showed similar results with improvement in the visualization of the gastric mucosa (OR, 3.43; 1.81–6.50), and a decrease in the need for a second-look endoscopy (OR, 0.47; 0.26–0.83).[27] Interestingly, the effects of pre-endoscopy IV erythromycin in decreasing units of blood transfused and reducing hospital duration of stay, attained significance when an additional trial that only included patients with variceal bleeding was added to the metaanalysis.[28]

Thus, the use of erythromycin (250 mg IV administered 30–120 minutes before endoscopy) may be the favored prokinetic agent based on current evidence.[26–28] It should be noted, however, that the QT-interval–prolonging effect of erythromycin should always be taken into consideration, and an electrocardiogram may be performed before initiation in suspected 'at-risk' patients. Although the routine use of prokinetic agents in all UGIB patients is not recommended, use in patients with a suspected high probability of having blood or clots in the stomach before undergoing endoscopy may result in improved endoscopic visualization, a higher diagnostic yield, and less need for repeat endoscopy, and therefore should be considered.[1–3]

SUMMARY

Upper GI endoscopy is the cornerstone of diagnosis and management of patients presenting with acute UGIB. Once hemodynamically resuscitated, early endoscopy (performed within 24 hours of patient presentation) ensures accurate identification of the bleeding source, facilitates risk stratification based on endoscopic stigmata, and allows endotherapy to be delivered where indicated. Moreover, the pre-endoscopy use of a prokinetic agent (eg, IV erythromycin), especially in patients with a suspected high probability of having blood or clots in the stomach before undergoing endoscopy, may result in improved endoscopic visualization, a higher diagnostic yield, and less need for repeat endoscopy.

REFERENCES

1. Gralnek IM, Barkun AM, Bardou M. Current concepts: management of acute bleeding from a peptic ulcer. N Engl J Med 2008;359:928–37.
2. Barkun AN, Bardou M, Kuipers EJ, et al. International consensus recommendations on the management of patients with non-variceal upper gastrointestinal bleeding. Ann Intern Med 2010;152:101–13.
3. Laine L, Jensen DM. Management of patients with ulcer bleeding. Am J Gastroenterol 2012;107:345–60.
4. Hwang JH, Fisher DA, Ben-Menachem T, et al. The role of endoscopy in the management of acute non-variceal upper GI bleeding. Gastrointest Endosc 2012;75: 132–8.
5. Esrailian E, Gralnek IM. Non-variceal upper gastrointestinal bleeding: epidemiology and diagnosis. Gastroenterol Clin North Am 2005;34:589–605.
6. Wilcox CM, Alexander LN, Cotsonis G. A prospective characterization of upper gastrointestinal hemorrhage presenting with hematochezia. Am J Gastroenterol 1997;92:231–5.
7. Hearnshaw SA, Logan RF, Palmer KR, et al. Outcomes following early red blood cell transfusion in acute upper gastrointestinal bleeding. Aliment Pharmacol Ther 2010;32:215–24.
8. Villanueva C, Colomo A, Bosch A, et al. Transfusion strategies for acute upper gastrointestinal bleeding. N Engl J Med 2013;368:11–21.
9. Stanley AJ, Ashley D, Dalton HR, et al. Outpatient management of patients with low-risk upper-gastrointestinal haemorrhage: multicentre validation and prospective evaluation. Lancet 2009;373:42–7.
10. Laine L, McQuaid KR. Endoscopic therapy for bleeding ulcers: an evidence-based approach based on meta-analyses of randomized controlled trials. Clin Gastroenterol Hepatol 2009;7:33–47.
11. Cooper GS, Chak A, Way LE, et al. Early endoscopy in upper gastrointestinal hemorrhage: associations with recurrent bleeding, surgery, and length of hospital stay. Gastrointest Endosc 1999;49:145–52.
12. Lee JG, Turnipseed S, Romano PS, et al. Endoscopy-based triage significantly reduces hospitalization rates and costs of treating upper GI bleeding: a randomized controlled trial. Gastrointest Endosc 1999;50:755–61.
13. Bjorkman DJ, Zaman A, Fennerty MB, et al. Urgent vs. elective endoscopy for acute non-variceal upper-GI bleeding: an effectiveness study. Gastrointest Endosc 2004;60:1–8.
14. Spiegel BM, Vakil NB, Ofman JJ. Endoscopy for acute nonvariceal upper gastrointestinal tract hemorrhage: is sooner better? A systematic review. Arch Intern Med 2001;161:1393–404.
15. Cipolletta L, Bianco MA, Rotondano G, et al. Outpatient management for low-risk nonvariceal upper GI bleeding: a randomized controlled trial. Gastrointest Endosc 2002;55:1–5.
16. Tsoi KK, Ma TK, Sung JJ. Endoscopy for upper gastrointestinal bleeding: how urgent is it? Nat Rev Gastroenterol Hepatol 2009;6:463–9.
17. Tai CM, Huang SP, Wang HP, et al. High-risk ED patients with nonvariceal upper gastrointestinal hemorrhage undergoing emergency or urgent endoscopy: a retrospective analysis. Am J Emerg Med 2007;25:273–8.

18. Lin HJ, Wang K, Perng CL, et al. Early or delayed endoscopy for patients with peptic ulcer bleeding. A prospective randomized study. J Clin Gastroenterol 1996;22:267–71.
19. Lim LG, Ho KY, Chan YH, et al. Urgent endoscopy is associated with lower mortality in high-risk but not low-risk nonvariceal upper gastrointestinal bleeding. Endoscopy 2011;43:300–6.
20. Hearnshaw SA, Logan RF, Lowe D, et al. Use of endoscopy for management of acute upper gastrointestinal bleeding in the UK: results of a nationwide audit. Gut 2010;59:1022–9.
21. Rosenstock SJ, Moller MH, Larsson H, et al. Improving quality of care in peptic ulcer bleeding: nationwide cohort study of 13,498 consecutive patients in the Danish Clinical Register of Emergency Surgery. Am J Gastroenterol 2013;108: 1449–57.
22. Gralnek IM. Evaluating the "weekend effect" on patient outcomes in upper GI bleeding. Gastrointest Endosc 2014;80:236–8.
23. Kanwal F, Barkun A, Gralnek IM, et al. Measuring quality of care in patients with nonvariceal upper gastrointestinal hemorrhage: development of an explicit quality indicator set. Am J Gastroenterol 2010;105:1710–8.
24. Enestvedt BK, Gralnek IM, Mattek N, et al. An evaluation of endoscopic indications and findings related to nonvariceal upper-GI hemorrhage in a large multicenter consortium. Gastrointest Endosc 2008;67:422–9.
25. Holster IL, Kuipers EJ. Management of acute nonvariceal upper gastrointestinal bleeding: current policies and future perspectives. World J Gastroenterol 2012; 18:1202–7.
26. Barkun AN, Bardou M, Martel M, et al. Prokinetics in acute upper GI bleeding: a meta-analysis. Gastrointest Endosc 2010;72:1138–45.
27. Szary NM, Gupta R, Choudhary A, et al. Erythromycin prior to endoscopy in acute upper gastrointestinal bleeding: a meta-analysis. Scand J Gastroenterol 2011;46: 920–4.
28. Bai Y, Guo JF, Li ZS. Meta-analysis: erythromycin before endoscopy for acute upper gastrointestinal bleeding. Aliment Pharmacol Ther 2011;34:166–71.

Management of Antiplatelet Agents and Anticoagulants in Patients with Gastrointestinal Bleeding

CrossMark

Neena S. Abraham, MD, MSCE[a,b,c],*

KEYWORDS

- Gastrointestinal hemorrhage • Upper gastrointestinal bleeding
- Lower gastrointestinal bleeding • Adverse effects • Thienopyridine
- Novel oral anticoagulant

KEY POINTS

- Antithrombotic drugs are associated with a clinically significant risk of gastrointestinal bleeding.
- An important consideration is if endoscopic hemostasis (in itself) constitutes a high vs. low-risk procedure.
- A better understanding of the pharmacology, mechanism of action and clinical indications for common antiplatelet drugs is imperative for sound decision-making regarding drug cessation or continuation in the peri-endoscopic period.
- Management of anticoagulant associated bleeding in the emergent and urgent setting is still grounded in the principles of A (airway), B (breathing), and C (circulation).
- There is remarkably little data to inform the endoscopist's decision of resumption of antithrombotic therapy.

INTRODUCTION

Current estimates of antithrombotic use in the United States are limited. The Reduction of Atherothrombosis for Continued Health (REACH) registry suggests that 70% of Americans (n = 25,686) are on acetylsalicylic acid (ASA) monotherapy; 13% are on ASA with a thienopyridine antiplatelet agent (ie, dual antiplatelet therapy [DAPT]), 8% are on anticoagulant or thienopyridine antiplatelet agent monotherapy, 4% are on ASA plus anticoagulant, and 1% are on thienopyridine agent plus anticoagulant or on all 3 antithrombotic agents

---

[a] Division of Gastroenterology and Hepatology, Department of Medicine, Mayo Clinic, 13400 East Shea Boulevard, Scottsdale, AZ 85259, USA; [b] Division of Health Care Policy and Research, Department of Health Services Research, 200 First Street SW, Rochester, MN 55905, USA; [c] Robert D. and Patricia E. Kern Center for the Science of Health Care Delivery, Mayo Clinic, 200 First Street SW, Rochester, MN 55905, USA
* Corresponding author. Mayo Clinic, 13400 East Shea Boulevard, Scottsdale, AZ 85259.
E-mail address: abraham.neena@mayo.edu

Gastrointest Endoscopy Clin N Am 25 (2015) 449–462
http://dx.doi.org/10.1016/j.giec.2015.02.002
1052-5157/15/$ – see front matter © 2015 Elsevier Inc. All rights reserved.

concurrently.[1] Data from the Department of Veterans' Affairs (n = 78,133) show that 50.5% are on DAPT, 29.3% are on ASA plus anticoagulant, 13.8% are on anticoagulant plus thienopyridine antiplatelet agent, and 6.3% are on triple therapy with ASA plus anti-coagulant plus thienopyridine agent.[2] It is projected that, by 2030, greater than 40% of US adults (>25 million individuals) will have at least 1 form of cardiovascular disease, accompanied by an expected aggressive increase in antithrombotic drug use for prevention of myocardial infarction (MI), stroke (cardiovascular accident [CVA]), and thromboembolic disorders (deep venous thromboembolism or pulmonary embolism) in patients who have already had a prior event (ie, for secondary cardioprophylaxis).[3]

These drugs are associated with an important and clinically relevant gastrointestinal bleeding (GIB) risk. Abraham and colleagues[2] showed the magnitude of risk associated with the use of antithrombotic drugs used in dual and triple combinations. The 1-year number needed to harm for common dual therapy strategies (ASA plus thieno-pyridine agent, ASA plus anticoagulant, or anticoagulant plus thienopyridine agent) as well as triple therapy (ASA plus thienopyridine agent plus anticoagulant) is less than 93 patients to incur 1 additional upper gastrointestinal (GI) bleed, less than 23 to incur 1 additional lower GI bleed, less than 51 to incur 1 additional blood transfusion, and less than 67 patients to incur 1 additional GI bleed–related hospitalization.

These estimates may represent just the "tip of the iceberg" because they fail to include the impact of GIB associated with the new oral anticoagulants, which are known to increase the risk of GIB 3-fold when combined with ASA and a thienopyridine agent.[4] Furthermore, with the aging US population, GIB is likely to increase because of the presence of multiple concomitant risk factors in this population: (1) advancing age, (2) multiple medical comorbidities, and (3) increased use of antiplatelet and anticoagulant agents in combination.[5] The synergism of these risk factors is likely to change the epidemiology of GIB in North America.[3]

This article focuses on the management of antithrombotic agents in the periendo-scopic period surrounding an acute, clinically significant GIB, requiring endoscopic intervention. These patients include those with hemodynamic compromise, greater than or equal to a 2-g reduction in hemoglobin, or overt signs of GIB (melena, hema-temesis, coffee-ground emesis, and hematochezia).

This article addresses the following clinical questions:

1. Is endoscopic hemostasis considered a high-risk or low-risk procedure?
2. How should antiplatelets be managed when the patient is bleeding?
3. How should anticoagulants be managed when the patient is bleeding?
   a. How should the novel oral anticoagulants (NOACs) be managed in the urgent setting?
   b. What are the new target-specific NOAC reversal agents?
4. Should the patient be bridged if stopping anticoagulation?
5. When should antithrombotics be restarted?

Is Endoscopic Hemostasis Considered a High-risk or Low-risk Procedure?

An important consideration is whether endoscopic hemostasis (in itself) constitutes a high-risk versus low-risk procedure. The American Society of Gastrointestinal Endos-copy considers a low-risk procedure to be a procedure that is associated with a clinical rate of bleeding of 1.5% or less, in the absence of antithrombotic therapy.[6] If a procedure with a risk greater than 1.5% is considered high risk, many of the commonly performed hemostatic procedures would be in this category.[7] Some pro-cedures (such as hemostatic clip placement, injection) remain ill-defined in terms of postprocedural bleeding risk (**Table 1**). However, few endoscopic procedures are

Table 1
Estimated risk of post-endoscopic bleeding risk

Endoscopic Procedure	Low-risk Bleeding (<1.5%)	High-risk Bleeding (>1.5%)
Diagnostic EGD or colonoscopy (with or without biopsy)	X	—
Nonthermal removal of small polyps (<1 cm)	X	—
Coagulation or ablation of tumors or vascular lesions (includes APC, bipolar cautery, and laser ablation)	—	X
Large (>1 cm) polypectomy	—	X
Variceal band ligation	—	X
Hemostatic clip placement	X (unknown risk)	—
Injection therapy	X (unknown risk)	—
Bipolar cautery	—	X

Abbreviations: APC, argon plasma coagulation; EGD, esophagogastroduodenoscopy.

associated with closed-space bleeding (ie, retroperitoneal, intrathoracic, or pericardial), unless a major perforation is incurred.

Consequences of the procedurally-induced bleed also need to be considered. Baron and colleagues[7] classified the severity of bleeding consequences based on expert consensus from a single institution and extrapolation from existing guidelines and consensus statements regarding endoscopic risk.[8] Mild consequences of postprocedural bleeding would include incomplete or aborted procedures, need for repeat endoscopy, transfusion or interventional radiology, the need for unplanned ventilation or anesthesia support, postprocedural medical consultation, or an unplanned hospital stay of less than 3 nights or intensive care admission of less than 1 night. Moderate consequences include an unplanned admission for 4 to 10 nights related to the procedural bleeding, intensive care unit admissions greater than 1 night, need for surgery, or permanent disability. Major consequences include admissions for greater than 10 nights, intensive care unit admissions greater than 1 night, and death.

What remains less clear is the underlying risk of performing endoscopic hemostasis in a patient in whom platelet dysfunction is expected because of the use of a pharmacologic agent, and in whom prompt resumption of the antithrombotic agent is necessary to prevent an adverse thromboembolic event. Endoscopic hemostasis should be considered an activity that carries with it a high risk of postprocedural bleeding.[9] The magnitude of risk is at least 1.5%, and possibly much higher, based on the patient's underlying antithrombotic regimen; preexisting nonpharmacologic coagulopathy and associated comorbidities, including renal and/or hepatic dysfunction; or the presence of carcinoma.

- Performing endoscopic procedures on patients currently prescribed antithrombotic regimens is both warranted and safe, providing clinicians consider the thrombotic risk of temporary interruption of drugs, and the relative risk of endoscopic maneuvers on subsequent bleeding, and promptly restart regimens when hemostasis is assured or provide temporary bridge therapy in patients in whom hemostasis is uncertain.[10]

How Should Antiplatelets Be Managed When the Patient Is Bleeding?

A better understanding of the pharmacology, mechanism of action, and clinical indications for common antiplatelet drugs is imperative for sound decision-making regarding drug cessation or continuation in the periendoscopic period. Commonly used antiplatelet agents include ASA; dipyridamole; and the thienopyridine drugs clopidogrel, prasugrel, and ticagrelor. ASA inhibits both cyclooxygenase (COX)-1 and COX-2 and causes irreversible inhibition of platelet function. Dipyridamole inhibits thrombus formation by inhibition of the phosphodiesterase enzymes that break down cAMP and cGMP, impairing platelet function and promoting arteriolar smooth muscle relaxation. The time required to recover adequate platelet function after ASA and dipyridamole use is ~7 to 10 days.

The thienopyridine agents, clopidogrel, prasugrel, and ticagrelor, inhibit the P2Y12 receptor on the platelet to inhibit platelet aggregation. Inhibition is irreversible for clopidogrel and prasugrel and reversible for ticagrelor. The antiplatelet effect can last between 3 and 9 days depending on the agent. The newer antiplatelet agents vorapaxar and atopaxar, inhibit the protease-activated receptor-1 on the platelet. These drugs are less commonly used because the increased risk of serious bleeding (especially intracranial bleeding) outweighs the modest finding of efficacy in randomized controlled trials (RCTs) among patients with acute coronary syndrome,[11] thus, they are not discussed further in this article.

Aspirin monotherapy
ASA is a COX inhibitor that is used alone or in combination with other antithrombotic therapies. It is the cornerstone of cardiac prevention strategies for patients at greater than 10% 5-year risk of heart attack or stroke[12] (ie, primary cardioprophylaxis) and for secondary prevention of cardioembolic events in patients who have had a prior acute coronary syndrome event or stroke.

Acetylsalicylic acid plus dipyridamole
Dipyridamole is commonly used in the United States as a combination pill with ASA (Aggrenox) for the secondary prevention of stroke and transient ischemic attack.[13] It is not approved as monotherapy for stroke prevention, and the use of ASA plus dipyridamole with the thienopyridine agent, clopidogrel, has generally been abandoned because of the high risk of bleeding adverse events.[14] Discontinuation of ASA plus dipyridamole for 7 to 10 days returns platelet function to normal, in the absence of other coagulopathies.

Dual antiplatelet therapy (acetylsalicylic acid plus thienopyridine agent)
Thienopyridine agents include clopidogrel [Plavix], prasugrel [Effient], ticlopidine [Ticlid], and ticagrelor [Brilinta]. Current national cardiology guidelines include prescription of clopidogrel, ticagrelor, and prasugrel plus ASA following acute coronary syndrome for up to 12 months following unstable angina or non–ST elevation MI managed without percutaneous coronary intervention (PCI) and for at least 14 days (12 months in some patients) following ST segment elevation myocardial infarction. Following a stent insertion, ASA must be continued indefinitely and clopidogrel or ticagrelor prescribed for up to 12 months following bare metal stent insertion and at least 12 months following drug-eluting stent placement.[15]

- When endoscopists are considering altering dual antiplatelet therapy (DAPT) with ASA plus thienopyridine agent, it is important to remember that thromboembolic risk depends on 3 factors:
  - The indication for the antiplatelet therapy
  - The consequences of thromboembolic event
  - The presence of additional thromboembolic risk factors

Low versus high thromboembolic risk conditions
Low thromboembolic risk conditions include uncomplicated or paroxysmal nonvalvular atrial fibrillation, bioprosthetic valves, a mechanical valve in the aortic position, and deep vein thrombosis. High-risk thromboembolic conditions include atrial fibrillation associated with one of the following: valvular heart disease and the presence of prosthetic valves, an ejection fraction less than 35%, hypertension, diabetes mellitus, age greater than 75 years, and a history of thromboembolic event. Additional high thromboembolic risk conditions include a mechanical valve in any position and previous thromboembolic event, prior stent occlusion, a recently placed coronary stent (~1 year), acute coronary syndrome, and PCI after MI.[9]

- Periods of time when thromboembolic risk are the highest in patients with coronary stents:
  - First 90 days following acute coronary syndrome
  - First 30 to 45 days after PCI and bare metal stent insertion
  - First 3 to 6 months following PCI and drug-eluting stent insertion

Following acute coronary syndrome, regardless of whether the patient has been medically treated or undergone PCI, the most dangerous period of time to alter DAPT is in the first 90 days following the event. In this time the risk is 2-fold higher for cardiac death or MI with clopidogrel discontinuation.[16] It is also important to remember that, after PCI and bare metal stent insertion, the highest risk of stent occlusion is in the first 30 to 45 days, and within the first 6 months of drug-eluting stent placement,[7] so this is not the time to alter DAPT. One in 5 patients who experience a first definite stent thrombosis experience a second stent thrombosis and that risk can remain at ~2.9% over the next 3 years.[17]

- For an endoscopic procedure with a high risk of GI bleeding, the thienopyridine can be discontinued for a short period of time (~5–7 days) as long as the ASA is continued.[18]

There is no increased risk of postprocedural bleeding associated with continued use of ASA and, in high-risk cardiac patients, discontinuation can increase 30-day mortality.[19]

- Premature and complete discontinuation of antithrombotic therapy in anticipation of an endoscopic procedure can result in stent occlusion, MI, and mortality in 50% of patients.[20,21]
- Elective diagnostic endoscopy can safely be performed without cessation of DAPT.

Glycoprotein IIb/IIIa receptor inhibitors
The intravenous agents abciximab (ReoPro), eptifibatide (Integrilin), and tirofiban (Aggrastat) are used following acute coronary syndrome in patients undergoing PCI or endovascular interventions. They prevent fibrinogen-mediated platelet aggregation, thrombus formation, and distal thromboembolism.[22] Associated adverse events include significant rates of major bleeding[23] and, with some, thrombocytopenia[24] that further exacerbate bleeding events. Duration of effect ranges from 1 to 2 seconds (tirofiban) to 4 to 24 hours, dictating their rate of intravenous infusion.

- In situations of major GI hemorrhage, aggressive volume resuscitation, the use of inotropes if necessary, transient discontinuation of the glycoprotein IIb/IIIa infusion, and platelet transfusion can be helpful to promote hemostasis in anticipation of endoscopic or surgical hemostatic interventions. In rare cases, hemodialysis may be required (tirofiban)

How Should Anticoagulants Be Managed When the Patient Is Bleeding?

Inhibition of single or multiple steps in the coagulation cascade is the mechanism of action associated with anticoagulants.

Heparin derivatives

Unfractionated heparin is administered parenterally and has a short half-life of 60 to 90 minutes. Complete dissipation of anticoagulant effect occurs after 3 to 4 hours. The risk of bleeding associated with parenteral unfractionated heparin is less than 3% in clinical trials (among patients with deep venous thrombosis [DVT]); a risk that increases with dose escalation and age greater than 70 years.[25] Low-molecular-weight heparin agents such as enoxaparin and dalteparin are administered subcutaneously and are frequently used for bridging therapy in patients during temporary interruption of oral anticoagulants. These agents are also used therapeutically in the treatment of DVT and have a lower risk of major bleeding than unfractionated heparin.[25]

Fondaparinux is specifically approved for perioperative thromboembolic prophylaxis and for the initial therapy for both DVT and pulmonary embolism. What differentiates this agent from others in this drug class is its high affinity for antithrombin III, which potentiates the inhibitory effect of factor Xa. Before a high-risk endoscopic procedure (eg, endoscopic mucosal resection, endoscopic ultrasonography with fine-needle aspiration, endoscopic submucosal dissection, variceal banding), a minimum of 36 hours of drug interruption is required.

Warfarin

For more than 80 years, warfarin was the only clinical choice for oral anticoagulation. This anticoagulant inhibits the vitamin K–dependent clotting factors II, VII, IX, and X, as well as proteins C and S. The risk of adverse bleeding events, unpredictable pharmacodynamic response, significant potential for drug-drug interactions, and delayed onset of action were drawbacks of this agent. The necessity for frequent monitoring, dose adjustment, and compliance with dietary restrictions has limited its popularity with patients.[10] The anticoagulant effect can be predictably reduced following temporary interruption; the International Normalized Ratio (INR) decreases to less than 1.5 in 93% of patients within 5 days.[26] This fact coupled with well-established algorithms for bridging therapy using low-molecular-weight heparin or unfractionated heparin products during periods of temporary interruption makes it a popular choice for clinical use.

The risk of warfarin-associated bleeding is determined by the intensity of the anticoagulant effect, baseline patient characteristics, and duration of therapy. A targeted INR of 2.5 (range, 2.0–3.0) is associated with a lower risk of bleeding than an INR greater than 3.0.[25] Reversal of warfarin-induced anticoagulant effect can be achieved by transfusion of hemostatic blood products, such as fresh frozen plasma, and provision of vitamin K. Normalization of the INR is unnecessary and does not reduce rebleeding risk, but does contribute to significant delays in endoscopy, which delays discovery of important endoscopic stigmata in 83% of cases.[27,28] Hemostatic therapy (injection therapy, heater probe, hemoclips) is very effective even with a moderately increased INR (up to 2.7).

- Endoscopic hemostasis can safely and reliably be performed in anticoagulated patients with INRs up to 2.7.
- No need to normalize the INR before proceeding with endoscopic therapy.
- Rebleeding rates are similar with and without anticoagulant reversal.

Novel oral anticoagulants

NOACs include direct thrombin inhibitor, dabigatran etexilate (Pradaxa), and direct oral factor Xa inhibitors, rivaroxaban (Xarelto), apixaban (Eliquis), and edoxaban

(Lixiana).[29] These agents, developed to overcome the limitations of warfarin with their rapid and predictable pharmacodynamic response and fixed once or twice daily dosing regimens, have quickly become popular with physicians and patients alike. Pivotal cardiac clinical trials have shown an unexpected increase in the risk of GI bleeding based on specific agents and indications for use.[30–37]

Apixaban seems to have the lowest risk of GI bleeding (hazard ratio [HR], 0.76; 95% confidence interval [CI], 0.98–1.15). A 46% increase in GI bleeding (HR, 1.46; 95% CI, 1.19–1.78) is observed with rivaroxaban.[36] Dabigatran, at 150 mg twice a day, is associated with a 50% increase in bleeding risk (HR, 1.50; 95% CI, 1.1.9–1.89), especially in the elderly.[30] When combined with DAPT,[38] a 3-fold increased risk of major bleeding is observed (HR, 3.03; 95% CI, 2.20–4.16) with a number needed to harm of 111 to generate 1 additional major bleed (which includes GI bleeds, intracranial hemorrhage, clinically overt signs of hemorrhage associated with a reduction in hemoglobin level ≥ 5 g/dL, and fatal bleeding that results in death within 7 days).[4] Lamberts and colleagues[39] report fatal NOAC-related intracranial hemorrhage in 48%, and fatal GI bleeds in 45.3%. Nonfatal GI bleeds are also common (33.8%) and represent the most common NOAC-related bleeding complication.

The large NOAC RCTs did not provide much guidance for periprocedural management of these drugs. A post-hoc analysis of the RE-LY (Randomized Evaluation of Long-term Anticoagulation Therapy) trial (dabigatran) identified 3033 patients who underwent surgery or invasive procedures during the observation period of the parent trial. The mean time of drug discontinuation before the procedure was 49 hours (range, 38–85 hours) and the observed rate of postprocedural bleeding was equivalent to that seen in the warfarin control group: 6.5% after elective major surgery and 17.7% after emergency surgery.[40] The most aggressive mucosal disruption caused by an endoscopic procedure would not be equivalent to a major elective surgical wound, so the predicted rate of bleeding following an endoscopic procedure is likely to be between 1.5% and 6.5%. Although the overall risk of postprocedural bleeding is similar to that of warfarin, a shorter period of drug cessation is required (with normal renal function); 2 days with dabigatran versus 5 days with warfarin.

Based on limited clinical data and pharmacodynamic studies of these agents, recommendations for NOAC management in the elective periendoscopic period have been proposed (**Table 2**). These data take advantage of the unique properties of the NOACs, which require less than 4 hours to achieve maximum effect, have a short half-life (<15 hours), and are excreted primarily through the kidneys. Timing of discontinuation of the drug before endoscopy is based on the patient's creatinine clearance (CrCl) and the anticipated bleeding risk of the endoscopic procedure.[9,41]

Most commonly performed diagnostic and hemostatic procedures, such as colonic polypectomy, diagnostic gastroscopy/colonoscopy/balloon-assisted enteroscopy,

Table 2
Periprocedural management of NOACs

Creatinine Clearance (mL/min)	Half-life (h)	Moderate Procedural Bleeding Risk; Discontinue Drug for 2–3 Half-lives (d)	High Procedural Bleeding Risk; Discontinue the Drug for 4–5 Half-lives (d)
>80	13 (11–22)	1–1.5	2–3
>50 to ≤80	15 (12–34)	1–2	2–3
>30 to ≤50	18 (13–23)	1.5–2	3–4
≤30	27 (22–35)	2–3	4–6

mechanical hemostasis, injection or cautery therapy for a mucosal lesion, have a low to moderate risk of postprocedural bleeding (<3.3%). Certain hemostatic procedures, such as endoscopic mucosal resection, variceal banding, and possibly argon plasma coagulation, are associated with a greater degree of sustained mucosal injury, and can incur bleeding in up to 22% of patients. These procedures are considered to have a higher risk of postprocedural bleeding.[9,19]

If the CrCl is normal (ie, >80 mL/min) the anticipated half-life of the drug is predictable and discontinuation of the drug can be scheduled 1 to 1.5 days before a low-risk endoscopic procedure and 2 to 2.5 days before a higher risk endoscopic procedure. The effect of impaired CrCl on the excretion of the drug and the anticoagulant effect is most observable in patients who are prescribed NOACs that are predominantly excreted by the kidneys (ie, dabigatran, edoxaban) versus those with lesser dependence on renal excretion (ie, rivaroxaban and apixaban) (**Table 3**). In situations with severe kidney disease (CrCl ≤ 30 mL/min), discontinuation of a NOAC for up to 3 to 4 days before a moderate-risk endoscopic procedure may be necessary.

The risk of temporary interruptions in NOAC has been studied and, although there are no data showing a rebound hypercoagulability effect,[40,42] the US Food and Drug Administration (FDA) has issued a black box warning for all 3 currently available agents (dabigatran, rivaroxaban, and apixaban) regarding the potential for increased thrombotic events following discontinuation of use. Current conservative approaches to minimize this risk include reinitiation of the drug as soon as hemostasis is assured, or using a short course of bridge therapy until hemostasis is established and full-dose NOAC can be resumed.

Management of Novel Oral Anticoagulants in the Nonurgent Setting

- Know the CrCl of the patient
- Know the specific NOAC prescribed and the time of the last dose
- Anticipate the bleeding risk of the endoscopic procedure that will be performed
- Time discontinuation of the NOAC based on the endoscopic postprocedural bleeding risk and the CrCl of the patient
- Restart the NOAC as soon as hemostasis has been achieved.

How Should the Novel Oral Anticoagulants Be Managed in the Urgent Setting?

Management of anticoagulant-associated bleeding in the emergent and urgent settings is still grounded in the principles of A (airway), B (breathing), and C (circulation). The importance of aggressive preendoscopic resuscitation is highlighted by the renal excretion of these drugs. By supporting the kidneys in a patient with normal renal function, the rapid excretion of the drug can be promoted. Given the short half-life of these agents, holding the next dose and promoting renal excretion is often sufficient to gain control of a clinically significant GI bleed.

In situations in which fluid resuscitation and withholding the drug are insufficient to cease active hemorrhage, consideration of transfusion of blood products such as fresh frozen plasma, activated factor VII, or prothrombin complex concentrate (activated or

Table 3	
Variation in renal excretion of common NOACs	
Dabigatran	80% renal clearance
Edoxaban	50% renal clearance
Rivaroxaban	35% renal clearance
Apixaban	27% renal clearance

not) can be considered. These products are best used in the setting of moderate or severe hemorrhage directly or indirectly related to the anticoagulant treatment.[43–45]

Activated prothrombin concentrate complex (PCC) contains the vitamin K–dependent factors II, VII, IX, and X either in nonactivated form (nonactivated PCCs) or partially activated form (activated PCCs; FEIBA). The nonactivated PCCs contain little factor VII and are referred to as 3-factor PCC (Bebulin, Profilnine). In 2012 the FDA approved a 4-factor PCC (Kcentra). The data supporting the use of PCC are mainly derived from small animal studies or based on partial or complete correction of laboratory parameters in healthy volunteers. Of these agents, activated PCC is most promising for the reversal of dabigatran, whereas nonactivated prothrombin concentrate is most useful for the reversal of anti–factor Xa agents.

In the setting of moderate to major GIB, prompt endoscopy to examine for underlying high-risk Forrest class stigmata becomes imperative. The optimal choice of endoscopic hemostatic strategy in this setting remains poorly defined. Mechanical hemostasis may be a safer option compared with thermal therapies for the treatment of mucosal defects among patients who require antithrombotic therapy because there is less risk of delayed bleeding following eschar sloughing with resumption of the anticoagulant or antiplatelet regimen. Further studies are required to inform best endoscopic practice in this setting.

What Are the New Target-specific Novel Oral Anticoagulant Reversal Agents?

Idarucizumab is a humanized monoclonal antibody expressed as a specific antibody fragment that has a very high affinity for the direct thrombin inhibitor dabigatran and prevents dabigatran inhibition of thrombin. This agent is unique in that it has no endogenous targets and no procoagulant or anticoagulant effects. Its short half-life and high affinity and specificity for the target drug contribute to the rapidity of its action. In early testing among human volunteers, complete reversal of the dabigatran anticoagulant effect was seen almost immediately (ie, within 5 minutes) of an intravenous infusion.[46] Clinical trials are underway to establish the efficacy of idarucizumab for the reversal of anticoagulant effect in the situation of life-threatening hemorrhage or need for emergency surgeries or procedures.

Another possible agent that may prove helpful is Perosphere (PER977). This small, synthetic, water-soluble, cationic molecule binds noncovalently to unfractionated and low-molecular-weight heparin. It has been found to bind in a similar fashion to the factor Xa inhibitors edoxaban, rivaroxaban, and apixaban, and to the direct thrombin inhibitor dabigatran.[47] Animal studies have shown reversal of NOACs with this agent and pharmacokinetic and pharmacodynamic studies using whole-blood clotting time are promising for the reversal of edoxaban, in particular. Preliminary studies showed reversal of the anticoagulant effect of edoxaban to 10% of baseline values within 10 minutes of drug delivery. Future studies are needed to show efficacy in human volunteers and within the clinical setting of major hemorrhage.

- Aggressively fluid resuscitate the patient to ensure maximal renal excretion of the drug.
- Hold the next dose in situations of mild to moderate bleeding.
- If there is evidence of continued hemodynamic compromise, early endoscopy is useful to identify important endoscopic stigmata requiring endoscopic hemostasis.
- Use of coagulation factors (fresh frozen plasma, prothrombin complex concentrates, or recombinant activated factor VII) may be helpful in reversing activity of the direct factor Xa inhibitors (rivaroxaban, apixaban, edoxaban).

- An antidote to the direct thrombin inhibitor dabigatran has been developed and is awaiting FDA approval (Idarucizumab). This agent will be helpful in rapid reversal of anticoagulation in life-threatening GI bleeding situations.
- Perosphere (PER977) may be a promising alternative for reversing the class of NOAC, in general. Further testing is required to establish efficacy.
- Consider the use of mechanical closure devices to limit postprocedural bleeding associated with hemostatic therapy of mucosal defects.

Should the Patient Be Bridged if Stopping Anticoagulation?

Bridge therapy is a subject steeped in dogma with little convincing evidence of its efficacy. Bridge therapy is suggested for patients at high risk (>10%/y) of thromboembolism related to atrial fibrillation, mechanical heart valve, or venous thromboembolism. However, it is often used in lower risk patients and has been shown to result in no thrombotic protection but increased risk of bleeding.[48] Evidence supporting the use of unfractionated heparin or low-molecular-weight heparin for bridge therapies in the periendoscopic period is limited to a small study of patients (N = 98) in whom bridge therapy was associated with no thromboembolic events and 2 major bleeds that were thought to be unrelated to endoscopy.[49] These data are consistent with a recent meta-analysis among warfarin users revealing that periprocedural heparin was associated with increased risk of overall and major bleeding events and a similar risk of thromboembolic events compared with nonbridged patients.[50–52]

The most recent guideline of the American College of Chest Physicians favors no bridging therapy in patients at low to moderate risk of thromboembolism and possible therapy for those at moderate to high risk of thromboembolism.[53] It is hoped that an ongoing RCT will better define the role of bridge therapy in anticoagulant users.[54] However, NOAC agents are excluded from this study, so results may not prove to be as informative as desired. It is also possible that NOAC may be used as bridge therapy given the similarity in the pharmacokinetics (ie, rapidity of onset and shortened half-lives) of traditional bridge agents enoxaparin and dalteparin; a hypothesis that is being tested in clinical studies.

- If endoscopic hemostasis has not been assured, consider a short bridge with low-molecular-weight heparin until hemostasis is established and a full dose of antithrombotic can be resumed.

When Should Antithrombotics Be Restarted?

There are few data to inform the endoscopist's decision of resumption of antithrombotic therapy. In general, once endoscopic hemostasis has been assured, antithrombotics should be restarted; on the same day of the procedure, in most cases. In situations in which hemostasis is uncertain, discussion with the patient's cardiologist, hematologist, or primary care physician is important to ensure an individualized approach for each patient. Risk of subsequent GIB needs to be carefully considered (based on the observed endoscopic stigmata) with the underlying thromboembolic risk of the patient, and the latter depends on the reason for which the antithrombotic strategy has been prescribed.

Following temporary discontinuation of warfarin, reinitiation of anticoagulant therapy should occur within 4 to 7 days of initial drug discontinuation to ensure that there is no increased risk of thromboembolic event.[55] If the patient requires dual antiplatelet coverage, discussion regarding the suitability of keeping the patient on ASA monotherapy may be appropriate as a temporary measure until hemostasis is achieved. Once hemostasis is assured, prompt resumption of the thienopyridine agent should occur; on the same day as the procedure, in most cases.

REFERENCES

1. Cannon CP, Rhee KE, Califf RM, et al. Current use of aspirin and antithrombotic agents in the United States among outpatients with atherothrombotic disease (from the REduction of Atherothrombosis for Continued Health [REACH] Registry). Am J Cardiol 2010;105(4):445–52.
2. Abraham NS, Hartman C, Richardson P, et al. Risk of lower and upper gastrointestinal bleeding, transfusions, and hospitalizations with complex antithrombotic therapy in elderly patients. Circulation 2013;128(17):1869–77.
3. Abraham NS. Gastrointestinal bleeding in cardiac patients: epidemiology and evolving clinical paradigms. Curr Opin Gastroenterol 2014;30(6):609–14.
4. Komocsi A, Vorobcsuk A, Kehl D, et al. Use of new-generation oral anticoagulant agents in patients receiving antiplatelet therapy after an acute coronary syndrome: systematic review and meta-analysis of randomized controlled trials. Arch Intern Med 2012;172(20):1537–45.
5. Crooks CJ, West J, Card TR. Comorbidities affect risk of nonvariceal upper gastrointestinal bleeding. Gastroenterology 2013;144(7):1384–93, 1393.e1–2.
6. Eisen GM, Baron TH, Dominitz JA, et al. Guideline on the management of anticoagulation and antiplatelet therapy for endoscopic procedures. Gastrointest Endosc 2002;55(7):775–9.
7. Baron TH, Kamath PS, McBane RD. Antithrombotic therapy and invasive procedures. N Engl J Med 2013;369(11):1079–80.
8. Cotton PB, Eisen GM, Aabakken L, et al. A lexicon for endoscopic adverse events: report of an ASGE workshop. Gastrointest Endosc 2010;71(3):446–54.
9. Anderson MA, Ben-Menachem T, Gan SI, et al. Management of antithrombotic agents for endoscopic procedures. Gastrointest Endosc 2009;70(6):1060–70.
10. Abraham NS, Castillo DL. Novel anticoagulants: bleeding risk and management strategies. Curr Opin Gastroenterol 2013;29(6):676–83.
11. Bhatt DL, Hulot JS, Moliterno DJ, et al. Antiplatelet and anticoagulation therapy for acute coronary syndromes. Circ Res 2014;114(12):1929–43.
12. D'Agostino RB Sr, Vasan RS, Pencina MJ, et al. General cardiovascular risk profile for use in primary care: the Framingham Heart Study. Circulation 2008;117(6): 743–53.
13. Halkes PH, van GJ, Kappelle LJ, et al. Aspirin plus dipyridamole versus aspirin alone after cerebral ischaemia of arterial origin (ESPRIT): randomised controlled trial. Lancet 2006;367(9523):1665–73.
14. Sprigg N, Gray LJ, England T, et al. A randomised controlled trial of triple antiplatelet therapy (aspirin, clopidogrel and dipyridamole) in the secondary prevention of stroke: safety, tolerability and feasibility. PLoS One 2008;3(8):e2852.
15. Jneid H, Anderson JL, Wright RS, et al. 2012 ACCF/AHA focused update of the guideline for the management of patients with unstable angina/non-ST-elevation myocardial infarction (updating the 2007 guideline and replacing the 2011 focused update): a report of the American College of Cardiology Foundation/ American Heart Association Task Force on Practice Guidelines. J Am Coll Cardiol 2012;60(7):645–81.
16. Ho PM, Peterson ED, Wang L, et al. Incidence of death and acute myocardial infarction associated with stopping clopidogrel after acute coronary syndrome. JAMA 2008;299(5):532–9.

17. van Werkum JW, Heestermans AA, de Korte FI, et al. Long-term clinical outcome after a first angiographically confirmed coronary stent thrombosis: an analysis of 431 cases. Circulation 2009;119(6):828–34.

18. Eisenberg MJ, Richard PR, Libersan D, et al. Safety of short-term discontinuation of antiplatelet therapy in patients with drug-eluting stents. Circulation 2009; 119(12):1634–42.

19. Becker RC, Scheiman J, Dauerman HL, et al. Management of platelet-directed pharmacotherapy in patients with atherosclerotic coronary artery disease undergoing elective endoscopic gastrointestinal procedures. Am J Gastroenterol 2009; 104(12):2903–17.

20. Grines CL, Bonow RO, Casey DE Jr, et al. Prevention of premature discontinuation of dual antiplatelet therapy in patients with coronary artery stents: a science advisory from the American Heart Association, American College of Cardiology, Society for Cardiovascular Angiography and Interventions, American College of Surgeons, and American Dental Association, with representation from the American College of Physicians. Circulation 2007;115(6):813–8.

21. Douketis JD, Spyropoulos AC, Spencer FA, et al. Perioperative management of antithrombotic therapy: Antithrombotic Therapy and Prevention of Thrombosis, 9th ed: American College of Chest Physicians Evidence-Based Clinical Practice Guidelines. Chest 2012;141(2 Suppl):e326S–50S.

22. Stangl PA, Lewis S. Review of currently available GP IIb/IIIa inhibitors and their role in peripheral vascular interventions. Semin Intervent Radiol 2010;27(4):412–21.

23. Boersma E, Harrington RA, Moliterno DJ, et al. Platelet glycoprotein IIb/IIIa inhibitors in acute coronary syndromes: a meta-analysis of all major randomised clinical trials. Lancet 2002;359(9302):189–98.

24. Kastrati A, Mehilli J, Neumann FJ, et al. Abciximab in patients with acute coronary syndromes undergoing percutaneous coronary intervention after clopidogrel pretreatment: the ISAR-REACT 2 randomized trial. JAMA 2006;295(13):1531–8.

25. Schulman S, Beyth RJ, Kearon C, et al. Hemorrhagic complications of anticoagulant and thrombolytic treatment: American College of Chest Physicians evidence-based clinical practice guidelines (8th edition). Chest 2008;133(6 Suppl):257S–98S.

26. Schulman S, Elbazi R, Zondag M, et al. Clinical factors influencing normalization of prothrombin time after stopping warfarin: a retrospective cohort study. Thromb J 2008;6:15.

27. Choudari CP, Rajgopal C, Palmer KR. Acute gastrointestinal haemorrhage in anticoagulated patients: diagnoses and response to endoscopic treatment. Gut 1994;35(4):464–6.

28. Wolf AT, Wasan SK, Saltzman JR. Impact of anticoagulation on rebleeding following endoscopic therapy for nonvariceal upper gastrointestinal hemorrhage. Am J Gastroenterol 2007;102(2):290–6.

29. Abraham NS. Novel oral anticoagulants and gastrointestinal bleeding: a case for cardiogastroenterology. Clin Gastroenterol Hepatol 2013;11(4):324–8.

30. Connolly SJ, Ezekowitz MD, Yusuf S, et al. Dabigatran versus warfarin in patients with atrial fibrillation. N Engl J Med 2009;361(12):1139–51.

31. Oldgren J, Budaj A, Granger CB, et al. Dabigatran vs placebo in patients with acute coronary syndromes on dual antiplatelet therapy: a randomized, double-blind, phase II trial. Eur Heart J 2011;32(22):2781–9.

32. Chung N, Jeon HK, Lien LM, et al. Safety of edoxaban, an oral factor Xa inhibitor, in Asian patients with non-valvular atrial fibrillation. Thromb Haemost 2011;105(3):535–44.

33. Granger CB, Alexander JH, McMurray JJ, et al. Apixaban versus warfarin in patients with atrial fibrillation. N Engl J Med 2011;365(11):981–92.
34. APPRAISE Steering Committee and Investigators, Alexander JH, Becker RC, et al. Apixaban, an oral, direct, selective factor Xa inhibitor, in combination with antiplatelet therapy after acute coronary syndrome: results of the Apixaban for Prevention of Acute Ischemic and Safety Events (APPRAISE) trial. Circulation 2009;119(22):2877–85.
35. Alexander JH, Lopes RD, James S, et al. Apixaban with antiplatelet therapy after acute coronary syndrome. N Engl J Med 2011;365(8):699–708.
36. Patel MR, Mahaffey KW, Garg J, et al. Rivaroxaban versus warfarin in nonvalvular atrial fibrillation. N Engl J Med 2011;365(10):883–91.
37. Mega JL, Braunwald E, Wiviott SD, et al. Rivaroxaban in patients with a recent acute coronary syndrome. N Engl J Med 2012;366(1):9–19.
38. Anderson JL, Halperin JL, Albert NM, et al. Management of patients with atrial fibrillation (compilation of 2006 ACCF/AHA/ESC and 2011 ACCF/AHA/HRS recommendations): a report of the American College of Cardiology/American Heart Association Task Force on Practice Guidelines. Circulation 2013;127(18):1916–26.
39. Lamberts M, Olesen JB, Ruwald MH, et al. Bleeding after initiation of multiple antithrombotic drugs, including triple therapy, in atrial fibrillation patients following myocardial infarction and coronary intervention: a nationwide cohort study. Circulation 2012;126(10):1185–93.
40. Healey JS, Eikelboom J, Douketis J, et al. Periprocedural bleeding and thromboembolic events with dabigatran compared with warfarin: results from the Randomized Evaluation of Long-Term Anticoagulation Therapy (RE-LY) randomized trial. Circulation 2012;126(3):343–8.
41. Weitz JI, Quinlan DJ, Eikelboom JW. Periprocedural management and approach to bleeding in patients taking dabigatran. Circulation 2012;126(20):2428–32.
42. Sherwood MW, Hellkamp A, Patel M, et al. Outcomes of temporary interruptions of rivaroxaban or warfarin in patients with atrial fibrillation in the ROCKET-AF trial. J Am Coll Cardiol 2013;61(10 Supplement):E316.
43. van RJ, Stangier J, Haertter S, et al. Dabigatran etexilate–a novel, reversible, oral direct thrombin inhibitor: interpretation of coagulation assays and reversal of anticoagulant activity. Thromb Haemost 2010;103(6):1116–27.
44. Majeed A, Hwang HG, Connolly SJ, et al. Management and outcomes of major bleeding during treatment with dabigatran or warfarin. Circulation 2013; 128(21):2325–32.
45. Majeed A, Schulman S. Bleeding and antidotes in new oral anticoagulants. Best Pract Res Clin Haematol 2013;26(2):191–202.
46. Glund S, Stangier J, Schmohl M, et al. A specific antidote for dabigatran: immediate, complete and sustained reversal of dabigatran induced anticoagulation in healthy male volunteers. Circulation 2013;128(Suppl) [abstract: 17765].
47. Ansell JE, Bakhru SH, Laulicht BE, et al. Use of PER977 to reverse the anticoagulant effect of edoxaban. N Engl J Med 2014;371(22):2141–2.
48. Wysokinski WE, McBane RD. Periprocedural bridging management of anticoagulation. Circulation 2012;126(4):486–90.
49. Constans M, Santamaria A, Mateo J, et al. Low-molecular-weight heparin as bridging therapy during interruption of oral anticoagulation in patients undergoing colonoscopy or gastroscopy. Int J Clin Pract 2007;61(2):212–7.
50. Fuster V, Ryden LE, Cannom DS, et al. 2011 ACCF/AHA/HRS focused updates incorporated into the ACC/AHA/ESC 2006 guidelines for the management of patients with atrial fibrillation: a report of the American College of Cardiology

Foundation/American Heart Association Task Force on Practice Guidelines. Circulation 2011;123(10):e269–367.

51. Nishimura RA, Otto CM, Bonow RO, et al. 2014 AHA/ACC guideline for the management of patients with valvular heart disease: a report of the American College of Cardiology/American Heart Association Task Force on Practice Guidelines. J Thorac Cardiovasc Surg 2014;148(1):e1–132.

52. Siegal D, Yudin J, Kaatz S, et al. Periprocedural heparin bridging in patients receiving vitamin K antagonists: systematic review and meta-analysis of bleeding and thromboembolic rates. Circulation 2012;126(13):1630–9.

53. Guyatt GH, Akl EA, Crowther M, et al. Introduction to the ninth edition: Antithrombotic Therapy and Prevention of Thrombosis, 9th ed: American College of Chest Physicians Evidence-Based Clinical Practice Guidelines. Chest 2012;141(2 Suppl):48S–52S.

54. BRIDGE study investigators. Bridging anticoagulation: is it needed when warfarin is interrupted around the time of a surgery or procedure? Circulation 2012; 125(12):e496–8.

55. Witt DM, Delate T, Garcia DA, et al. Risk of thromboembolism, recurrent hemorrhage, and death after warfarin therapy interruption for gastrointestinal tract bleeding. Arch Intern Med 2012;172(19):1484–91.

Role of Medical Therapy for Nonvariceal Upper Gastrointestinal Bleeding

Kyle J. Fortinsky, MD[a], Marc Bardou, MD, PhD[b],*,
Alan N. Barkun, MD, MSc[c]

KEYWORDS

- Nonvariceal upper gastrointestinal bleeding • Red blood cell transfusions
- Proton pump inhibitors • Erythromycin • Tranexamic acid • Nasogastric lavage
- Iron replacement therapy

KEY POINTS

- Optimal resuscitation should be initiated before any diagnostic or therapeutic procedure.
- Red blood cell transfusion should be offered to patients with a hemoglobin level less than 70 g/L, unless they have preexisting cardiac disease or evidence of an acute coronary syndrome, in which case more liberal transfusion may be appropriate.
- The use of intravenous erythromycin approximately 30 minutes before endoscopy may be useful to improve visualization.
- Preendoscopic high-dose intravenous proton pump inhibitor (PPI) therapy should be offered to all patients, but should not precede adequate resuscitation with crystalloid and/or blood products as necessary.
- Postendoscopic intravenous PPI therapy for 72 hours followed by double-dose oral PPI treatment of 14 days of the next 1 to 2 months prevents recurrence of bleeding in high-risk patients.

INTRODUCTION

The annual incidence of upper gastrointestinal bleeding (UGIB) is 48 to 160 events per 100,000 adults in the United States, where it is the cause of approximately 300,000 hospital admissions per year.[1,2] In Europe, the annual incidence of UGIB in the general population ranges from 19.4[3,4] to 57.0[3,5] events per 100,000 individuals. There is no formal explanation for the breadth of the range between countries, although

Conflicts of interest: A.N. Barkun declares associations with the following companies: AstraZeneca, Takeda Canada. The other authors declare no competing interests.
[a] Department of Medicine, Toronto General Hospital, University of Toronto, 200 Elizabeth Street, Toronto, Ontario M5G 2C4, Canada; [b] Gastroenterology Department & Centre d'Investigations Clinique CIC1432, CHU de Dijon, 14 rue Gaffarel BP77908, Dijon, Cedex 21079, France; [c] Gastroenterology Department, McGill University Health Centre, Montreal General Hospital Site, Room D7-346, 1650 Cedar Avenue, Montréal, Québec H3G 1A4, Canada
* Corresponding author.
E-mail address: marc.bardou@u-bourgogne.fr

differences in health care systems and case recording capacities may be substantial.[4,5] Additional contributing factors may include alcohol intake and *Helicobacter pylori* prevalence. In both North America and Europe, around 80% to 90% of acute UGIB episodes have a nonvariceal cause, with peptic ulcers and gastroduodenal erosions accounting for most such lesions.[6,7]

UGIB-related mortalities have slightly decreased in the past 2 decades, but still range from 2% to 15%.[8–10] Two studies conducted in the United Kingdom highlighted that, despite a notable decrease in mortality in patients with UGIB from 1993 to 2007, mortality from peptic ulcer bleeding is still 10% to 13%.[7,9] A multidisciplinary group of 34 experts from 15 countries published international guidelines in 2010, which were modified and expanded from initial guidelines published in 2003, to help inform clinicians on the optimal management of patients with nonvariceal UGIB.[2]

This article discusses the various management principles of medical therapy in nonvariceal UGIB put forth by guidelines from the multidisciplinary international consensus group in 2010, and the American College of Gastroenterology in 2012.[2,11] When applicable, more recent evidence is included. This article presents the most current evidence and provides recommendations for practice. Overall, this article focuses on providing an evidence-based approach to initial resuscitation, the role of blood transfusion, and both preendoscopic and postendoscopic pharmacologic and nonpharmacologic therapies in patients presenting with nonvariceal UGIB.

REVIEW CRITERIA

We conducted a literature search using the OVID, MEDLINE, EMBASE, PubMed, and ISI Web of Knowledge 4.0 databases to identify articles published in the English or French languages up until December 2014. A highly sensitive search strategy was used to identify randomized controlled trials, cohort studies, and case-control studies conducted in adults, using combinations of search terms, including "UGIB"; "epidemiology," "motility agents," "prokinetics," "erythromycin," "nasogastric," "tranexamic acid," "transfusion," "iron replacement," "*Helicobacter pylori*," "endoscopy," and "proton pump inhibitors" (PPIs). In addition, recursive searches and cross-referencing were performed and manual searches of the reference lists of articles identified in the initial search were completed.

PREENDOSCOPIC MEDICAL MANAGEMENT
Initial Resuscitation

The immediate priority in management is to secure the patient's airway, and tend to breathing and circulation (**Fig. 1**). The patient should be placed in a monitored setting, at which point large-bore venous access should be established. All pertinent blood work (eg, complete blood count, renal function, liver function tests, coagulation testing) should be obtained, in addition to typing and cross-matching.[11] Resuscitation should be initiated for patients with UGIB before any other procedure, and should include stabilization of the blood pressure with appropriate infusion of sufficient fluid volumes.[12,13] In intensive care units, saline or Ringer acetate must be preferred to hydroxyethyl starch (HES), because HES has been shown to increase the need for renal-replacement therapy in intensive care unit patients, and may even increase the risk for severe bleeding.[14] The primary objectives of resuscitation are to restore blood volume and to maintain adequate tissue perfusion, in the hope of preventing hypovolemic shock and ultimately death. No data suggest that any particular type of colloid solution is safer or more effective than any other in patients needing volume

---

Initial resuscitation
- Maintain airway, breathing, and circulation
- Ensure large-bore intravenous access and consider monitored setting
- Resuscitate initially with crystalloid solution
- Send blood work including CBC, coagulation studies, and type and cross-matching

Transfusion requirements
- Transfuse red blood cells only if hemoglobin <70g/L, unless symptoms of anemia or significant cardiac disease
- Transfuse platelets only if platelet count <50 x 10^9/L or <100 x 10^9/L with suspected platelet dysfunction

Pre-endoscopic therapy
- Provide erythromycin intravenously 30 minutes prior to endoscopy
- High-dose intravenous proton pump inhibitors should be initiated
- The routine use of nasogastric lavage and/or tranexamic acid is not recommended

---

Fig. 1. Preendoscopic medical management of nonvariceal UGIB. CBC, complete blood count.

replacement.[15] Certain patients require resuscitation with blood products, including red blood cells, platelets, and rarely clotting factors (eg, fresh frozen plasma).

Red Blood Cell Transfusion

The decision whether to transfuse red blood cells is based largely on the presenting hemoglobin level, coupled with symptoms of anemia, patient comorbidities such as cardiac disease, and the initial hemodynamic status. A large Cochrane Review questioned the benefits of red blood cell transfusions in UGIB, showing no overall survival benefit.[16] A recent randomized controlled trial of 921 patients with acute UGIB found a restrictive transfusion strategy (transfusion threshold <70 g/L with target hemoglobin 70–90 g/L) significantly decreased 6-week mortality, length of stay, and transfusion-related adverse events compared with a liberal transfusion strategy (transfusion threshold <90 g/L with target hemoglobin 90 to 110 g/L).[17] The overall mortality benefit conferred by the restrictive transfusion strategy seems to have been driven by results obtained in patients with Child-Pugh class A and B cirrhosis. The subgroup of patients with nonvariceal UGIB did not show a significant decrease in their overall mortality with a restrictive transfusion policy, although there was no suggestion of harm. Moreover, this study excluded all patients presenting with severe hemorrhagic shock, in keeping with consensus guidelines suggesting higher hemoglobin targets for these patients. In addition, patients with acute coronary syndrome, symptomatic peripheral vasculopathy, stroke, transient ischemic attack, or blood transfusion within 30 days were excluded from the study.

The current guidelines suggest that patients with hemoglobin levels less than or equal to 70 g/L should receive blood transfusions to reach a target hemoglobin level of 70 to 90 g/L, provided that the individual has no coronary artery disease, evidence of tissue hypoperfusion, or acute hemorrhage.[2] In patients with acute coronary syndrome, UGIB is associated with a markedly increased mortality, and a higher hemoglobin target level (>100 g/L) may be required to prevent decompensation.[2,18] In contrast, avoidance of unnecessary transfusions reduces the small but real risks attributable to administration of blood components, such as infectious or immune diseases. As part of a recent UK audit, despite 73% of patients with UGIB presenting with a hemoglobin level greater than 80 g/L, approximately 43% nonetheless received red blood cell transfusions.[7,19] A recently published meta-analysis, not restricted to nonvariceal UGIB, suggests that a restrictive transfusion approach reduces health care–associated infections.[20] Additional randomized trials are needed to address the issue of hemoglobin transfusion thresholds in patients with nonvariceal UGIB, and those with preexisting cardiac disease. One large multicentre randomized trial is currently being completed in the United Kingdom, which may help to answer these uncertainties.[21]

Platelet Transfusion

A recent systematic review of 18 studies of platelet transfusion thresholds in patients with UGIB found insufficient evidence supporting an optimal platelet count.[22] However, based primarily on expert opinion, the investigators proposed a platelet transfusion threshold of 50×10^9/L (or 100×10^9/L if altered platelet function is suspected). Additional high-quality data are needed to confirm these recommendations.

Nasogastric Lavage

The routine placement of a nasogastric tube (NGT) in patients with UGIB remains controversial and is not recommended by current guidelines.[2,11] Overall, studies have failed to show any improvement in clinical outcomes attributable to the insertion of an NGT.[23–26] However, there are certain patients in whom the source of gastrointestinal bleeding is unclear and who may benefit from placement of an NGT in order to confirm an upper gastrointestinal source.[27] A recent study investigated the utility of NGT aspirate at predicting UGIB in 64 patients presenting with hematemesis.[28] By using fecal occult blood testing on the aspirate, they were able to accurately identify all cases of UGIB later confirmed on endoscopy, while maintaining a specificity of 94%.[28] Although this study does lend support to the practice of obtaining an NGT aspirate to identify the source of bleeding in certain cases, it is unclear whether the same results would hold true in patients presenting with either coffee-ground emesis or melena. One recent retrospective study of 166 patients was able to predict active bleeding at endoscopy by combining NGT aspirate results with blood pressure and heart rate parameters.[29] Overall, opinions vary because high-quality evidence is lacking to decide whether certain patients benefit from NGT aspiration and lavage to help aid in diagnosing UGIB as well as improving visualization during endoscopy.[30–33]

Prokinetic Agents

The use of prokinetic agents (such as erythromycin) before gastrointestinal endoscopy has been shown to significantly shorten the duration of endoscopy, reduce the need for repeat endoscopy, and decrease the need for blood transfusions.[34–38] In a large, multicentre, randomized controlled trial involving 253 patients presenting with either melena or hematemesis, erythromycin alone was equally efficacious at improving endoscopic visualization as NGT aspirate alone or in combination with erythromycin.[26]

A separate randomized, placebo-controlled trial that involved patients with bleeding esophageal varices found that an erythromycin infusion significantly increased the proportion of empty stomachs at gastroscopy compared with placebo (48.9% with erythromycin vs 23.3% with placebo), reduced the mean endoscopy duration (19 minutes vs 26 minutes), and shortened durations of hospital stay (3.4 days vs 5.1 days).[39]

More recently, another small, low-quality, randomized trial compared NGT aspirate alone versus NGT aspirate with erythromycin, and the combination provided superior visualization, reduced hospital admissions, and decreased blood transfusions.[34] No data suggest that the administration of prokinetic agents can decrease mortality, the risk of rebleeding, or the need for surgery.[35–37,40] Nonetheless, given improved visibility at endoscopy and other potential benefits discussed earlier, especially in light of the favorable benefit-harm profile of erythromycin, current guidelines suggest that, after ruling out contraindications to these agents (such as hypokalemia or a prolonged QT interval), a 250-mg bolus of erythromycin should be administered approximately 30 to 45 minutes before endoscopy in patients with clinical evidence of active hemorrhage (hematemesis or melena) or acute anemia requiring resuscitation, or in those who have recently eaten.[2,26]

Proton Pump Inhibitor Therapy

Despite theoretic pharmacologic differences between the different PPIs, no data support the use of a particular intravenous PPI rather than another when treating patients with UGIB. In this article, "PPI" is therefore used as a generic term for all such agents.

Starting PPI treatment before endoscopy for UGIB remains a controversial practice. A meta-analysis that included 2223 participants from 6 randomized clinical trials found that preendoscopic PPI treatment reduces the proportion of patients identified as having high-risk lesions (active bleeding, nonbleeding visible vessel, and adherent clot) at early endoscopy and the resultant need for endoscopic therapy (ie, there is downstaging of high-risk endoscopic lesions).[41] Despite these advantages, there is no evidence that preendoscopic PPI treatment affects mortality, the risk of rebleeding, or the need for surgery. For this reason, current guidelines recommend initiating PPI therapy on presentation to hospital, although it should never delay optimal resuscitation.[2] PPI therapy is cost-effective in scenarios in which there is an anticipated delay in endoscopy or a high likelihood of a nonvariceal source of bleeding. Current guidelines advise against the use of histamine2 receptor antagonists in acute ulcer bleeding.[2]

No recommendations can be made regarding the optimal dose of PPIs administered preendoscopy. A reasonable strategy may be to adopt a regimen of a high-dose intravenous bolus (eg, Pantoprazole 80 mg) followed by a continuous infusion (eg, Pantoprazole 8 mg/h).[42] This infusion can be continued until endoscopy, at which point reassessment is required, depending on the appearance of the bleeding lesion and the need for therapeutic intervention (discussed later).

Although there is insufficient high-quality evidence to recommend intravenous PPI versus oral PPI, current guidelines suggest high-dose intravenous PPI preendoscopically because this administration has been well studied in multiple randomized controlled trials.[42–44]

A meta-analysis of randomized trials in patients not receiving endoscopic therapy discovered that PPI therapy reduced rebleeding rates and the need for surgery, and may decrease mortality in certain high-risk patients.[45] This approach could be cost-effective if endoscopy is delayed to greater than 16 hours after admission, or if patients have a high likelihood of nonvariceal bleeding, especially in those with high-risk symptoms, such as hematemesis.[46,47] These findings suggest a definite benefit of PPI therapy when endoscopy may be unavailable or delayed.

Somatostatin and Octreotide

Although usually reserved for patients with variceal UGIB, both somatostatin and octreotide may be used in patients presenting with nonvariceal UGIB. One meta-analysis consisting of 1829 patients from 14 randomized controlled trials found that both somatostatin and octreotide reduced the risk of continued nonvariceal UGIB (relative risk [RR], 0.53, 0.43–0.63; number needed to treat [NNT], 5).[48] These trials only compared somatostatin and octreotide with H2-blockers and placebo and none of these patients were on PPI therapy. Current guidelines recommend the use of octreotide or somatostatin in nonvariceal UGIB only as the last resort in patients who are bleeding uncontrollably while waiting for more definitive therapy.[2] Its use in the treatment of gastrointestinal bleeding of unknown origin is controversial.[49]

Tranexamic Acid

The efficacy of tranexamic acid, an antifibrinolytic, has been explored in several randomized trials and a recent meta-analysis.[50] Although the meta-analysis found a significant overall reduction in mortality, there was no reduction in rebleeding rates, the need for surgery, or blood transfusion. Importantly, the mortality benefit of tranexamic acid was absent when current therapy with PPIs and endoscopy were instituted. Although there are currently 2 randomized trials underway (one vs placebo [NCT01713101] and one vs esomeprazole [NCT02071316]) that are investigating the benefit of tranexamic acid in combination with current therapy in UGIB, current guidelines do not support its routine use in UGIB.[51]

POSTENDOSCOPIC MEDICAL MANAGEMENT
Intravenous Proton Pump Inhibitor Therapy

Opinions differ about the optimal time to begin intravenous PPI infusion after endoscopic hemostasis (**Fig. 2**).[13,42,52] The goal of PPI therapy is to increase the gastric pH sufficiently to promote clot stability and to reduce the effect of pepsin and gastric acid.[53] In a study designed to identify the lowest effective dose of PPI, rather than using a high (or low) dose, continuous infusion was the key to maintaining an intragastric pH greater than 6.[54] Two meta-analyses have confirmed that an intravenous PPI bolus followed by continuous PPI infusion over 72 hours reduces the rates of mortality (RR, 0.40, 0.28–0.59; NNT, 12), rebleeding (RR, 0.40, 0.28–0.59; NNT, 12), and surgery (RR, 0.43, 0.24–0.76; NNT, 28). Mortality was only reduced in patients who had previously undergone successful endoscopic hemostasis.[45,55]

A placebo-controlled, randomized trial showed that, in patients with Forrest class Ia to IIb bleeding lesions,[56] intravenous esomeprazole administered as an 80-mg intravenous bolus over 30 minutes followed by continuous infusion of 8 mg/h for 71.5 hours, which was started after successful endoscopic hemostasis and followed by a 40-mg esomeprazole oral regimen for 27 days, significantly reduced rates of rebleeding at 72 hours (5.9% in esomeprazole group compared with 10.3% in the placebo group; RR, 0.57; 95% confidence interval [CI], 0.35–0.94; NNT, 23). The difference in rebleeding rates remained significant at 7 days and 30 days after initial presentation.[57] However, the 30-day mortality was not significantly reduced by the use of a PPI. Because mortality was lower than expected in the placebo group (2.1%), this finding might reflect the exclusion of patients with life-threatening systemic disease (American Society of Anesthesiologists class >3). Cost-effectiveness analyses have shown the economic dominance of high-dose intravenous PPI compared with no treatment strategies.[58]

More recently, a systematic review and meta-analysis compared intermittent versus continuous PPI therapy for the treatment of high-risk bleeding ulcers after endoscopic

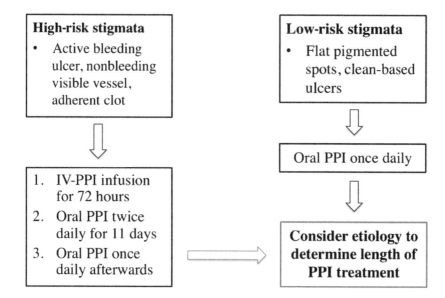

Fig. 2. Postendoscopic medical management of peptic ulcer disease. ASA, acetylsalicylic acid; COX-2, cyclooxygenase-2; IV, intravenous.

therapy.[59] This study revealed that intermittent PPI therapy may be as effective as continuous-infusion high-dose therapy in these high-risk patients, which may have benefits in terms of cost-savings, and the investigators firmly concluded that guidelines should be revised to recommend intermittent PPI therapy. However, overall, current guidelines remain ambivalent toward optimal postendoscopy PPI dosing because of an overall low quality of evidence secondary to a high risk of bias and imprecision in the aforementioned systematic review.[11]

Oral Proton Pump Inhibitor Therapy

High-dose oral PPI treatment after endoscopy was efficacious in early trials conducted in India and Iran, but differences in the physiologic and pharmacokinetic characteristics of the patients, as well as local high H pylori carriage rate and limited comorbidities, make the results of these studies difficult to apply to other populations. The endoscopic treatment administered was also not the current recommended standard.[60]

A study published in 2009 assessed gastric pH in patients receiving a 90-mg oral dose of lansoprazole followed by 30 mg every 3 hours (total dose, 300 mg in 24 hours), following successful endoscopic treatment of peptic ulcer bleeding.[61] The primary end point was the proportion of the 24-hour period that the patients had a gastric pH greater than 6 (median, 55%). However, large differences in this value were evident between individuals (range, 6%–99%), and only 1 of the 14 included patients (7%) reached a pH of more than 6 in at least 80% of this time period.[61]

Accordingly, the evidence is currently insufficient to support the use of oral PPI therapy immediately after endoscopy in high-risk patients. However, current recommendations do recommend oral PPI therapy in patients with lower-risk stigmata on endoscopy, such as a clean-based ulcer or a flat pigmented spot. In these lower-risk patients, the rates of significant rebleeding remain low.[62]

A recent randomized controlled trial of 293 patients investigated the efficacy of double-dose oral PPI (esomeprazole 40 mg orally twice daily for 11 days followed by once-daily dosing for another 14 days) compared with single-dose oral PPI (esomeprazole 40 mg orally once daily for 25 days) after 3 days of intravenous PPI infusion.[63] Patients with a Rockall score greater than or equal to 6 had significantly less rebleeding rates with twice-daily PPI compared with single-dose PPI (10.8% rebleeding in the twice-daily group vs 28.7% in once-daily group; $P = .002$). Surprisingly, rebleeding rates in an earlier study were much lower, whereby patients were randomized to intravenous esomeprazole or placebo for the first 72 hours, followed by oral esomeprazole 40 mg once a day, and reported rebleeding rates were only 1.9% and 5.1%, respectively.[57]

We recommend routinely prescribing double-dose PPI for at least 14 days following intravenous PPI infusion in these high-risk patients and single-dose PPI thereafter. The decision to continue oral PPIs past 28 days must be judged on an individualized basis because there is insufficient evidence to guide practice, and it is determined by the nature of the bleeding lesion. For example, longer courses of PPI therapy may be warranted for patients with bleeding erosive esophagitis compared with patients with duodenal ulcers.

The optimal duration of treatment with oral PPI is unknown and also depends on patient ongoing risk factors, and sometimes the severity of the presentation. For example, a patient treated for peptic ulcer disease related to either H pylori or nonsteroidal antiinflammatory drug (NSAID) use may only require a short course of PPI so long as the H pylori is eradicated or the NSAID discontinued.[2,11] The benefits and risks of ongoing PPI therapy should be discussed with individual patients.

Long-term Safety of Proton Pump Inhibitors

Many patients remain on PPI therapy long after the initial episode of UGIB. The 2 main concerns that have been raised about the long-term safety profile of PPI therapy include infections, such as Clostridium difficile–associated diarrhea (CDAD) and pneumonia, as well as metabolic bone disease.[64]

Gastric acid inhibition predisposes patients to an increased risk of enteric infections because normally the gastric acidity protects against these pathogens. It has been proposed that there is an increased risk of CDAD in patients on PPI therapy, even without exposure to antibiotics.[65] However, a systematic review and meta-analysis recently found only a weak relationship between exposure to PPI therapy and CDAD.[66]

Some evidence suggests that PPI therapy increases the risk of pneumonia, presumably through increased bacteria in the upper gastrointestinal tract that can migrate into the pulmonary system.[67] More recently, a meta-analysis found no increased risk of

CDAD with the use of PPIs.[68] A separate meta-analysis comparing PPI with H2-receptor antagonists for stress ulcer prophylaxis found no difference in rates of nosocomial pneumonia or mortality.[69]

PPI therapy in postmenopausal women has been associated with an increased risk of hip fracture (RR, 1.30, 1.19–1.43), spine fracture (RR, 1.56, 1.31–1.85), and any-site fracture (RR, 1.16, 1.02–1.32) in the Nurses' Health Study.[70] In the same study, current and former smokers on PPI therapy had a 51% increased risk of hip fracture (hazard ratio, 1.52, 1.20–1.91). Similarly, another meta-analysis found that PPIs increased fracture risk, whereas histamine2 receptor antagonists did not.[71] PPI therapy may directly alter bone metabolism via the vacuolar H^+-ATPase in osteoclasts.[72] Although a recent meta-analysis suggests that PPIs may be linked to a slightly increased risk of fracture (RR, 1.30; 95% CI, 1.13–1.49), this association may be caused by confounding factors such as frailty.[73,74]

Other potential consequences of PPI therapy include hypomagnesaemia, vitamin B_{12} malabsorption, and acute interstitial nephritis.[75–77] The most current US Food and Drug Administration warnings suggest routine screening of magnesium levels before initiating PPI therapy, and occasional monitoring of serum magnesium, especially in those patients at higher risk who are taking digoxin or diuretics. Moreover, interactions with medications, most notably clopidogrel, are a concern, although the most recent high-quality data suggest no clinically significant clopidogrel-PPI interaction.[78–80] Although there are risks involved with long-term PPI therapy, the absolute risks are small. Monitoring magnesium levels periodically, as well as encouraging patients- to stop smoking, may mitigate some of the risk. Overall, physicians should aim to minimize the dose and duration of PPI therapy whenever possible.

Secondary Prophylaxis to Prevent Recurrent Bleeding

In patients with *H pylori*–associated bleeding ulcers, continuing PPI therapy after *H pylori* eradication is not required unless there are other ongoing risk factors, including NSAID use or antithrombotic therapy. Similarly, patients with NSAID-induced ulcers do not require long-term PPI therapy unless the ongoing NSAID therapy is warranted. Should NSAID treatment be necessary, the authors recommend considering a cyclo-oxygenase-2–selective NSAID at the lowest possible dose along with daily PPI therapy. Similarly, in patients with low-dose aspirin–related ulcers, long-term PPI therapy is required if acetylsalicylic acid (ASA) must be continued (eg, secondary prevention of cardiovascular disease).[11,81,82]

Pooled results of 2 randomized trials have shown that ASA with PPI has significantly less risk of rebleeding than clopidogrel alone (OR, 0.06; 95% CI, 0.01–0.32).[2,83,84] Recent guidelines suggest long-term PPI therapy in patients who have idiopathic ulcers (non–*H pylori*, non-NSAID), in whom the incidence of recurrent ulcer bleeding has been reported at 42%.[11,85]

Helicobacter pylori Eradication

All patients should be tested for infection with *H pylori*, which is one of the principal causes of bleeding ulcers. Several testing methods are available.[86,87] The low prevalence reported for *H pylori* infection in patients with UGIB might be related to delay in testing, which is often not performed until 4 weeks after the bleeding episode.[88] Urea breath tests (UBTs) are widely used, but serology is preferable in acute settings because it has the best diagnostic accuracy in this specific condition.[89,90] A second test should be performed if a negative index result is obtained at the time of acute UGIB because false-negative rates in the acute setting reach 55% and are increased for all diagnostic modalities.[2] Real-time polymerase chain reaction (PCR) might improve *H pylori* detection in patients with peptic ulcer bleeding. Real-time PCR testing for a combination of *H pylori* 16S ribosomal RNA and urease A had a sensitivity of 64% and a specificity of 80% in tissue samples that had previously been considered negative by histologic testing alone.[91]

After the completion of antibiotic and PPI treatment, a UBT might be the most convenient approach to assess the effectiveness of *H pylori* eradication treatment, unless repeat endoscopy is indicated, at which time gastric biopsies can be performed. Regardless of the method being used, checking for eradication is mandatory because *H pylori* infection is a major cause of gastric cancer, specifically noncardia gastric cancer.[92,93]

Iron Replacement Therapy

Patients who present with UGIB should have iron studies performed after the acute bleeding episode. Anemic patients and even nonanemic patients with evidence of iron deficiency should be offered iron replacement therapy on discharge from hospital because it may improve their quality of life and cognitive function.[94,95] In one study, only 16% of anemic patients after UGIB were prescribed oral supplementation on discharge from hospital.[96] Correcting anemia rapidly after discharge may be crucial in minimizing both mortality risk and possible need for a transfusion during a rebleeding episode. In a large prospective study, patients discharged after UGIB with hemoglobin values less than 100 g/L had twice the mortality of patients with hemoglobin levels greater than 100 g/L.[97]

However, current international consensus and American College of Gastroenterology guidelines do not discuss the role of iron replacement after UGIB.[2,11] A recent randomized controlled trial of 97 patients highlighted the importance of iron replacement by comparing intravenous iron, oral iron, and placebo in patients with anemia secondary to nonvariceal UGIB.[98] Patients receiving iron therapy had significantly lower rates of anemia (hemoglobin level <120 g/L for women and hemoglobin level <130 g/L for men) compared with patients receiving placebo at 3 months after UGIB (17% on iron therapy vs 70% on placebo; $P<.01$). Importantly, there was no difference in efficacy between 1 dose of intravenous iron and 3 months of oral iron replacement, although compliance in patients taking oral iron was only 56%.

The primary limitation to oral iron supplementation seems to be gastrointestinal tolerability, which is likely attributable to nonabsorbed iron.[99] All iron salts (ferrous sulfate, ferrous fumarate, and ferrous gluconate) showed similar efficacy and side effect profiles in a randomized trial.[100] A certain controlled-release iron preparation (extended-release ferrous sulfate with mucoproteose) has fewer gastrointestinal side effects than the iron salts according to a large meta-analysis.[101] There are currently no studies evaluating the tolerability of the newer polysaccharide-iron complexes, although previous studies evaluating similar formulations (eg, ferric-dextrin complex) have not shown any clear benefit.[102]

SUMMARY

The acute management of patients with nonvariceal UGIB has evolved considerably over the past 10 years, mostly because of earlier endoscopy, improved endoscopic techniques, and enhanced multidisciplinary management of these patients including gastroenterologists, intensivists, radiologists and surgeons. Application of the existing recommendations should lead to improved outcomes. Clinicians are encouraged to monitor ongoing controversies, such as optimal PPI dosing before and after endoscopic therapy, as well as the appropriate use of blood products. All patients should be screened and treated for Helicobacter Pylori and anemic patients should be offered iron therapy upon discharge from hospital.

REFERENCES

1. Button LA, Roberts SE, Evans PA, et al. Hospitalized incidence and case fatality for upper gastrointestinal bleeding from 1999 to 2007: a record linkage study. Aliment Pharmacol Ther 2011;33:64–76.
2. Barkun AN, Bardou M, Kuipers EJ, et al. International consensus recommendations on the management of patients with nonvariceal upper gastrointestinal bleeding. Ann Intern Med 2010;152:101–13.
3. Lau JY, Sung J, Hill C, et al. Systematic review of the epidemiology of complicated peptic ulcer disease: incidence, recurrence, risk factors and mortality. Digestion 2011;84:102–13.
4. Bardhan KD, Williamson M, Royston C, et al. Admission rates for peptic ulcer in the Trent region, UK, 1972–2000. Changing pattern, a changing disease? Dig Liver Dis 2004;36:577–88.
5. Soplepmann J, Peetsalu A, Peetsalu M, et al. Peptic ulcer haemorrhage in Tartu County, Estonia: epidemiology and mortality risk factors. Scand J Gastroenterol 1997;32:1195–200.
6. Barkun A, Sabbah S, Enns R, et al. The Canadian Registry on Nonvariceal Upper Gastrointestinal Bleeding and Endoscopy (RUGBE): endoscopic hemostasis and proton pump inhibition are associated with improved outcomes in a real-life setting. Am J Gastroenterol 2004;99:1238–46.
7. Hearnshaw SA, Logan RF, Lowe D, et al. Acute upper gastrointestinal bleeding in the UK: patient characteristics, diagnoses and outcomes in the 2007 UK audit. Gut 2011;60:1327–35.
8. Liu NJ, Lee CS, Tang JH, et al. Outcomes of bleeding peptic ulcers: a prospective study. J Gastroenterol Hepatol 2007;23(8 Pt 2):e340–7.
9. Crooks C, Card T, West J. Reductions in 28-day mortality following hospital admission for upper gastrointestinal hemorrhage. Gastroenterology 2011;141:62–70.
10. Lanas A, Carrera-Lasfuentes P, Garcia-Rodriguez LA, et al. Outcomes of peptic ulcer bleeding following treatment with proton pump inhibitors in routine clinical practice: 935 patients with high- or low-risk stigmata. Scand J Gastroenterol 2014;49:1181–90.
11. Laine L, Jensen DM. Management of patients with ulcer bleeding. Am J Gastroenterol 2012;107:345–60 [quiz: 61].
12. Greenspoon J, Barkun A. A summary of recent recommendations on the management of patients with nonvariceal upper gastrointestinal bleeding. Pol Arch Med Wewn 2010;120:341–6.
13. Wee E. Management of nonvariceal upper gastrointestinal bleeding. J Postgrad Med 2011;57:161–7.
14. Myburgh JA, Finfer S, Bellomo R, et al. Hydroxyethyl starch or saline for fluid resuscitation in intensive care. N Engl J Med 2012;367:1901–11.
15. Bunn F, Trivedi D, Ashraf S. Colloid solutions for fluid resuscitation. Cochrane Database Syst Rev 2011;(3):CD001319.
16. Jairath V, Hearnshaw S, Brunskill SJ, et al. Red cell transfusion for the management of upper gastrointestinal haemorrhage. Cochrane Database Syst Rev 2010;(9):CD006613.
17. Villanueva C, Colomo A, Bosch A. Transfusion for acute upper gastrointestinal bleeding. N Engl J Med 2013;368:1362–3.

18. Shalev A, Zahger D, Novack V, et al. Incidence, predictors and outcome of upper gastrointestinal bleeding in patients with acute coronary syndromes. Int J Cardiol 2012;157:386–90.
19. Jairath V, Kahan BC, Logan RF, et al. Red blood cell transfusion practice in patients presenting with acute upper gastrointestinal bleeding: a survey of 815 UK clinicians. Transfusion 2011;51:1940–8.
20. Rohde JM, Dimcheff DE, Blumberg N, et al. Health care-associated infection after red blood cell transfusion: a systematic review and meta-analysis. JAMA 2014;311:1317–26.
21. Kahan BC, Jairath V, Murphy MF, et al. Update on the transfusion in gastrointestinal bleeding (TRIGGER) trial: statistical analysis plan for a cluster-randomised feasibility trial. Trials 2013;14:206.
22. Razzaghi A, Barkun AN. Platelet transfusion threshold in patients with upper gastrointestinal bleeding: a systematic review. J Clin Gastroenterol 2012;46:482–6.
23. Pallin DJ, Saltzman JR. Is nasogastric tube lavage in patients with acute upper GI bleeding indicated or antiquated? Gastrointest Endosc 2011;74:981–4.
24. Witting MD. You wanna do what?! Modern indications for nasogastric intubation. J Emerg Med 2007;33:61–4.
25. Palamidessi N, Sinert R, Falzon L, et al. Nasogastric aspiration and lavage in emergency department patients with hematochezia or melena without hematemesis. Acad Emerg Med 2010;17:126–32.
26. Pateron D, Vicaut E, Debuc E, et al. Erythromycin infusion or gastric lavage for upper gastrointestinal bleeding: a multicenter randomized controlled trial. Ann Emerg Med 2011;57:582–9.
27. Barkun A, Bardou M, Marshall JK. Consensus recommendations for managing patients with nonvariceal upper gastrointestinal bleeding. Ann Intern Med 2003; 139:843–57.
28. Colak S, Erdogan MO, Sekban H, et al. Emergency diagnosis of upper gastrointestinal bleeding by detection of haemoglobin in nasogastric aspirate. J Int Med Res 2013;41:1825–9.
29. Iwasaki H, Shimura T, Yamada T, et al. Novel nasogastric tube-related criteria for urgent endoscopy in nonvariceal upper gastrointestinal bleeding. Dig Dis Sci 2013;58(9):2564–71.
30. Aljebreen AM, Fallone CA, Barkun AN. Nasogastric aspirate predicts high-risk endoscopic lesions in patients with acute upper-GI bleeding. Gastrointest Endosc 2004;59:172–8.
31. Gralnek IM, Barkun AN, Bardou M. Management of acute bleeding from a peptic ulcer. N Engl J Med 2008;359:928–37.
32. Pitera A, Sarko J. Just say no: gastric aspiration and lavage rarely provide benefit. Ann Emerg Med 2010;55:365–6.
33. Anderson RS, Witting MD. Nasogastric aspiration: a useful tool in some patients with gastrointestinal bleeding. Ann Emerg Med 2010;55:364–5.
34. Javad Ehsani Ardakani M, Zare E, Basiri M, et al. Erythromycin decreases the time and improves the quality of EGD in patients with acute upper GI bleeding. Gastroenterol Hepatol Bed Bench 2013;6:195–201.
35. Frossard JL, Spahr L, Queneau PE, et al. Erythromycin intravenous bolus infusion in acute upper gastrointestinal bleeding: a randomized, controlled, double-blind trial. Gastroenterology 2002;123:17–23.
36. Barkun AN, Bardou M, Martel M, et al. Prokinetics in acute upper GI bleeding: a meta-analysis. Gastrointest Endosc 2010;72:1138–45.

37. Bai Y, Guo JF, Li ZS. Meta-analysis: erythromycin before endoscopy for acute upper gastrointestinal bleeding. Aliment Pharmacol Ther 2011;34:166–71.
38. Szary NM, Gupta R, Choudhary A, et al. Erythromycin prior to endoscopy in acute upper gastrointestinal bleeding: a meta-analysis. Scand J Gastroenterol 2011;46:920–4.
39. Altraif I, Handoo FA, Aljumah A, et al. Effect of erythromycin before endoscopy in patients presenting with variceal bleeding: a prospective, randomized, double-blind, placebo-controlled trial. Gastrointest Endosc 2011;73:245–50.
40. Coffin B, Pocard M, Panis Y, et al. Erythromycin improves the quality of EGD in patients with acute upper GI bleeding: a randomized controlled study. Gastrointest Endosc 2002;56:174–9.
41. Sreedharan A, Martin J, Leontiadis GI, et al. Proton pump inhibitor treatment initiated prior to endoscopic diagnosis in upper gastrointestinal bleeding. Cochrane Database Syst Rev 2010;(7):CD005415.
42. Lau JY, Leung WK, Wu JC, et al. Omeprazole before endoscopy in patients with gastrointestinal bleeding. N Engl J Med 2007;356:1631–40.
43. Laine L, Shah A, Bemanian S. Intragastric pH with oral vs intravenous bolus plus infusion proton-pump inhibitor therapy in patients with bleeding ulcers. Gastroenterology 2008;134:1836–41.
44. Lin HJ, Lo WC, Cheng YC, et al. Role of intravenous omeprazole in patients with high-risk peptic ulcer bleeding after successful endoscopic epinephrine injection: a prospective randomized comparative trial. Am J Gastroenterol 2006;101:500–5.
45. Leontiadis GI, Sharma VK, Howden CW. Proton pump inhibitor therapy for peptic ulcer bleeding: Cochrane collaboration meta-analysis of randomized controlled trials. Mayo Clin Proc 2007;82:286–96.
46. Al-Sabah S, Barkun AN, Herba K, et al. Cost-effectiveness of proton-pump inhibition before endoscopy in upper gastrointestinal bleeding. Clin Gastroenterol Hepatol 2008;6:418–25.
47. Barkun AN, Bardou M, Kuipers EJ, et al. How early should endoscopy be performed in suspected upper gastrointestinal bleeding? Am J Gastroenterol 2012;107:328–9.
48. Imperiale TF, Birgisson S. Somatostatin or octreotide compared with H2 antagonists and placebo in the management of acute nonvariceal upper gastrointestinal hemorrhage: a meta-analysis. Ann Intern Med 1997;127:1062–71.
49. Arabi Y, Al Knawy B, Barkun AN, et al. Pro/con debate: octreotide has an important role in the treatment of gastrointestinal bleeding of unknown origin? Crit Care 2006;10:218.
50. Bennett C, Klingenberg SL, Langholz E, et al. Tranexamic acid for upper gastrointestinal bleeding. Cochrane Database Syst Rev 2014;(11):CD006640.
51. Manno D, Ker K, Roberts I. How effective is tranexamic acid for acute gastrointestinal bleeding? BMJ 2014;348:g1421.
52. Bardou M, Martin J, Barkun A. Intravenous proton pump inhibitors: an evidence-based review of their use in gastrointestinal disorders. Drugs 2009;69:435–48.
53. Ghassemi KA, Kovacs TO, Jensen DM. Gastric acid inhibition in the treatment of peptic ulcer hemorrhage. Curr Gastroenterol Rep 2009;11:462–9.
54. Vorder Bruegge WF, Peura DA. Stress-related mucosal damage: review of drug therapy. J Clin Gastroenterol 1990;12(Suppl 2):S35–40.
55. Laine L, McQuaid KR. Endoscopic therapy for bleeding ulcers: an evidence-based approach based on meta-analyses of randomized controlled trials. Clin Gastroenterol Hepatol 2009;7:33–47 [quiz: 1–2].

56. Forrest JA, Finlayson ND, Shearman DJ. Endoscopy in gastrointestinal bleeding. Lancet 1974;2:394–7.
57. Sung JJ, Barkun A, Kuipers EJ, et al. Intravenous esomeprazole for prevention of recurrent peptic ulcer bleeding: a randomized trial. Ann Intern Med 2009;150: 455–64.
58. Barkun AN, Adam V, Sun-g JJ, et al. Cost effectiveness of high-dose intravenous esomeprazole for peptic ulcer bleeding. Pharmacoeconomics 2010;28:217–30.
59. Sachar H, Vaidya K, Laine L. Intermittent vs continuous proton pump inhibitor therapy for high-risk bleeding ulcers: a systematic review and meta-analysis. JAMA Intern Med 2014;174:1755–62.
60. Leontiadis GI, Sharma VK, Howden CW. Systematic review and meta-analysis: enhanced efficacy of proton-pump inhibitor therapy for peptic ulcer bleeding in Asia–a post hoc analysis from the Cochrane Collaboration. Aliment Pharmacol Ther 2005;21:1055–61.
61. Hoie O, Stallemo A, Matre J, et al. Effect of oral lansoprazole on intragastric pH after endoscopic treatment for bleeding peptic ulcer. Scand J Gastroenterol 2009;44:284–8.
62. Laine L, Peterson WL. Bleeding peptic ulcer. N Engl J Med 1994;331:717–27.
63. Cheng HC, Wu CT, Chang WL, et al. Double oral esomeprazole after a 3-day intravenous esomeprazole infusion reduces recurrent peptic ulcer bleeding in high-risk patients: a randomised controlled study. Gut 2014;63:1864–72.
64. Yang YX, Metz DC. Safety of proton pump inhibitor exposure. Gastroenterology 2010;139:1115–27.
65. Dial S, Delaney JA, Barkun AN, et al. Use of gastric acid-suppressive agents and the risk of community-acquired Clostridium difficile-associated disease. JAMA 2005;294:2989–95.
66. Tleyjeh IM, Bin Abdulhak AA, Riaz M, et al. Association between proton pump inhibitor therapy and Clostridium difficile infection: a contemporary systematic review and meta-analysis. PLoS One 2012;7:e50836.
67. Eom CS, Jeon CY, Lim JW, et al. Use of acid-suppressive drugs and risk of pneumonia: a systematic review and meta-analysis. CMAJ 2011;183:310–9.
68. Filion KB, Chateau D, Targownik LE, et al. Proton pump inhibitors and the risk of hospitalisation for community-acquired pneumonia: replicated cohort studies with meta-analysis. Gut 2014;63:552–8.
69. Barkun AN, Bardou M, Pham CQ, et al. Proton pump inhibitors vs. histamine 2 receptor antagonists for stress-related mucosal bleeding prophylaxis in critically ill patients: a meta-analysis. Am J Gastroenterol 2012;107:507–20 [quiz: 21].
70. Khalili H, Huang ES, Jacobson BC, et al. Use of proton pump inhibitors and risk of hip fracture in relation to dietary and lifestyle factors: a prospective cohort study. BMJ 2012;344:e372.
71. Yu EW, Bauer SR, Bain PA, et al. Proton pump inhibitors and risk of fractures: a meta-analysis of 11 international studies. Am J Med 2011;124:519–26.
72. Jo Y, Park E, Ahn SB, et al. A proton pump inhibitor's effect on bone metabolism mediated by osteoclast action in old age: a prospective randomized study. Gut Liver 2014. [Epub ahead of print].
73. Moayyedi P, Yuan Y, Leontiadis G, et al. Canadian Association of Gastroenterology position statement: hip fracture and proton pump inhibitor therapy–a 2013 update. Can J Gastroenterol 2013;27:593–5.
74. Leontiadis GI, Moayyedi P. Proton pump inhibitors and risk of bone fractures. Curr Treat Options Gastroenterol 2014;12:414–23.

75. Hess MW, Hoenderop JG, Bindels RJ, et al. Systematic review: hypomagnesae-mia induced by proton pump inhibition. Aliment Pharmacol Ther 2012;36:405–13.
76. Lam JR, Schneider JL, Zhao W, et al. Proton pump inhibitor and histamine 2 re-ceptor antagonist use and vitamin B12 deficiency. JAMA 2013;310:2435–42.
77. Muriithi AK, Leung N, Valeri AM, et al. Biopsy-proven acute interstitial nephritis, 1993–2011: a case series. Am J Kidney Dis 2014;64:558–66.
78. Ghebremariam YT, LePendu P, Lee JC, et al. Unexpected effect of proton pump inhibitors: elevation of the cardiovascular risk factor asymmetric dimethylargi-nine. Circulation 2013;128:845–53.
79. Lima JP, Brophy JM. The potential interaction between clopidogrel and proton pump inhibitors: a systematic review. BMC Med 2010;8:81.
80. Schneider-Lindner V, Filion KB, Brophy JM. Adverse outcomes associated with use of proton pump inhibitors and clopidogrel. JAMA 2009;302:29–30 [author reply: 1].
81. Lai KC, Lam SK, Chu KM, et al. Lansoprazole for the prevention of recurrences of ulcer complications from long-term low-dose aspirin use. N Engl J Med 2002; 346:2033–8.
82. Sung JJ, Lau JY, Ching JY, et al. Continuation of low-dose aspirin therapy in peptic ulcer bleeding: a randomized trial. Ann Intern Med 2010;152:1–9.
83. Lai KC, Chu KM, Hui WM, et al. Esomeprazole with aspirin versus clopidogrel for prevention of recurrent gastrointestinal ulcer complications. Clin Gastroenterol Hepatol 2006;4:860–5.
84. Chan FK, Ching JY, Hung LC, et al. Clopidogrel versus aspirin and esomepra-zole to prevent recurrent ulcer bleeding. N Engl J Med 2005;352:238–44.
85. Wong GL, Wong VW, Chan Y, et al. High incidence of mortality and recurrent bleeding in patients with Helicobacter pylori-negative idiopathic bleeding ulcers. Gastroenterology 2009;137:525–31.
86. Talley NJ, Li Z. Helicobacter pylori: testing and treatment. Expert Rev Gastroenterol Hepatol 2007;1:71–9.
87. Sfarti C, Stanciu C, Cojocariu C, et al. 13C-urea breath test for the diagnosis of Helicobacter pylori infection in bleeding duodenal ulcer. Rev Med Chir Soc Med Nat Iasi 2009;113:704–9.
88. Sanchez-Delgado J, Gene E, Suarez D, et al. Has H. pylori prevalence in bleeding peptic ulcer been underestimated? A meta-regression. Am J Gastroenterol 2011;106:398–405.
89. Gisbert JP, Abraira V. Accuracy of Helicobacter pylori diagnostic tests in patients with bleeding peptic ulcer: a systematic review and meta-analysis. Am J Gastroenterol 2006;101:848–63.
90. Stenstrom B, Mendis A, Marshall B. Helicobacter pylori–the latest in diagnosis and treatment. Aust Fam Physician 2008;37:608–12.
91. Ramirez-Lazaro MJ, Lario S, Casalots A, et al. Real-time PCR improves Helico-bacter pylori detection in patients with peptic ulcer bleeding. PLoS One 2011;6: e20009.
92. Fock KM. Review article: the epidemiology and prevention of gastric cancer. Aliment Pharmacol Ther 2014;40:250–60.
93. Plummer M, Franceschi S, Vignat J, et al. Global burden of gastric cancer attrib-utable to Helicobacter pylori. Int J Cancer 2015;136:487–90.
94. Verdon F, Burnand B, Stubi CL, et al. Iron supplementation for unexplained fatigue in non-anaemic women: double blind randomised placebo controlled trial. BMJ 2003;326:1124.

95. Bruner AB, Joffe A, Duggan AK, et al. Randomised study of cognitive effects of iron supplementation in non-anaemic iron-deficient adolescent girls. Lancet 1996;348:992–6.

96. Bager P, Dahlerup JF. Lack of follow-up of anaemia after discharge from an upper gastrointestinal bleeding centre. Dan Med J 2013;60:A4583.

97. Rockall TA, Logan RF, Devlin HB, et al. Risk assessment after acute upper gastrointestinal haemorrhage. Gut 1996;38:316–21.

98. Bager P, Dahlerup JF. Randomised clinical trial: oral vs. intravenous iron after upper gastrointestinal haemorrhage–a placebo-controlled study. Aliment Pharmacol Ther 2014;39:176–87.

99. Bayraktar UD, Bayraktar S. Treatment of iron deficiency anemia associated with gastrointestinal tract diseases. World J Gastroenterol 2010;16:2720–5.

100. Hallberg L, Ryttinger L, Solvell L. Side-effects of oral iron therapy. A double-blind study of different iron compounds in tablet form. Acta Med Scand Suppl 1966;459:3–10.

101. Cancelo-Hidalgo MJ, Castelo-Branco C, Palacios S, et al. Tolerability of different oral iron supplements: a systematic review. Curr Med Res Opin 2013;29:291–303.

102. Sas G, Nemesanszky E, Brauer H, et al. On the therapeutic effects of trivalent and divalent iron in iron deficiency anaemia. Arzneimittelforschung 1984;34:1575–9.

The Role of Medical Therapy for Variceal Bleeding

Abdul Q. Bhutta, MD[a,b], Guadalupe Garcia-Tsao, MD[c,d,*]

KEYWORDS

- Cirrhosis • Variceal hemorrhage • Drug therapy • Pharmacologic bases
- Nonselective β-blockers • Octreotide • Terlipressin • Somatostatin

KEY POINTS

- Variceal hemorrhage is a complication of cirrhosis that is mostly due to portal hypertension.
- Pharmacologic therapy for portal hypertension consists of splanchnic vasoconstrictors that decrease portal venous inflow or intrahepatic vasodilators that decrease intrahepatic resistance.
- Pharmacologic therapy for acute variceal hemorrhage consists of intravenous vasoconstrictors and antibiotics.
- Pharmacologic therapy to prevent recurrent variceal hemorrhage is based mainly on the use of nonselective β-blockers with or without nitrates.

INTRODUCTION

Acute variceal hemorrhage (AVH) is a medical emergency, and one of the complications of portal hypertension that define the development of decompensated cirrhosis. Approximately half of the patients with cirrhosis have gastroesophageal varices and one-third of all patients with varices will develop AVH, a complication that still carries a mortality of up to 15% to 20% despite all recent medical advances.[1] This review summarizes the current standard pharmacologic management of AVH in the context of cirrhosis-related portal hypertension. Discussed is not only treatment of the acute

Grant Support: NIH P-30DK 034989.
[a] Department of Internal Medicine, Yale University, 330 Cedar St, Boardman 110 P.O. Box 208056, New Haven, CT 06520-8056, USA; [b] Section of Hospital Medicine, Yale-New Haven Hospital, 20 York Street, CB-2041, New Haven, CT 06520, USA; [c] Section of Digestive Diseases, Yale University School of Medicine, 333 Cedar St, 1080 LMP, P.O. Box 208019, New Haven, CT 06520-8019, USA; [d] Section of Digestive Diseases, VA-CT Healthcare System, 950 Campbell Avenue, West Haven, CT 06516, USA
* Corresponding author. Section of Digestive Diseases, Yale University School of Medicine, 333 Cedar Street–1080 LMP, P.O. Box 208019, New Haven, CT 06520-8019.
E-mail address: guadalupe.garcia-tsao@yale.edu

Gastrointest Endoscopy Clin N Am 25 (2015) 479–490
http://dx.doi.org/10.1016/j.giec.2015.03.001

episode of variceal hemorrhage but also the prevention of recurrent variceal hemorrhage, which is an integral part of the management of any patient with AVH. The recommendations made are mostly based on evidence in literature that has been summarized and prioritized at consensus conferences.[2-4]

PATHOPHYSIOLOGY OF PORTAL HYPERTENSION

An understanding of pathophysiology of portal hypertension is important to understand the basis for the pharmacologic management of variceal hemorrhage. An increase in intrahepatic resistance is the initial mechanism of portal hypertension. Intrahepatic resistance results mainly from progressive architectural distortion (a fixed component), but one-third is due to intrahepatic vasoconstriction secondary to endothelial dysfunction with a deficiency in nitric oxide (NO) being the predominant abnormality.[5] As intrahepatic resistance increases, portal flow is diverted through portosystemic collaterals that develop through pre-existing vessels that would normally drain blood into the portal vein and probably also through vessels that are newly formed (neoangiogenesis through an increase in vascular endothelial growth factor).[6,7] Despite diversion of blood through collaterals and some attenuation of portal pressure, increased portal venous inflow sustains and progressively worsens portal hypertension. Portal inflow results from splanchnic vasodilatation, and the main contributor is an increase in NO. Therefore, in cirrhosis, NO is low in the intrahepatic circulation (vasoconstricted) but elevated in the splanchnic circulation (vasodilated).[8,9]

In patients with cirrhosis, mostly of an alcoholic or viral cause, indirect measurement of portal pressure by hepatic vein catheterization and determination of the hepatic venous pressure gradient (HVPG) has been shown to be the best predictor of different stages in the development of varices and variceal hemorrhage.[10] Normal HVPG is 3 to 5 mm Hg. An HVPG between 5 and 9.5 mm Hg indicates the presence of a silent stage of portal hypertension. Once the HVPG reaches and surpasses a threshold of 10 mm Hg (the so-called clinically significant portal hypertension), patients are at a higher risk of developing varices[10] and cirrhosis decompensation.[11] Almost all patients with gastroesophageal varices have reached an HVPG threshold of at least 12 mm Hg.[1,3] In patients who present with AVH, a threshold of greater than 20 mm Hg identifies those with a higher risk for treatment failure and death.[12,13] Conversely, decreases in HVPG are predictive of favorable outcomes. A decrease greater than 10% from baseline identifies a subgroup of patients without varices that is less likely to develop varices over time[10] and identifies a subgroup of patients with large varices that is less likely to develop variceal hemorrhage.[14] Patients with a history of variceal hemorrhage, a decrease in HVPG to less than 12 mm Hg, or a decrease greater than 20% from baseline (the so-called HVPG responders), are at a significantly reduced risk of recurrent variceal hemorrhage and show improved survival.[1,13,15]

Therefore, reduction in portal pressure is the main goal of therapy in patients with variceal hemorrhage. Targets of pharmacologic therapy consist of drugs that will reduce portal pressure by decreasing portal venous inflow or by decreasing intrahepatic resistance. In the following section, drugs used in the treatment of AVH and in the prevention of recurrent variceal hemorrhage are described.

DRUGS USED IN THE TREATMENT OF ACUTE VARICEAL HEMORRHAGE BY MECHANISM OF ACTION
Drugs That Act by Decreasing Portal Flow

Splanchnic vasoconstrictors decrease portal flow by constricting arterioles that feed the intestine and thereby reduce blood flow into the portal vein. Intravenous vasoconstrictors, such as vasopressin and analogues (terlipressin) and somatostatin analogues (octreotide, vapreotide), are used in the acute intrahospital therapy for AVH. Splanchnic vasoconstrictors used in long-term treatment of primary and secondary prophylaxis of variceal hemorrhage are nonselective β-adrenergic blockers (NSBB). Antibiotics are another category of drugs that possibly act by decreasing portal flow.

Vasopressin and analogues
Vasopressin is a potent vasoconstrictor of both systemic and splanchnic circulation. In a study, an intravenous vasopressin injection resulted in a reduction of HVPG of 23% and intravariceal pressure of 14%.[16] Addition of nitroglycerin has been shown to reduce many side effects of vasopressin and has a synergistic effect in reducing portal pressure.[17] However, vasopressin use has been abandoned in the therapy for AVH because of its numerous side effects, including arterial hypertension, myocardial and peripheral vascular ischemia, limb gangrene, hyponatremia, and fluid retention.

Terlipressin is a long-acting triglycyl lysine derivative of vasopressin. Clinical studies have shown that the frequency and severity of side effects are lower with terlipressin compared with vasopressin. The most common side effect is abdominal pain. The overall efficacy of terlipressin in controlling AVH is 75% to 80% at 48 hours[18] and of 67% at 5 days.[19] Terlipressin is currently not approved for use in the United States.

Somatostatin and analogues
Somatostatin and analogues (octreotide, vapreotide) cause splanchnic vasoconstriction by inhibiting the release of vasodilator glucagon and also by a local mesenteric vasoconstrictive effect.[20] However, the primary mechanism for the control of AVH may be through blunting of postprandial splanchnic hyperemia.[21]

Intravenous boluses of somatostatin and octreotide cause significant transient reductions in portal pressure. Continuous infusion of somatostatin has a mild but sustained effect in reduction of portal pressure,[22] but octreotide does not result in a sustained reduction in portal pressure. This rapid desensitization to the effects of octeriotide infusion may explain the divergent effects achieved with octreotide in acute variceal bleeding.[23] These drugs have a short half-life and are used in a continuous intravenous infusion for AVH. Unlike other vasoactive drugs, somatostatin and analogues have fewer side effects. Octreotide is the only vasoactive drug available in the United States for control of acute variceal bleeding, although its use in this setting is off-label.

Antibiotics
Bacterial infections by inducing the production of vasodilating cytokines that cause vasodilatation can theoretically lead to an increase in portal pressure, and the development of infections has been shown to increase the rate of treatment failure in patients with AVH.[24] Infections can also precipitate renal and liver failure through worsening of effective hypovolemia and impaired oxygen utilization. Antibiotics used in the setting of AVH have been shown to improve survival after AVH likely due to decreased infections and rebleeding.[24]

Nonselective β-blockers
In the setting of AVH, these drugs are used in the prevention of recurrent variceal hemorrhage not in the management of AVH because they can cause hypotension in potentially hemodynamically unstable patients. NSBB decrease portal pressure by unopposed α-adrenergic-mediated splanchnic vasoconstriction (β-2 antagonist effect) and by reducing cardiac output (β-1 antagonist effect).

NSBB use is associated with a median reduction in HVPG of approximately 15%, with only 37% of the patients being hemodynamic responders (ie, achieving a reduction in HVPG to <12 mm Hg or a reduction >20% from baseline).[25] The high percentage of HVPG nonresponders on NSBB, despite adequate β-blockade, may be due to a concomitant increase in portocollateral resistance.[26]

In many randomized clinical trials (RCTs), the dose of NSBB was adjusted to obtain a 25% decrease in heart rate; however, because a change in heart rate is not predictive of a decrease in portal pressure,[27] recent guidelines have recommended the adjustment of NSBB to the highest tolerated dose or to a heart rate of 50 to 55 beats per minute.[3] Measuring the hemodynamic response to a β- blocker is the best way to determine a pharmacologic effect on portal hypertension, and this could actually be done by determining the acute HVPG response to intravenous propranolol.[27] However, the HVPG technique is not adequately practiced or standardized in most sites and therefore cannot be widely recommended.

NSBB commonly used clinically are nadolol and propranolol. Nadolol is longer acting, can be given once a day, is not metabolized by the liver, crosses blood-brain barrier to a lesser extent, and is better tolerated. The disadvantage of NSBB is that approximately 15% of patients may have relative or absolute contraindications to therapy, and that another 15% require dose reduction or discontinuation because of its common side effects (including fatigue, shortness of breath, and hypotension).[25]

Drugs That Act by Reducing Intrahepatic Resistance

Drugs that will act on the intrahepatic circulation by causing vasodilation can reduce portal pressure and can potentially lead to increased flow through the liver and an improved liver function.

Nitrates

In the setting of AVH, and as mentioned above, nitrates have been used in combination with vasopressin. The addition of nitrates not only decreases the rate of side effects of vasopressin related to vasoconstriction, but also has an additive effect in reducing portal pressure.[17,25] Nitrates alone seem to decrease portal pressure by their systemic hypotensive effect with a resultant reduction in cardiac output rather than by intrahepatic vasodilation. Therefore, nitrates used alone have no role in the treatment of portal hypertension because this hypotensive effect is potentially deleterious.

Nitrates can also be used in combination with NSBB for the prevention of rebleeding after AVH. Isosorbide-5-mononitrate (ISMN) is the long-acting nitrate of choice in patients with cirrhosis because of minimal first-pass metabolism. Compared with HVPG reduction of 15% with NSBB alone, combining either ISMN or prazosin with NSBB results in HVPG reduction of around 20% to 24%.[25,28] The rate of HVPG responders with NSBB plus ISMN is 44%, a rate that is significantly higher than that observed with NSBB alone (37%).[25] However, this combination is associated with more side effects and most patients cannot tolerate it.

Simvastatin

Simvastatin decreases intrahepatic vascular resistance resulting in vasodilation of liver vasculature in cirrhotic liver; this occurs because of upregulation of NO production through an enhancement in endothelial NO synthase activity as shown recently in both animals and humans.[29,30] In a placebo-controlled double-blind RCT of 59 patients, 1-month simvastatin administration was associated with a significant reduction in HVPG 8%, with 32% of hemodynamic responders. These effects were additive with those of β-blockers.[30]

A recent RCT compared the addition of simvastatin versus placebo in patients receiving standard therapy (ligation and drugs) and, although it showed a lacking effect on recurrent variceal hemorrhage, it showed a beneficial effect on survival.[31]

Drugs That Act by Reducing Both Flow and Resistance

As mentioned previously, nitrates have been used in combination with vasopressin (in the control of AVH) and in combination with NSBB for the prevention of variceal rebleeding.

Carvedilol is a drug that is NSBB with additional vasodilating effect due to a weak α-1 antagonist activity that has been mostly tested in the prevention of first variceal hemorrhage, where low doses have a greater portal pressure-reducing effect than β-blockers, particularly in Child class A patients.[32] In a recent RCT, carvedilol was as effective as nadolol plus ISMN in the secondary prophylaxis with fewer severe side effects and similar survival.[33]

However, as these patients are more decompensated, the vasodilatory effect of carvedilol may cause further hypotension and potentially lead to fluid retention and renal injury as has been shown to occur in proof-of-concept studies.[25] Therefore, until more data are available, carvedilol should be used cautiously in this setting.

PHARMACOLOGIC THERAPY IN THE DIFFERENT CLINICAL SETTINGS
Control of Acute Variceal Hemorrhage

AVH is associated with significant mortality, morbidity, and health care cost and should be suspected in every patient with cirrhosis presenting with upper gastrointestinal bleed.

Initial resuscitation

These patients generally require management in the intensive care setting. The initial resuscitation follows basic principles of ABC (airway, breathing, and circulation) to achieve hemodynamic stability. The goal is to correct or prevent hypovolemic shock (crystalloids, transfusion) and complications associated with gastrointestinal bleed (bacterial infections, renal failure, hepatic decompensation). Intubation is required if the risk of aspiration is high as in deeply encephalopathic patients. In patients who are hemodynamically stable, transfusion of packed red blood cells should be done conservatively at a target hemoglobin levels between 7 and 8 g/dL because a recent RCT in patients with acute upper gastrointestinal hemorrhage showed that a restrictive transfusion strategy (transfusion when hemoglobin decreases to <7 g/dL) is associated with a better survival than a liberal transfusion strategy (transfusion when hemoglobin decreases to <9 g/dL) to restrictive strategy (transfusion when the hemoglobin decreased to <7 g/dL).[34] In a subset of patients with cirrhosis, the restrictive strategy was associated with significantly less rebleeding and improved survival, particularly in those belonging to Child class A and B.[34] Portal pressure increased in those in the liberal transfusion group but not in those in the restrictive transfusion group.

The prothrombin time/international normalized ratio is not a reliable indicator of the coagulation status in patients with cirrhosis because of a concomitant decrease of both procoagulants and anticoagulants.[35] Proof of this is a multicenter randomized, placebo-controlled trial of recombinant factor VIIa that showed no benefit regarding the ability to control 24-hour bleeding or to prevent rebleeding or death at day 5 in Child class B and C patients with AVH.[36]

Prophylactic antibiotics

Bacterial infections occur in up to 35% to 66% of patients with AVH depending on the severity of liver disease.[37] Infection is an independent prognostic indicator of rebleeding within 7 days. In a meta-analysis of 5 trials, prophylactic antibiotics were found to significantly decrease the risk of infections and rebleeding and improve the survival rate.[24] Therefore, prophylactic antibiotics are currently recommended in all cirrhotic patients with AVH (**Table 1**). The preferred antibiotic for most patients is an oral quinolone, although intravenous ceftriaxone is preferable in patients with advanced cirrhosis or high prevalence of quinolone resistance or in patients already on quinolone prophylaxis.[38] However, given the increasing rate of infections due to multi-drug-resistant organisms and their close relationship with the widespread use of antibiotics, high-risk populations that will benefit from antibiotics should be identified. A recent retrospective study suggests that Child class A patients with AVH may not require prophylactic antibiotics because they are shown have a low risk of infection and death even in the absence of antibiotic prophylaxis.[37]

Hemostatic therapy

In AVH, the treatment of choice is a combination of vasoactive drugs (started before esophagogastroduodenoscopy [EGD]) and emergency endoscopic therapy (within the first 12 hours). A meta-analysis of RCTs for the specific management of AVH shows that a combination of endoscopic and pharmacologic therapy is significantly better than endoscopic therapy alone.[39] Another meta-analysis showed that vasoactive drugs in general are associated with an improvement in control of bleeding and a decrease in mortality.[40] A recent prospective, multicenter, randomized, noninferiority trial compared the 3 most commonly used drugs, terlipressin, somatostatin, and octreotide, and showed that they were identical in terms of hemostatic effects and safety.[18] Thus, any of the vasoactive drugs can be used during AVH depending on the local availability and should be continued until the achievement of 24-hour bleed-free period and up to 5 days (see **Table 1**).

Rescue therapy

The above-mentioned combined approach with vasoactive drugs, prophylactic antibiotics, and endoscopic techniques is the recommended current standard of care for patients with AVH. However, 10% to 15% of patients fail this combined approach because either the initial bleeding continues or the early rebleeding occurs in first 5 days.[41] The transjugular intrahepatic portosystemic shunt (TIPS) is the therapy of choice for patients who fail standard therapy with combination vasoactive drugs and endoscopic therapy.[2,3] However, mortality remains very high in these patients even after TIPS placement. These high-risk patients are specifically those with an HVPG greater than 20 mm Hg[42] or Child class C with a score between 9 and 13 or Child class B with persistent bleeding at endoscopy.[43] A recent RCT examined the effect of "early" (preemptive) TIPS (within 24 to 48 hours of admission) versus standard therapy inpatients at high risk of treatment failure. In the early TIPS group, the 1-year probability of remaining free of rebleeding and 1-year survival was 97% and 86% compared with 50% and 61% with the pharmacotherapy-endoscopic variceal ligation (EVL) group. The survival benefit was maintained in the long term (at least up to 2 years) without an increase in the rate of hepatic encephalopathy.[44]

In refractory AVH, balloon tamponade may be used as a temporary bridge to TIPS but is associated with serious complications in more than 20% of patients. The use of a safer self-expanding esophageal metal stent may be an option in refractory variceal bleeding, although further evaluation is needed.[45]

Secondary Prophylaxis (Prevention of Recurrent Variceal Hemorrhage)

The rebleeding risk in patients who survive an episode of AVH is very high; 63% at 1 to 2 years with a mortality of 33%.[46] Therefore, therapy to prevent rebleeding should be

Table 1
Pharmacologic therapy in the management of acute esophageal variceal hemorrhage

Regimen	Dose	Duration	Follow-up	Comments
Vasoconstrictor				
Octreotide	Intravenous 50-μg bolus, followed by infusion of 50 μg/h	2–5 d	Bolus can be repeated in first hour if variceal hemorrhage uncontrolled; if rebleeding occurs during therapy, consider TIPS	Available in the United States
Terlipressin	2 mg given intravenously every 4 h for first 48 h, followed by 1 mg given intravenously every 4 h	2–5 d	If rebleeding occurs during therapy, consider TIPS	Not available in the United States
Somatostatin	Intravenous 250-μg bolus, followed by infusion of 250–500 μg/h	2–5 d	Bolus can be repeated in first hour if variceal hemorrhage uncontrolled; if rebleeding occurs during therapy, consider TIPS	Not available in the United States
Antibiotic				
Ceftriaxone	Intravenous ceftriaxone at a dose of 1 g once a day	5–7 d or until discharge	No long-term antibiotics unless spontaneous bacterial peritonitis develops	Used in patients with advanced liver disease, high probability of quinolone resistance, or both
Norfloxacin	400 mg given orally twice a day	5–7 d or until discharge	No long-term antibiotics unless spontaneous bacterial peritonitis develops	Used in patients with low probability of quinolone-resistant organisms

Only one vasoconstrictor plus one antibiotic plus endoscopic therapy should be used.

Table 2
Pharmacologic therapy for the prevention of recurrent variceal hemorrhage

Regimen	Dose	Goal	Duration	Follow-up
β-Blocker				
Propranolol	Start at 20 mg orally twice a day Maximum 320 mg/d	Increase to maximally tolerated dose or once heart rate is 50–55 beats/min	Indefinite	Ensure heart-rate goals are met at each clinic visit
Nadolol	Start at 40 mg orally once a day Maximum 240 mg/d	Increase to maximally tolerated dose or once heart rate is 50–55 beats/min	Indefinite	Ensure heart-rate goals are met at each clinic visit; no need for follow-up endoscopy
Isosorbide mononitrate[a]	10 mg given orally every night, with stepwise increase to a maximum of 20 mg twice a day	Increase to maximally tolerated dose with maintenance of blood pressure at >95 mm Hg	Indefinite	Ensure compliance with medication regimen at each visit
Carvedilol[b]	6.25 mg given orally once a day Maximum 12.5 mg/d	Increase to 12.5 mg/d in 2 wk provided systolic blood pressure >100 mm Hg	Indefinite	Ensure compliance with medication regimen at each visit

β-Blockers are used in combination with variceal ligation.
[a] Isosorbide mononitrate should only be used in combination with a β-blocker and in patients who are intolerant to variceal ligation.
[b] Under investigation, has only been used compared with β-blockers plus isosorbide mononitrate.

initiated while the patient is still in the hospital, as soon as AVH is controlled and the intravenous vasoactive drug is discontinued.

Several studies and meta-analyses have shown that a combination of EVL and drug therapy (NSBB $\pm$ ISMN) is better than single therapy alone in preventing variceal rebleeding. However, a recent meta-analysis shows that although combination therapy is more effective than EVL alone in preventing recurrent variceal hemorrhage and all-cause rebleeding, drug therapy alone is not significantly different from combination therapy in preventing all-cause rebleeding.[47] Similarly, a more recent meta-analysis shows that adding drugs to EVL reduces all-cause rebleeding with a tendency for a reduced mortality, whereas adding EVL to drug therapy was only marginally more effective than drugs alone with a tendency for a better survival with drugs alone,[48] indicating that there may be a role for drug therapy alone in the secondary prophylaxis of variceal hemorrhage but the specific population that would benefit from it remains to be determined. Another issue is whether NSBB should be used alone or in combination with nitrates. Although combination nitrates plus NSBB results in greater portal pressure reduction and higher rate of HVPG responders, most patients cannot tolerate this combination because of a higher rate of adverse effects.[25,28] Carvedilol has been shown to be similar to a combination of NSBB plus nitrates in the prevention of recurrent variceal hemorrhage with a lower rate of side effects.[33] In this study, carvedilol was used at a dose of 6.25 mg/d increased to a maximum of 12.5 mg/d provided the systolic blood pressure was greater than 100 mm Hg. Carvedilol can be potentially deleterious in patients with ascites (worsening vasodilatation) and should not be used routinely in the prevention of recurrent variceal hemorrhage.

Therefore, the current standard of care for prevention of rebleeding is a combination of EVL and NSBB (**Table 2**).

Recently, the benefits of NSBB in decompensated liver cirrhosis have been questioned. A single-center observational study suggested that NSBB are associated with a poorer survival in patients with refractory ascites but groups were mismatched at baseline.[49] In addition, a recent study that used propensity score matching showed entirely opposite results with a significantly better survival in patients with refractory ascites on propranolol compared with those patients not on propranolol, with carvedilol having an intermediate survival.[50] A deleterious effect of NSBB in patients with refractory ascites is potentially possible if they would cause hypotension and worsen the already altered hemodynamics in these patients. Until this is further investigated, the recommendation is that NSBB should be used in these patients unless associated with hypotension.

Other special populations in whom alternative therapies should be investigated are patients who have bled from varices despite being on adequate primary prophylaxis with NSBB. In a retrospective study, these patients were shown to have higher rebleeding and mortality compared with patients who had not been on NSBB before AVH.[51]

REFERENCES

1. Garcia-Tsao G, Bosch J. Management of varices and variceal hemorrhage in cirrhosis. N Engl J Med 2010;362:823–32.
2. de Franchis R. Revising consensus in portal hypertension: report of the Baveno V consensus workshop on methodology of diagnosis and therapy in portal hypertension. J Hepatol 2010;53:762–8.
3. Garcia-Tsao G, Sanyal AJ, Grace ND, et al. Prevention and management of gastroesophageal varices and variceal hemorrhage in cirrhosis. Hepatology 2007;46:922–38.

4. Garcia-Tsao G, Bosch J, Groszmann RJ. Portal hypertension and variceal bleeding—unresolved issues: summary of an American Association for the Study of Liver Diseases and European Association for the Study of the Liver single topic conference. Hepatology 2008;47:1764–72.
5. Bhathal PS, Grossman HJ. Reduction of the increased portal vascular resistance of the isolated perfused cirrhotic rat liver by vasodilators. J Hepatol 1985;1:325–37.
6. Fernandez M, Mejias M, Garcia-Pras E, et al. Reversal of portal hypertension and hyperdynamic splanchnic circulation by combined vascular endothelial growth factor and platelet-derived growth factor blockade in rats. Hepatology 2007;46:1208–17.
7. Fernandez M, Mejias M, Angermayr B, et al. Inhibition of VEGF receptor-2 decreases the development of hyperdynamic splanchnic circulation and portal-systemic collateral vessels in portal hypertensive rats. J Hepatol 2005;43:98–103.
8. Iwakiri Y, Groszmann RJ. Vascular endothelial dysfunction in cirrhosis. J Hepatol 2007;46:927–34.
9. Wiest R, Groszmann RJ. The paradox of nitric oxide in cirrhosis and portal hypertension: too much, not enough. Hepatology 2002;35:478–91.
10. Groszmann RJ, Garcia-Tsao G, Bosch J, et al. Beta-blockers to prevent gastroesophageal varices in patients with cirrhosis. N Engl J Med 2005;353:2254–61.
11. Ripoll C, Groszmann R, Garcia-Tsao G, et al. Hepatic venous pressure gradient predicts clinical decompensation in patients with compensated cirrhosis. Gastroenterology 2007;133:481–8.
12. Moitinho E, Escorsell A, Bandi JC, et al. Prognostic value of early measurements of portal pressure in acute variceal bleeding. Gastroenterology 1999;117(3):626–31.
13. Abraldes JG, Tarantino I, Turnes J, et al. Hemodynamic response to pharmacological treatment of portal hypertension and long-term prognosis of cirrhosis. Hepatology 2003;37:902–8.
14. Villanueva C, Aracil C, Colomo A, et al. Acute hemodynamic response to beta-blockers and prediction of long-term outcome in primary prophylaxis of variceal bleeding. Gastroenterology 2009;137:119–28.
15. D'Amico G, Garcia-Pagan JC, Luca A, et al. HVPG reduction and prevention of variceal bleeding in cirrhosis: a systematic review. Gastroenterology 2006;131:1611–24.
16. Bosch J, Bordas JM, Mastai R, et al. Effects of vasopressin on the intravariceal pressure in patients with cirrhosis: comparison with the effects on portal pressure. Hepatology 1988;8:861–5.
17. Groszmann RJ, Kravetz D, Bosch J, et al. Nitroglycerin improves the hemodynamic response to vasopressin in portal hypertension. Hepatology 1982;2:757–62.
18. Seo YS, Park SY, Kim MY, et al. Lack of difference among terlipressin, somatostatin, and octreotide in the control of acute gastroesophageal variceal hemorrhage. Hepatology 2014;60(3):954–63.
19. Escorsell A, Ruiz dA, Planas R, et al. Multicenter randomized controlled trial of terlipressin versus sclerotherapy in the treatment of acute variceal bleeding: the TEST study. Hepatology 2000;32(3):471–6.
20. Wiest R, Tsai MH, Groszmann RJ. Octreotide potentiates PKC-dependent vasoconstrictors in portal-hypertensive and control rats. Gastroenterology 2000;120:975–83.
21. Buonamico P, Sabba C, Garcia-Tsao G, et al. Octreotide blunts post-prandial splanchnic hyperemia in cirrhotic patients: a double-blind randomized echo-Doppler study. Hepatology 1995;21:134–9.

22. Cirera I, Feu F, Luca A, et al. Effects of bolus injections and continuous infusions of somatostatin and placebo in patients with cirrhosis and portal hypertension. A double-blind hemodynamic investigation. Hepatology 1995;22: 106–11.
23. Escorsell A, Bandi JC, Andreu V, et al. Desensitization to the effects of intravenous octreotide in cirrhotic patients with portal hypertension. Gastroenterology 2001;120:161–9.
24. Bernard B, Grange JD, Khac EN, et al. Antibiotic prophylaxis for the prevention of bacterial infections in cirrhotic patients with gastrointestinal bleeding: a meta-analysis. Hepatology 1999;29:1655–61.
25. Miñano C, Garcia-Tsao G. Clinical pharmacology of portal hypertension. Gastroenterol Clin North Am 2010;39:681–95.
26. Kroeger RJ, Groszmann RJ. Increased portal venous resistance hinders portal pressure reduction during the administration of beta-adrenergic blocking agents in a portal hypertensive model. Hepatology 1985;5:97–101.
27. La Mura V, Abraldes JG, Raffa S, et al. Prognostic value of acute hemodynamic response to i.v. propranolol in patients with cirrhosis and portal hypertension. J Hepatol 2009;51:279–87.
28. Albillos A, Garcia-Pagan JC, Iborra J, et al. Propranolol plus prazosin compared with propranolol plus isosorbide-5-mononitrate in the treatment of portal hypertension. Gastroenterology 1998;115:116–23.
29. Abraldes JG, Rodríguez-Vilarrupla A, Graupera M, et al. Simvastatin treatment improves liver sinusoidal endothelial dysfunction in CCl4 cirrhotic rats. J Hepatol 2007;46(6):1040–6.
30. Abraldes JG, Albillos A, Banares R, et al. Simvastatin lowers portal pressure in patients with cirrhosis and portal hypertension: a randomized controlled trial. Gastroenterology 2009;136:1651–8.
31. Abraldes JG, Villanueva C, Aracil C, et al. Addition of simvastatin to standard treatment improves survival after variceal bleeding in patients with cirrhosis: a double-blind randomized trial [abstract]. J Hepatol 2014;60(1):S525.
32. Reiberger T, Ulbrich G, Ferlitsch A, et al. Vienna Hepatic Hemodynamic Lab. Carvedilol for primary prophylaxis of variceal bleeding in cirrhotic patients with haemodynamic non-response to propranolol. Gut 2013;62(11):1634–41.
33. Lo GH, Chen WC, Wang HM, et al. Randomized, controlled trial of carvedilol versus nadolol plus isosorbide mononitrate for the prevention of variceal rebleeding. J Gastroenterol Hepatol 2012;27(11):1681–7.
34. Villanueva C, Colomo A, Bosch A, et al. Transfusion strategies for acute upper gastrointestinal bleeding. N Engl J Med 2013;368(1):11–21.
35. Tripodi A, Mannucci PM. The coagulopathy of chronic liver disease. N Engl J Med 2011;365(2):147–56.
36. Bosch J, Thabut D, Albillos A, et al. Recombinant factor VIIa for variceal bleeding in patients with advanced cirrhosis: a randomized, controlled trial. Hepatology 2008;47:1604–14.
37. Tandon P, Abraldes JG, Keough A, et al. Risk of bacterial infection in patients with cirrhosis and acute variceal hemorrhage, based on Child-Pugh class, and effects of antibiotics. Clin Gastroenterol Hepatol 2014. pii: S1542-3565(14)01710-8. http://dx.doi.org/10.1016/j.cgh.2014.11.019. [Epub ahead of print].
38. Fernandez J, Ruiz d A, Gomez C, et al. Norfloxacin vs ceftriaxone in the prophylaxis of infections in patients with advanced cirrhosis and hemorrhage. Gastroenterology 2006;131:1049–56.

39. Banares R, Albillos A, Rincon D, et al. Endoscopic treatment versus endoscopic plus pharmacologic treatment for acute variceal bleeding: a meta-analysis. Hepatology 2002;35:609–15.

40. Wells M, Chande N, Adams P, et al. Meta-analysis: vasoactive medications for the management of acute variceal bleeds. Aliment Pharmacol Ther 2012;35(11): 1267–78.

41. D'Amico G, de Franchis R. Upper digestive bleeding in cirrhosis: post-therapeutic outcome and prognostic indicators. Hepatology 2003;38:599–612.

42. Monescillo A, Martínez-Lagares F, Ruiz-del-Arbol L, et al. Influence of portal hypertension and its early decompression by TIPS placement on the outcome of variceal bleeding. Hepatology 2004;40:793–801.

43. Garcia-Pagán JC, Caca K, Bureau C, et al. An early decision for PTFE-TIPS improves survival in high risk cirrhotic patients admitted with an acute variceal bleeding: a multicenter RCT [abstract]. Hepatology 2008;48(Suppl):373A–4A.

44. García-Pagán JC, Caca K, Bureau C, et al, Early TIPS (Transjugular Intrahepatic Portosystemic Shunt) Cooperative Study Group. Early use of TIPS in patients with cirrhosis and variceal bleeding. N Engl J Med 2010;362(25):2370–9.

45. Hubmann R, Bodlaj G, Czompo M, et al. The use of self-expanding metal stents to treat acute esophageal variceal bleeding. Endoscopy 2006;38:896–901.

46. D'Amico G, Pagliaro L, Bosch J. The treatment of portal hypertension: a meta-analytic review. Hepatology 1995;22(1):332–54.

47. Thiele M, Krag A, Rohde U, et al. Meta-analysis: banding ligation and medical interventions for the prevention of rebleeding from oesophageal varices. Aliment Pharmacol Ther 2012;35(10):1155–65.

48. Puente A, Hernández-Gea V, Graupera I, et al. Drugs plus ligation to prevent rebleeding in cirrhosis: an updated systematic review. Liver Int 2014;34(6):823–33.

49. Sersté T, Melot C, Francoz C, et al. Deleterious effects of β-blockers on survival in patients with cirrhosis and refractory ascites. Hepatology 2010;52:1017–22.

50. Leithead JA, Rajoriya N, Tehami N, et al. Non-selective β-blockers are associated with improved survival in patients with ascites listed for liver transplantation. Gut 2014. pii: gutjnl-2013-306502. http://dx.doi.org/10.1136/gutjnl-2013-306502. [Epub ahead of print].

51. De Souza AR, La Mura V, Reverter E, et al. Patients whose first episode of bleeding occurs while taking a β-blocker have high long-term risks of rebleeding and death. Clin Gastroenterol Hepatol 2012;10(6):670–6.

Endoscopic Diagnosis and Therapy in Gastroesophageal Variceal Bleeding

Ashwani Kapoor, MBBS[1], Narayan Dharel, MBBS, PhD[1],
Arun J. Sanyal, MBBS, MD*

KEYWORDS

- Variceal hemorrhage • Esophageal varices • Gastric varices • Endoscopy
- Endoscopic band ligation • Endoscopic sclerotherapy
- Endoscopic variceal obturation • Cirrhosis

KEY POINTS

- Gastroesophageal variceal hemorrhage is a medical emergency with high morbidity and mortality.
- Endoscopic therapy is the mainstay of management of bleeding varices.
- It requires attention to technique and the appropriate choice of therapy for a given patient at a given point in time.
- Subjects must be monitored continuously after initiation of therapy for control of bleeding, and second-line definitive therapies must be introduced quickly if endoscopic and pharmacologic treatment fails.
- An appropriate surveillance plan must be established for prevention of future bleedings.

INTRODUCTION

Gastroesophageal varices (GOVs) are present in approximately 50% of patients with cirrhosis, more so with Child C cirrhosis (up to 85%). Rupture of these varices

Grant support: This article was supported in part by NIH T32 DK 07150-038 to Dr A.J. Sanyal.
Conflicts of Interest: None to report (Dr A. Kapoor, Dr N. Dharel); Dr A.J. Sanyal: has stock options in Genfit. He has served as a consultant to AbbVie, Astra Zeneca, Nitto Denko, Nimbus, Salix, Tobira, Takeda, Fibrogen, Immuron, Exhalenz, and Genfit. He has been an unpaid consultant to Intercept and Echosens. His institution has received grant support from Gilead, Salix, Tobira, and Novartis.
Division of Gastroenterology, Department of Internal Medicine, Virginia Commonwealth University School of Medicine, MCV Box 980341, Richmond, VA 23298-0341, USA
[1] Both Drs A. Kapoor and N. Dharel contributed equally to this article and are co-primary authors.
* Corresponding author.
E-mail address: asanyal@mcvh-vcu.edu

Gastrointest Endoscopy Clin N Am 25 (2015) 491–507
http://dx.doi.org/10.1016/j.giec.2015.03.004
1052-5157/15/$ – see front matter © 2015 Elsevier Inc. All rights reserved.

constitutes a medical emergency and can be rapidly fatal unless quickly controlled. Acute variceal bleeding occurs in a yearly rate of about 5% to 15% in subjects with varices and, despite advancement in diagnostics and therapy, the 6-week mortality from variceal bleeding can be as high as 20%.[1] Prompt diagnosis is a key factor in effective and timely management of these patients. Focused history, directed physical examination, and basic laboratory measurements are important parts of the triage to plan resuscitative measures, timing of endoscopy, other therapies, and for prognostication. In later discussion, the role of endoscopy in the diagnosis and management of bleeding gastr-esophageal varices is discussed.

ENDOSCOPIC DIAGNOSIS OF VARICEAL HEMORRHAGE

The key objectives of the initial evaluation of a subject with suspected variceal bleed include assessment of the severity of bleeding, identification of the source of bleeding, and risk assessment of prognosis, including the presence of infection and complications. Once therapy is initiated, ongoing assessment of bleeding control is required to determine the need for second-line interventions. Endoscopy plays a critical role in these processes and is central to the management of active variceal bleeding.

Any upper gastrointestinal bleeding in a patient with known cirrhosis or evidence of portal hypertension should be considered and managed as a case of variceal bleeding until proven otherwise by endoscopy. Esophagogastroduodenoscopy is considered the gold standard for the diagnosis of gastroesophageal variceal bleeding. It can be performed at the bedside in the emergency department, and therapy can be provided at the same time when diagnostic assessment is performed. In the setting of active bleeding, a diagnosis of variceal hemorrhage is based on demonstration of bleeding varices, stigmata of recent bleeding (eg, an adherent clot over a varix or a platelet plug [white nipple sign]), or the presence of varices and upper gastrointestinal bleeding without other obvious identifiable sources of bleeding (**Box 1**).[2] The location of the varices is also identifiable at the time of endoscopy along with assessment of the size of the varices. These data are needed for both the diagnosis and the determination of the optimal approach for long-term bleeding control.

Box 1
Diagnosis of gastroesophageal variceal bleeding

Esophagogastroduodenoscopy is the gold standard for the diagnosis of acute variceal bleeding. A diagnosis of gastroesophageal variceal bleeding is made if any of the following criteria is satisfied:

1. Direct visualization of blood (spurting or oozing) arising from an esophageal or gastric varix.

2. Presence of gastroesophageal varix with signs of recent bleed (stigmata) such as white nipple sign or overlying clot.

3. Presence of varix with red signs plus presence of blood in the stomach in the absence of another source of bleeding.

4. Presence of varix with red signs (cherry red spots: small, ~2 mm, red, spotty flat spot on the variceal surface, red wale signs, longitudinal read streaks on the variceal surface, hematocystic spots, large, >3 mm, round, discrete, red raised spots on the variceal surface) and clinical signs of upper gastrointestinal bleeding, without blood in the stomach.

Adapted from Sarin SK, Kumar A, Angus PW, et al. Diagnosis and management of acute variceal bleeding: Asian Pacific Association for study of the liver recommendations. Hepatol Int 2011;5:619; with permission.

Timing of Endoscopy

Ideally, endoscopy should be performed as soon as the proper resuscitation has taken place and hemodynamics have been stabilized. American Association for the Study of Liver Diseases guidelines suggest timing of endoscopy to be within 12 hours for acute variceal bleeding.[3,4] In a retrospective study of patients who presented with acute variceal bleeding but were hemodynamically stable, there was no significant difference in mortality in patients with endoscopy performed within 4 hours versus 8 hours or 12 hours.[5] In contrast, another study found delayed endoscopy (endoscopy time >15 hours) as a risk factor for increased mortality in acute variceal bleeding.[6] It is the authors' opinion that the urgency is dictated by the severity of bleeding and the clinical setting. For example, a patient who is exsanguinating needs immediate therapy to stop bleeding, whereas care could be delayed until hemodynamics are fully stabilized in those with less severe bleeding. Also, the presence of comorbidities, such as cardiac disease and such, and the ability to tolerate hemorrhagic anemia must also be taken in to account when making the decision to proceed rapidly versus not so rapidly toward endoscopy.

Utility of Endoscopy for Diagnosis of Variceal Hemorrhage

Endoscopy provides direct visualization of varices and is the cornerstone of the diagnostic approach to confirm the presence of variceal hemorrhage. There are, however, occasional situations wherein it may be difficult to visualize bleeding varices. The most common situation is a large clot in the fundus of the stomach that prevents an adequate retroflexed view of the cardia and the gastroesophageal junction. Several modalities can be attempted to improve the ability to diagnose variceal bleeding in this setting. If the blood pressure permits, one may raise the head end of the bed to allow the clot to pass to the antrum. There are only anecdotal reports of the utility of this maneuver. More commonly, a prokinetic agent such as erythromycin has been used for this purpose. A recent meta-analysis suggests that this may improve visualization of gastric varices.[7] It must be noted, however, that none of the published trials are of very high quality.

Is Airway Protection Required for Urgent Endoscopy for Bleeding Varices?

This topic is frequently debated. Airway compromise can occur before endoscopy, during endoscopy, and in the period after endoscopy when the subject may not have fully recovered from sedation. One retrospective study did not find any benefit for prophylactic airway intubation before endoscopy.[8] However, this study did not address the expertise of the intubators and the potential for selection bias. In a previous uncontrolled study, prevention of aspiration was associated with a substantial improvement in mortality in a subset of patients with severe uncontrolled variceal bleeding despite first-line therapies.[9] Based on these first-line therapies, the authors currently recommend airway protection in those subjects with severe active hematemesis and those who are unable to protect their airway and are at high risk in the periprocedural period.

SPECIFIC THERAPIES FOR ESOPHAGEAL VARICEAL BLEEDING
Endoscopic Variceal Band Ligation

Principles of band ligation

Endoscopic variceal band ligation (EVBL) is the cornerstone for the management of acute variceal bleeding. The principle for band ligation is based on the venous drainage system in the esophagus. Vianna and colleagues[10] described 4 zones in the esophagus: gastric, palisade, perforating, and truncal zones. The gastric zone extends 2 to 3 cm below the gastroesophageal junction and drains in short gastric and left gastric veins. The palisade zone extends 2 to 3 cm superior to the gastric zone and is a watershed area between portal and systemic circulation. The perforating zone extends 2 cm further above the palisade zone and has perforating veins joining submucosal venous plexuses to paraesophageal venous plexuses. The truncal zone is 8 to 10 cm long and has perforating veins joining submucosal veins to extraesophageal veins. The palisade and perforating zones are important for esophageal varices ligation. The objective is to obliterate the submucosal veins in the palisade zone, which is followed by thrombosis and obliteration of the perforating veins that connect the submucosal varices to extraesophageal collaterals.

Consequences of endoscopic variceal band ligation

The pathologic changes after EVBL have been evaluated in canine models and humans. Variceal ligation results in ischemic necrosis of banded tissue and thrombosis of varices (24–48 hours). The resultant mucosal ulceration takes 2 to 3 weeks for complete re-epithelialization.[11,12] It has been reported that with complete variceal obliteration, the risk of portal vein thrombosis may be increased and the development of gastric varices may be facilitated.[13] Portal hypertensive gastropathy may also worsen after successful esophageal variceal eradication by EVBL.[13]

Technique

Initially, single-band devices were used. It was cumbersome to use single-band devices because it involved reloading and reintubating the esophagus multiple times. To overcome this limitation, multiple band shooters, including the Saeed Multiple Ligator (Wilson-Cook Medical, Inc, Winston-Salem, NC, USA) and the Speedband (Boston Scientific Corporation, Natick, MA, USA), were developed. The Saeed Six-Shooter is a safe and effective method to eradicate varices.[14] The band ligator is attached to the shaft of endoscope. After advancing the endoscope toward the varix that needs to be banded, suction is applied until "red out" occurs and then the band is fired. It is important at this point not to release suction until after a band has been successfully applied; this is required to minimize the risk of iatrogenic bleeding. The bands are placed in distal 5 cm of the esophagus in a spiral fashion from the gastroesophageal junction and moving upwards. This placement is dictated by the thickness of the overlying mucosa, which is the least at the gastroesophageal junction, thereby making this region particularly prone to bleeding.

Efficacy

In 1991, Stiegmann and colleagues[15] published a landmark study on the superiority of EVBL over endoscopic injection sclerotherapy (EIS) for active variceal bleeding. EVBL had fewer complications and rebleeding rates compared with EIS. The 2 techniques were equally effective (approximately 90%). EVBL required a smaller mean number of sessions (3.5 sessions) compared with EIS (4 sessions). A recent meta-analysis showed better bleeding control and low mortality with EVBL compared with EIS.[16] In another meta-analysis, a combination of EVBL with EIS offered no advantage over EVBL alone in the prevention of rebleeding or reducing mortality. On the other hand, stricture formation was higher after EIS compared with EVBL alone.[17]

Complications

Risk of complications after banding varies from 2% to 23%. Chest pain, infection, stricture, and ulcers are complications seen. The incidence of ulcer bleeding after banding is 2.6% to 7.3%[18] and has been associated with Child B or C cirrhosis. In the absence of active bleeding, it can be managed conservatively. For actively bleeding ulcers, one needs to consider alternate endoscopic therapies including sclerotherapy or transjugular intrahepatic portosystemic shunt (TIPS). Pantoprazole given for 10 days has been shown to decrease the size of the ulcers. It does not affect symptoms like chest pain and dysphagia, however.[19]

Combination endoscopic treatment with pharmacologics is better than either treatment alone for active bleeding and has been confirmed in numerous trials, which have now been assessed by meta-analyses. Combination therapy was associated with improved bleeding-related outcomes (relative risk [RR] = 1.21, confidence interval [CI] −1.13 to 1.30, $P<.001$) and survival advantage (RR 0.74, 95% CI 0.57–0.95, $P = .02$) compared with EVBL alone.[20]

Endoscopic Injection Sclerotherapy

Sclerosants are chemical agents that are an oily or an aqueous solution when injected in or around the varices, inducing sclerosis. Several such agents have been used to induce phlebitis and thrombosis of varices with subsequent obliteration. Sodium tetradecyl sulfate, sodium morrhuate (5%), sodium ethanolamine (5%), polidocanol, and absolute alcohol have all been used for control of variceal hemorrhage. Only sodium tetradecyl sulfate is US Food and Drug Administration (FDA) approved for this indication.

Technique

The type of needle used is usually a 23 G or 25 G. Injections can be made in to the varices (intravariceal injection) or around the varices (paravariceal injection).[21] For the intravariceal technique, the first injection is usually made just below the bleeding site in the varix. Subsequent injections are made at all the varices around the gastro-esophageal junction. Proximal injections are made at 2-cm intervals up to 5 to 6 cm from the gastroesophageal junction. For the paravariceal technique, the injection is made adjacent to the varix. There is no convincing evidence that one technique is better than the other. Also, even in expert hands, intravariceal injections often result in paravariceal spillover.

Efficacy

EIS is 60% to 100% effective in controlling active esophageal variceal bleeding.[22] Treatment is repeated at 1- to 3-week intervals until obliteration and then every 3 months. EIS is not recommended for primary prophylaxis. Effectiveness of different sclerosants has been studied. From currently available data, one agent cannot be recommended over the others.[23–25] Currently, EIS is generally restricted to the very uncommon situation wherein EVBL is not technically feasible, mainly due to its adverse event profile noted in later discussion. Nonetheless, EIS can and should be considered a rescue therapy if EVBL is not successful or results in further bleeding. However, TIPS should be the preferred alternate whenever feasible because it has been shown to improve survival.

Complications

Chest pain is noted in about 10% of patients after sclerotherapy. Ulcer formation is noted in 20% to 60% of cases. The volume of sclerosant and Child C cirrhosis has been associated with the risk of ulcer formation. When performed, the volume of sclerosant per site should not exceed the recommended amount (volume injected depends on sclerosant used) to avoid the risks associated with EIS. Ranitidine has been shown to hasten healing of ulcers but does not prevent ulcer formation.[26] Stricture formation may occur in up to 40% of cases. Most strictures are asymptomatic.

Symptomatic strictures respond well to endoscopic dilation. Risk of rebleeding is 15% to 50% in the first 24 hours. Other rare complications include perforation, mediastinitis, pericarditis, pneumothorax, spinal cord paralysis, and mesenteric vein thrombosis. There are few case reports of esophageal squamous cell carcinoma after sclerotherapy.[27]

Esophageal Stents

Endoscopic stent placement for control of active esophageal bleeding

Over the last 5 years, several studies have demonstrated the feasibility of controlling active bleeding from esophageal varices with an endoscopically placed stent in the esophagus. Initial bleeding control rates of 80% to 90% have been reported with minimal side effects.[28] Also, the stent placement can occur at the bedside, can come in handy as a rescue therapy, and can buy time for those with severe bleeding who will need a more definitive treatment such as TIPS. One of the stents evaluated in such settings is a fully covered self-expandable metal stent, SX-Ella Danis stent (135 × 25 mm; ELLA-CS, Hradec Kralove, Czech Republic). It has atraumatic edges and is a fully covered metal stent. The stent can be easily removed after 7 days.

Endoscopic Therapy for Secondary Prophylaxis of Esophageal Variceal Hemorrhage

Left untreated, survivors of an index bleed have a 70% probability of rebleeding within a year; this is associated with a high mortality as well. It is therefore imperative to plan treatment to prevent subsequent bleeds. TIPS is rapidly becoming a front-line approach for secondary prophylaxis and should be considered especially among patients with high risks of treatment failure with EVBL.[29–31] In its absence, a combination of EVBL and nonselective β-blockers constitutes the standard of care of prevention of variceal rebleeding. Multiple trials have evaluated and demonstrated that combination therapy is superior to either EVBL alone or pharmacologic therapy alone for secondary prophylaxis.[4,32] Combination therapy reduces the risk of esophageal variceal rebleeding by more than 20%.[32] EVBL is generally performed at 2- to 4-week intervals until varices are obliterated. Generally about 3 to 5 sessions are needed for complete obliteration.[33] There are, however, rare instances where varices persist despite 5 to 6 sessions. In such cases, it has been the authors' personal experience that one should suspect underlying portal vein thrombosis and, in the absence thereof, move toward TIPS.

Once varices are obliterated, repeat endoscopy is indicated at 3- to 6-month intervals to detect recurrent varices. When present, EVBL should be used again to obliterate these varices. Endoscopic ultrasound was at one time advocated for early diagnosis of recurrent varices. However, currently its use is not supported by evidence from clinical trials. The authors typically perform endoscopy at 2- to 4-week intervals until obliteration of varices. Surveillance endoscopy is performed at 3 to 6 months and then every 6 to 12 months to check for variceal recurrence.

ENDOSCOPIC MANAGEMENT OF GASTRIC VARICEAL HEMORRHAGE
Anatomy of Gastric Varices

Gastric varices occur approximately 20% of the time among patients with cirrhotic portal hypertension. Unlike esophageal varices, gastric varices are a rather heterogeneous group of disorders and their cause and pathophysiology can be different. Gastric varices can also develop in the absence of cirrhosis, primarily due to splenic vein thrombosis or other thrombophilic conditions, such as polycythemia vera and other hypercoagulable conditions.[34,35]

Classification of Gastric Varices

The most widely used classification system is the Sarin classification, which categorizes gastric varices into 4 types based on location and in relation to esophageal varices.[36] Gastric varices in the presence of esophageal varices are defined as GOVs. GOVs are thought to be an extension of the esophageal varices. Type 1 GOVs (GOV1) are gastric varices that occur along the lesser curvature, whereas gastric varices present along the fundus are defined as type 2 GOVs (GOV2). Gastric varices with no concurrent esophageal varices are called isolated gastric varices (IGVs). IGVs are further classified into type 1 (IGV1) when they are present in the gastric fundus or type 2 (IGV2) if present elsewhere in the stomach or first portion of the duodenum. GOV2 and IGV1 are sometimes grouped together and referred to as "fundic varices" (**Fig. 1**).

Clinical Correlates of Gastric Varices

Almost 70% of gastric varices are GOV1. Fundic varices (GOV2 and IGV1) account for the rest and IGV2 are quite rare. Although GOV1 are the most common type of varices present, fundic varices bleed more often, accounting for almost 80% of all gastric variceal bleeding. Gastric varices are often large and have numerous shunts present. Although gastric varices tend to bleed less commonly than esophageal varices, such

Gastroesophageal varices (GOV)

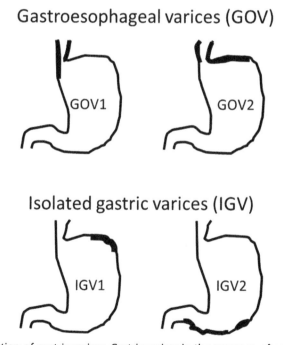

Isolated gastric varices (IGV)

Fig. 1. Classification of gastric varices. Gastric varices in the presence of esophageal varices are defined as GOVs. GOV1 are gastric varices that occur along the lesser curvature, whereas GOVs present along the fundus are defined as GOV2. Gastric varices with no concurrent esophageal varices are called IGVs. IGVs are further classified into IGV1 when they are present in the gastric fundus or IGV2 if present elsewhere in the stomach or first portion of the duodenum. GOV2 and IGV1 are sometimes grouped together and referred to as fundic varices. (*Adapted from* Sarin SK, Kumar A. Gastric varices: profile, classification, and management. Am J Gastroenterol 1989;84:1244–9; with permission.)

bleedings are more severe, are technically difficult, and are less amenable to therapy. They tend to bleed at a lower portal pressure than esophageal varices and bleeding can be massive owing to the increased blood flow from the gastric bed in these patients. The risks of rebleeding from gastric variceal bleeds are higher, and mortality can be as high as 30%.[33] Also, it is important to note that eradication of esophageal varices by variceal ligation or sclerotherapy can exacerbate gastric fundic varices.[13,33]

Diagnosis of Gastric Varices

The diagnosis of gastric varices by endoscopy can be difficult because gastric varices lie in the submucosa and are often indistinguishable from the gastric rugae. Examination of gastric varices is best done with full insufflation of the stomach in both direct and retroflexed view. When in doubt, a Doppler probe should be used to confirm the presence of venous hum. The Doppler probe should be gently applied directly on top of the varix. A continuous venous hum will confirm the presence of venous flow in the varix. Note should be made of the location of the varices, size (small, <5 mm, or large, ≥5 mm), presence of high-risk stigmata (cherry red spot, red wale sign, hematocystic spot), active or recent bleeding (white nipple sign, overlying clot), as well as the presence or absence of esophageal varices.[37]

Specific Endoscopic Therapies for Gastric Variceal Bleeding

Endoscopic therapies for gastric variceal bleeding include band ligation, sclerotherapy, and variceal obturation with cyanoacrylate glue. Novel approaches include thrombin/fibrin adhesives, detachable snares, and hemostatic sprays. The choice of therapy is primarily determined by the location of the varix, and the presence or absence of esophageal varices (summarized in **Table 1**). In the case of torrential bleeding, salvage therapy with balloon tamponade (Sengstaken-Blakemore or Linton tubes) is used as a bridge to more definitive treatment, such as placement of TIPS or balloon-occluded retrograde transvenous obliteration (BRTO).

The quality of the literature on endoscopic management of gastric varices is not as robust as that for esophageal variceal hemorrhage. In general, GOV1 is regarded as an extension of esophageal varices and is managed the same way as esophageal varices. EVBL is not as effective for GOV2 and is not suitable for IGV1. Management of the fundic varices is different and generally involves use of cyanoacrylate glue.[3,4]

Endoscopic variceal obturation

First described by Soehendra and colleagues,[38] endoscopic variceal obturation (EVO) using tissue adhesives such as N-butyl-2-cyanoacrylate (Histoacryl; Brau Medical, Bethlehem, PA, USA; Indermil; Covedien, Mansfield, MA, USA) or 2-octyl cyanoacrylate (Dermabond; Johnson and Johnson, New Brunswick, NJ, USA) is an effective means of hemostasis in bleeding gastric varices. Cyanoacrylate is a liquid polymer that on coming in contact with plasma instantly polymerizes and can lead to obliteration of the varices. EVO with N-butyl-2-cyanoacrylate injections is widely performed across Europe and Asia with excellent outcomes but is not widely used in the United States.

Technique Cyanoacrylate (glue) injections are performed along the same principles as injection sclerotherapy, but extra precautions are required to protect the endoscope from glue damage. Use of personal protective devices including goggles is recommended while handling glue because this can lead to potential eye injury. Once a gastric varix to be glued is identified, the endoscope is withdrawn. The tip of the endoscope is coated with silicon oil and a few drops of the oil is applied to the channel and

Table 1
Summary of endoscopic therapies for esophagogastric variceal hemorrhage

Treatment Modality	Comment
EVBL	Therapy of choice for EV, and GOV1, alternate for non-GOV1 *Primary hemostasis:* 71%–100% *Rebleeding:* 3%–36% *Complications:* overall (2%–23%), band ulcers (2.6%–7.3%), stricture formation (2%), chest pain
EVO	Therapy of choice for fundic varices (GOV2 and IGV1) *Primary hemostasis:* >90% *Rebleeding:* ∼15% *Complications:* distant emboli (0.7%), sepsis (1.3%), ulcer formation (0.1%), fever, abdominal pain, chances of scope damage
EIS	Second-line therapy for both esophageal and gastric varices *Primary hemostasis:* 60%–100% *Rebleeding:* 5%–10% in EV, 37%–89% in GV (half caused by therapy-induced ulcers) *Complications:* chest pain (10%), ulcers and perforation (20%–60%), strictures up to 40%
Detachable snare	No controlled studies Small uncontrolled studies shown as effective as band ligation
Thrombin/fibrin injection	*Primary hemostasis:* up to 92% *Rebleeding:* thought minimal because it will not cause ulcers *Complications:* anaphylactic reactions, infection risk, high cost No controlled studies to date
Hemostatic spray	No controlled studies, potential role as a rescue agent when primary modality fails Potential complications include allergic reactions, embolization, small bowel obstructions from foreign body impaction
Esophageal stent	*Hemostasis:* 80%–90% Potential role as a rescue agent when primary modality fails in place of balloon tamponade No controlled studies

Abbreviations: EV, esophageal varices; GV, gastric varices.

flushed to protect the scope from glue damage. The scope is reinserted. A 23- to 25-gauge needle with a metal hub is used for the injection. The needle is primed with sterile water (or saline if using octyl-cyanoacrylate). The needle is inserted directly onto the varix and 1 to 2 mL of the glue solution is rapidly injected directly into the varix (intravariceal injection) followed by a sterile water flush (∼1 mL) to clear the glue remaining in the scope channel. The needle should be quickly withdrawn from the varix and continuously flushed to keep open for repeat use if necessary. Injection can be repeated until the varix is completely obliterated as evident by a feeling of "hardness" on probing. The authors routinely use a Doppler probe to confirm the absence of the venous hum, indicating complete variceal obliteration. They generally limit their treatment to 1 to 2 injections per varix. A larger volume of injection may increase the risk of embolization. Treatment can be repeated to control recurrent bleeding. Once an acute bleeding episode is controlled, follow-up treatment should be performed every 3 to 4 weeks until complete eradication of the varices is achieved. The role of endoscopic ultrasound guidance for cyanoacrylate glue injection or placement of coils is evolving and remains to be defined.[36]

Efficacy The reported success rate of EVO in fundic variceal bleeding is in the range of 90% with a complication rate of about 15%.[39,40] Kang and colleagues[41] performed EVO in 127 gastric varices (100 cases with active bleeding) and reported a primary hemostasis rate of 98% and a 1-year bleeding recurrence rate of 18%. There have been at least 3 controlled studies comparing EVO to EVBL or EIS with favorable outcomes of EVO in terms of primary hemostasis, rebleeding rates, and complications (summarized in **Table 2**).[42–44] In a recent meta-analysis involving 648 patients with bleeding gastric varices (all types), pooled analysis suggested better efficacy of EVO in achieving primary hemostasis, and lower rebleeding rates (odds ratio [OR] 2.32; 95% CI 1.19–4.51).[45] There was no difference between EVO and EVBL in terms of mortality, complications, and number of treatment sessions required for complete variceal eradication. There was significant heterogeneity among the studies in terms of techniques used, type and dose of cyanoacrylate, and number of injections, however. Most importantly, most the subjects in these trials were with GOV1, which could be managed by EVBL. It is important to note that EVBL is not suitable as a treatment of IGV1 and the response rates of EVBL for GOV2 are poorer than that for GOV1.

Complications Although safe and effective, severe complications related to embolization of cyanoacrylate glue have been reported including systemic embolization (pulmonary, cerebral, splenic; 0.7%), recurrent sepsis (1.3%), recurrent bleeding from glue extrusions (4.4%), and ulcer formation (0.1%).[46,47] Most common complications are transient fever, chest and abdominal pain, and such. In studies comparing EVO with EIS or EVBL, the overall complication rates were similar. Complications related to technical issues such as adherence of needle into the varix and scope damage due to glue adherence have been anecdotally reported. Of note, cyanoacrylate glue has not been approved by the FDA for use in variceal bleeding. However, all other modalities for variceal hemostasis have not been FDA approved as well.

Endoscopic sclerotherapy

Similar to esophageal varices, sclerotherapy can be performed in gastric variceal bleeding but with much lower initial hemostasis rates and higher rebleeding rates. A larger volume of injection is required as gastric varices are larger and consequently can induce more adverse events. In their 11-year experience with ethanol-based sclerotherapy, Sarin and colleagues[48] reported a hemostatic rate of 66% in acute gastric variceal bleeding with sclerotherapy using absolute alcohol. Likewise, in a prospective nonrandomized trial, sclerotherapy with ethanolamine achieved initial hemostasis in 67% cases of fundic varices, far less than with cyanoacrylate injections (93%).[49] High rates of recurrent bleeding (up to 90%) have been reported with EIS for gastric varices.[50,51] Moreover, sclerotherapy is also associated with increased complications, such as fever, abdominal and chest pain, dysphagia, ulceration, and rebleeding, including ulcer-related bleeding. Sclerotherapy has therefore fallen out of favor in the management of gastric as well as esophageal varices.

Fibrin Sealant/Thrombin

Thrombin promotes the conversion of fibrinogen to fibrin, producing a local fibrin clot. As a liquid preparation delivered topically via a catheter, thrombin has been shown to be effective in achieving primary hemostasis of 75% to 94% among patients with gastric variceal bleeding in a few small uncontrolled studies.[52–54] In an earlier randomized trial, however, thrombin plus ethanolamine was not superior to ethanolamine alone in controlling bleeding esophageal varices.[55] Both bovine- and human-derived thrombin products are commercially available. Likewise, fibrin sealant has

Table 2
Randomized controlled studies comparing endoscopic variceal band ligation with endoscopic variceal obturation

Study	Description	N (Active Bleeding)	GOV1/GOV2/IGV	Primary Hemostasis OR (95% CI)	Rebleeding Rate HR (95% CI)	1y Mortality	Comment
Lo et al,[42] 2001	RCT Taiwan single center EVBL vs EVO	29 vs 31 (11 vs 15 with active bleeding)	13/33/14	45% vs 87% 7.8 (1.16, 52.35)	48% vs 29% 0.44 (0.19, 1.00)	62% vs 42%	EVO more effective and safer than EVBL in gastric variceal bleeding
Tan et al,[43] 2006	RCT Taiwan single center EVBL vs EVO	48 vs 49 (15 vs 15 with active bleeding)	25/51/21	93% vs 93% 1.00 (0.06, 17.62)	42% vs 22% 0.41 (0.20, 0.82)	44% vs 42%	No difference between EVO and EVBL in efficacy, survival, or severe complications EVO associated with less rebleeding
El Amin et al,[44] 2010	RCT Egypt multicenter EVBL vs EVO	75 vs 75 (All GOV1)	150/0/0	81% vs 91% 2.23 (0.84, 5.89)	16% vs 6%	1.3% vs 7% mortality at 6 mo, most died from HRS	All pts with GOV1, EVBL performed better in junctional varices EVO can be an alternate therapy

Abbreviations: HR, hazard ratio; HRS, hepatorenal syndrome; RCT, randomized controlled trial; NS, nonsignificant; PVT, portal vein thrombosis.

been anecdotally used with some success in gastric variceal bleeding, but their use at this point remains largely experimental.[56,57] These agents are largely safe, but complications, including anaphylaxis, antibody formations, transmission of infections, and systemic embolization, are possible. Of note, product labeling states that intravascular injection of fibrin glue is contraindicated because of the risk of embolization.

Detachable Snares

Detachable snares (Endoloop; Olympus, Tokyo, Japan) in conjunction with a transparent endcap applied at the tip of the endoscope have been tried in bleeding esophageal varices with varied outcomes. Their application on gastric varices is limited. In an earlier study of 41 patients with large (>2 cm) gastric varices (12 with active bleeding, and 29 with red signs), endoscopic ligation using detachable snares and elastic bands reported an overall hemostasis of 82.9%.[58] Repeated treatment resulted in eradication of varices in more than 91%. Likewise, Naga and colleagues[59] compared detachable snares with EVBL in patients with bleeding esophageal varices (25 each group) and found a lower rate of recurrent bleeding (12% vs 28%) with detachable snares. The difference was not, however, statistically significant. EVBL and detachable snares were comparable in terms of primary hemostasis (100% with both techniques), variceal eradication rate, number of sessions required for eradication, and cost.[59] Others have reported similar outcomes.[60] Although the detachable snares along with endcap seems to have an appeal because it will give better visualization and can be applied without needing withdrawal and reinsertion of the endoscope, it has not yet gained popularity. Controlled trials are needed to demonstrate its utility for bleeding GOV2 and IGV1 varices.

Hemostatic Sprays

Various mineral- and plant-based hemostatic granules or powders have been used for the control of external hemorrhages. These agents are now also incorporated in first aid kits. Their use in control of gastrointestinal bleedings including variceal bleeding remains experimental, however. There have been a few case reports with successful use of Ankaferd Blood Stopper (ABS, a plant alkaloid extract) in acute upper gastrointestinal bleedings including gastric variceal bleeding.[61,62] Such agents may prove handy as a rescue agent in difficult cases that fail the standard approach of band ligation or glue injections. Potential complications include embolization, allergic reactions, and small bowel obstruction from foreign body impaction. Larger and controlled studies are required to establish their safety and efficacy.

In summary, GOV1 are thought to be an extension of esophageal varices and their management should follow the same principles as for the esophageal varices, especially if they are limited within 3 cm of the gastroesophageal junction. As for bleeding esophageal varices, the preferred approach for GOV1 is EVL. Hemostasis and rebleeding rates for GOV1 are comparable to esophageal varices following EVBL. However, the efficacy of EVBL has not been proven for the rest of the gastric variceal bleedings, including GOV2, IGV1, and IGV2. The choice of endoscopic therapy for bleeding fundic varices (GOV2 and IGV1) is EVO with cyanoacrylate glue. TIPS should be considered in situations where EVO is not available. TIPS should also be considered in cases of treatment failures as a rescue therapy. BRTO is an alternate modality and is generally considered a second-line treatment (**Fig. 2**).

Endoscopic Therapy for Secondary Prophylaxis of Gastric Variceal Hemorrhage

As noted above, gastric varices are at high risk for rebleeding. GOV1 are managed by EVBL of esophageal varices and the associated GOV1. They should be followed by

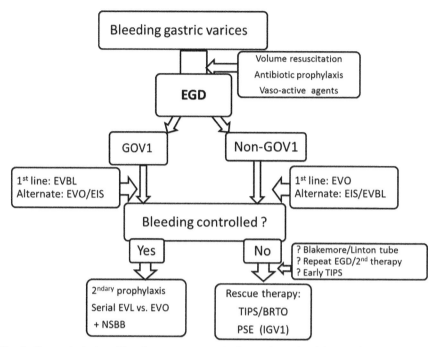

Fig. 2. Suggested algorithm for management of gastric variceal hemorrhage. GOV1 are thought to be an extension of esophageal varices and are best treated with band ligation. Cyanoacrylate glue can be applied as an alternate therapy. The choice of endoscopic therapy for bleeding fundic varices is EVO with cyanoacrylate glue. Although EIS and thrombin may come as an alternate, TIPS should be considered in situations where EVO is not available. Alternately, BRTO should be considered when TIPS is not suitable. If splenic vein thrombosis is identified as the cause of bleeding fundic varices, either splenectomy or partial splenic embolization should be considered. NSBB, nonselective β-blocker; PSE, partial splenic embolization.

repeat banding until eradication, followed by a periodic surveillance endoscopy as described above. In contrast, management of GOV2 and IGV1 can prove to be challenging. TIPS should be considered in situations where EVO is not available. Alternately, serial EVO should be performed to obliterate such varices. The role of β-blockers for the prevention of gastric variceal rebleeding is controversial. BRTO is an alternate modality and is generally considered a second-line treatment. If splenic vein thrombosis is identified as the cause of bleeding fundic varices, splenectomy should be considered.[3,4]

SUMMARY

In summary, endoscopic treatment of variceal hemorrhage is the mainstay of management of bleeding varices. It requires attention to technique and the appropriate choice of therapy for a given patient at a given point in time. Subjects must be monitored continuously after initiation of therapy for control of bleeding, and second-line definitive therapies must be introduced quickly if endoscopic and pharmacologic treatment fails.

REFERENCES

1. de Franchis R, Primignani M. Natural history of portal hypertension in patients with cirrhosis. Clin Liver Dis 2001;5:645–63.
2. de Franchis R, Pascal JP, Ancona E, et al. Definitions, methodology and therapeutic strategies in portal hypertension. A consensus development workshop, Baveno, Lake Maggiore, Italy, April 5 and 6, 1990. J Hepatol 1992;15:256–61.
3. de Franchis R. Evolving consensus in portal hypertension. Report of the Baveno IV consensus workshop on methodology of diagnosis and therapy in portal hypertension. J Hepatol 2005;43:167–76.
4. Garcia-Tsao G, Sanyal AJ, Grace ND, et al, Practice Guidelines Committee of the American Association for the Study of Liver Diseases, Practice Parameters Committee of the American College of Gastroenterology. Prevention and management of gastroesophageal varices and variceal hemorrhage in cirrhosis. Hepatology 2007;46:922–38.
5. Cheung J, Soo I, Bastiampillai R, et al. Urgent vs. non-urgent endoscopy in stable acute variceal bleeding. Am J Gastroenterol 2009;104:1125–9.
6. Hsu YC, Chen CC, Wang HP. Endoscopy timing in acute variceal hemorrhage: perhaps not the sooner the better, but delay not justified. Am J Gastroenterol 2009;104:2629–30.
7. Bai Y, Guo JF, Li ZS. Meta-analysis: erythromycin before endoscopy for acute upper gastrointestinal bleeding. Aliment Pharmacol Ther 2011;34:166–71.
8. Rudolph SJ, Landsverk BK, Freeman ML. Endotracheal intubation for airway protection during endoscopy for severe upper GI hemorrhage. Gastrointest Endosc 2003;57:58–61.
9. Sanyal AJ, Freedman AM, Luketic VA, et al. Transjugular intrahepatic portosystemic shunts for patients with active variceal hemorrhage unresponsive to sclerotherapy. Gastroenterology 1996;111:138–46.
10. Vianna A, Hayes PC, Moscoso G, et al. Normal venous circulation of the gastroesophageal junction. A route to understanding varices. Gastroenterology 1987; 93:876–89.
11. Polski JM, Brunt EM, Saeed ZA. Chronology of histological changes after band ligation of esophageal varices in humans. Endoscopy 2001;33:443–7.
12. Stiegmann GV, Sun JH, Hammond WS. Results of experimental endoscopic esophageal varix ligation. Am Surg 1988;54:105–8.
13. Yuksel O, Koklu S, Arhan M, et al. Effects of esophageal varices eradication on portal hypertensive gastropathy and fundal varices: a retrospective and comparative study. Dig Dis Sci 2006;51:27–30.
14. Saeed ZA. The Saeed Six-Shooter: a prospective study of a new endoscopic multiple rubber-band ligator for the treatment of varices. Endoscopy 1996;28:559–64.
15. Stiegmann GV, Goff JS, Michaletz-Onody PA, et al. Endoscopic sclerotherapy as compared with endoscopic ligation for bleeding esophageal varices. N Engl J Med 1992;326:1527–32.
16. Laine L, Cook D. Endoscopic ligation compared with sclerotherapy for treatment of esophageal variceal bleeding. A meta-analysis. Ann Intern Med 1995;123:280–7.
17. Singh P, Pooran N, Indaram A, et al. Combined ligation and sclerotherapy versus ligation alone for secondary prophylaxis of esophageal variceal bleeding: a meta-analysis. Am J Gastroenterol 2002;97:623–9.
18. Tierney A, Toriz BE, Mian S, et al. Interventions and outcomes of treatment of postbanding ulcer hemorrhage after endoscopic band ligation: a single-center case series. Gastrointest Endosc 2013;77:136–40.

19. Shaheen NJ, Stuart E, Schmitz SM, et al. Pantoprazole reduces the size of postbanding ulcers after variceal band ligation: a randomized, controlled trial. Hepatology 2005;41:588–94.
20. Wells M, Chande N, Adams P, et al. Meta-analysis: vasoactive medications for the management of acute variceal bleeds. Aliment Pharmacol Ther 2012;35: 1267–78.
21. Sarin SK, Nanda R, Sachdev G, et al. Intravariceal versus paravariceal sclerotherapy: a prospective, controlled, randomised trial. Gut 1987;28:657–62.
22. Memon MA, Jones WF. Injection therapy for variceal bleeding. Gastrointest Endosc Clin N Am 1999;9:231–52.
23. Sarin SK, Kumar A. Sclerosants for variceal sclerotherapy: a critical appraisal. Am J Gastroenterol 1990;85:641–9.
24. Andreani T, Poupon RE, Balkau BJ, et al. Preventive therapy of first gastrointestinal bleeding in patients with cirrhosis: results of a controlled trial comparing propranolol, endoscopic sclerotherapy and placebo. Hepatology 1990;12: 1413–9.
25. Paquet KJ. Prophylactic endoscopic sclerosing treatment of the esophageal wall in varices—a prospective controlled randomized trial. Endoscopy 1982;14:4–5.
26. Tamura S, Shiozaki H, Kobayashi K, et al. Prospective randomized study on the effect of ranitidine against injection ulcer after endoscopic injection sclerotherapy for esophageal varices. Am J Gastroenterol 1991;86:477–80.
27. Baillie J, Yudelman P. Complications of endoscopic sclerotherapy of esophageal varices. Endoscopy 1992;24:284–91.
28. Cardenas A, Fernandez-Simon A, Escorcell A. Endoscopic band ligation and esophageal stents for acute variceal bleeding. Clin Liver Dis 2014;18:793–808.
29. Monescillo A, Martínez-Lagares F, Ruiz-del-Arbol L, et al. Influence of portal hypertension and its early decompression by TIPS placement on the outcome of variceal bleeding. Hepatology 2004;40:793–801.
30. García-Pagán JC, Caca K, Bureau C, et al, Early TIPS (Transjugular Intrahepatic Portosystemic Shunt) Cooperative Study Group. Early use of TIPS in patients with cirrhosis and variceal bleeding. N Engl J Med 2010;362:2370–9.
31. Khan S, Tudur Smith C, Williamson P, et al. Portosystemic shunts versus endoscopic therapy for variceal rebleeding in patients with cirrhosis. Cochrane Database Syst Rev 2006;(4):CD000553.
32. de Franchis R. Somatostatin, somatostatin analogues and other vasoactive drugs in the treatment of bleeding oesophageal varices. Dig Liver Dis 2004;36(Suppl 1): S93–100.
33. Stiegmann GV, Goff JS, Sun JH, et al. Endoscopic variceal ligation: an alternative to sclerotherapy. Gastrointest Endosc 1989;35:431–4.
34. Sarin SK, Lahoti D, Saxena SP, et al. Prevalence, classification and natural history of gastric varices: a long-term follow-up study in 568 portal hypertension patients. Hepatology 1992;16:1343–9.
35. Ryan BM, Stockbrugger RW, Ryan JM. A pathophysiologic, gastroenterologic, and radiologic approach in the management of gastric varices. Gastroenterology 2004;126:1175–89.
36. Sarin SK, Kumar A. Gastric varices: profile, classification, and management. Am J Gastroenterol 1989;84:1244–9.
37. Kim T, Shijo H, Kokawa H, et al. Risk factors for hemorrhage from gastric fundal varices. Hepatology 1997;25:307–12.
38. Soehendra N, Griomm H, Nam V. N-butyl-2-cyanoacrylate: a supplement to endoscopic sclerotherapy. Endoscopy 1986;19:221–4.

39. Weilert F, Binmoeller KF. Endoscopic management of gastric variceal bleeding. Gastroenterol Clin North Am 2014;43:807–18.
40. Sarin SK, Kumar A. Endoscopic treatment of gastric varices. Clin Liver Dis 2014; 18:809–27.
41. Kang EJ, Jeong SW, Jang JY, et al. Long-term result of endoscopic Histoacryl (N-butyl-2-cyanoacrylate) injection for treatment of gastric varices. World J Gastroenterol 2011;17:1494–500.
42. Lo GH, Lai KH, Cheng JS, et al. A prospective, randomized trial of butyl cyanoacrylate injection versus band ligation in the management of bleeding gastric varices. Hepatology 2001;33:1060–4.
43. Tan PC, Hou MC, Lin HC, et al. A randomized trial of endoscopic treatment of acute gastric variceal hemorrhage: N-butyl-2-cyanoacrylate injection versus band ligation. Hepatology 2006;43:690–7.
44. El Amin H, Abdel Baky L, Sayed Z, et al. A randomized trial of endoscopic variceal ligation versus cyanoacrylate injection for treatment of bleeding junctional varices. Trop Gastroenterol 2010;31:279–84.
45. Ye X, Huai J, Chen Y. Cyanoacrylate injection compared with band ligation for acute gastric variceal hemorrhage: a meta-analysis of randomized controlled trials and observational studies. Gastroenterol Res Pract 2014;2014:806586.
46. Binmoeller KF, Borsatto R. Variceal bleeding and portal hypertension. Endoscopy 2000;32:189–99.
47. Cheng LF, Wang ZQ, Li CZ, et al. Low incidence of complications from endoscopic gastric variceal obturation with butyl cyanoacrylate. Clin Gastroenterol Hepatol 2010;9:760–6.
48. Sarin SK. Long-term follow-up of gastric variceal sclerotherapy: an eleven-year experience. Gastrointest Endosc 1997;46:8–14.
49. Oho K, Iwao T, Sumino M, et al. Ethanolamine oleate versus butyl cyanoacrylate for bleeding gastric varices: a nonrandomized study. Endoscopy 1995;27: 349–54.
50. Sarin SK, Sachdev G, Nanda R, et al. Endoscopic sclerotherapy in the treatment of gastric varices. Br J Surg 1988;75:747–50.
51. Gimson AE, Westaby D, Williams R. Endoscopic sclerotherapy in the management of gastric variceal hemorrhage. J Hepatol 1991;13:274–8.
52. Yang WL, Tripathi D, Therapondos G, et al. Endoscopic use of human thrombin in bleeding gastric varices. Am J Gastroenterol 2002;97:1381–5.
53. Przemioslo RT, McNair A, Williams R. Thrombin is effective in arresting bleeding from gastric variceal hemorrhage. Dig Dis Sci 1999;44:778–81.
54. Ramesh J, Limdi JK, Sharma V, et al. The use of thrombin injections in the management of bleeding gastric varices: a single-center experience. Gastrointest Endosc 2008;68:877–82.
55. Kitano S, Hashizume M, Yamaga H, et al. Human thrombin plus 5 percent ethanolamine oleate injected to sclerose oesophageal varices: a prospective randomized trial. Br J Surg 1989;76:715–8.
56. Heneghan MA, Byrne A, Harrison PM. An open pilot study of the effects of human fibrin glue for endoscopic treatment of patients with acute bleeding from gastric varices. Gastrointest Endosc 2002;56:422–6.
57. Datta D, Vlavianos P, Alisa A, et al. Use of fibrin glue (beriplast) in the management of bleeding gastric varices. Endoscopy 2003;35:675–8.
58. Lee MS, Cho JY, Cheon YK, et al. Use of detachable snares and elastic bands for endoscopic control of bleeding from large gastric varices. Gastrointest Endosc 2002;56:83–8.

59. Naga MI, Okasha HH, Foda AR, et al. Detachable endoloop vs. elastic band ligation for bleeding esophageal varices. Gastrointest Endosc 2004;59:804–9.
60. Shim CS, Cho JY, Park YJ, et al. Mini-detachable snare ligation for the treatment of esophageal varices. Gastrointest Endosc 1999;50:673–6.
61. Kurt M, Disibeyaz S, Akdogan M, et al. Endoscopic application of ankaferd blood stopper as a novel experimental treatment modality for upper gastrointestinal bleeding: a case report. Am J Gastroenterol 2008;103:2156–8.
62. Tuncer I, Doganay L, Ozturk O. Instant control of fundal variceal bleeding with a folkloric medicinal plant extract: Ankaferd Blood Stopper. Gastrointest Endosc 2010;71:873–5.

Injection and Cautery Methods for Nonvariceal Bleeding Control

Cristina Bucci, MD, PhD[a], Gianluca Rotondano, MD[b],
Riccardo Marmo, MD[c],*

KEYWORDS

- Nonvariceal gastrointestinal bleeding • Injection therapy • Thermal coagulation
- Hemostasis • Endoscopic methods

KEY POINTS

- Epinephrine remains the most used method to achieve initial hemostasis, but it should only be used in conjunction with a second endoscopic hemostatic procedure.
- Sclerosants and acrylate glue injection might be used as rescue therapy in selected cases.
- Hemostasis with argon plasma coagulation is easy to perform, allows treating lesions in awkward positions with a reduced depth of penetration, and has been proven to be effective in controlling nonvariceal upper gastrointestinal bleeding, especially extended superficial vascular lesions.
- All cautery methods are equally effective tools and the choice depends essentially on the experience of the operator, the type, and the site of the bleeding lesion.

INTRODUCTION

Upper gastrointestinal bleeding (UGIB) is predominantly nonvariceal in origin and remains one of the most common challenges faced by gastroenterologists and endoscopists in daily clinical practice. Endoscopic management of nonvariceal upper gastrointestinal bleeding (NVUGIB) has been shown to improve clinical outcomes, with significant reduction of recurrent bleeding, need for surgery, and mortality.[1–5] Different methods of endoscopic interventions can be categorized on their mechanism of action and include injection therapy, thermal coagulation, or mechanical therapy. Several meta-analyses have consistently shown that cautery devices and clips are effective methods for securing hemostasis in peptic ulcer bleeding, with no single

The authors disclose no commercial or financial conflicts of interest or any funding sources.
[a] Gastroenterology Unit, University of Salerno, Via Allende, 84081, Baronissi-Salerno, Italy;
[b] Division of Gastroenterology, Maresca Hospital, Via Montedoro, 80059, Torre del Greco, NA, Italy; [c] Endoscopy Unit, Division of Gastroenterology, L.Curto Hospital, Via Luigi Curto, 84035, Polla- Salerno, Italy
* Corresponding author.
E-mail address: ricmarmo1@virgilio.it

modality proven superior.[6–11] Both thermal and mechanical methods can be preceded by injection therapy, an approach known as combination therapy, to slow or stop bleeding before the application of subsequent definitive therapy.

INDICATIONS/CONTRAINDICATIONS

Early upper gastrointestinal (GI) endoscopy is recommended in all patients presenting with UGIB within 24 hours of presentation.[1–5] At urgent endoscopy, recognition of high-risk endoscopic signs is essential for proper therapeutic planning. Endoscopic treatment is indicated for patients found to have spurting or oozing active bleeding and for those with a nonbleeding exposed vessel in an ulcer.[1–4] Overlying adherent clots should be irrigated to evaluate and potentially treat the underlying lesion. However, the management of peptic ulcers with adherent clots that are resistant to removal by irrigation is still controversial.[2] Ulcers with low-risk stigmata (ie, those with pigmented spots of hematin or fibrin-covered clean base) do not warrant any endoscopic intervention.

Appropriate resuscitation and stabilization of hemodynamic parameters are essential. No endoscopic procedure should be done at the expense of adequate resuscitation.

TECHNIQUE/PROCEDURE
Preparation, Patient Positioning, and Approach

Upper endoscopy in patients with GI bleeding should be carried out in an adequately equipped setting, be it the endoscopy suite or the operating theater, by qualified operators. A therapeutic endoscope with a 3.7-mm operative channel should be used, if available. Scopes with 6-mm "jumbo" channels or double-channel scopes may occasionally be required. All devices for endoscopic hemostasis (injection needles and solutions, monopolar or bipolar thermal probes, and mechanical devices such as hemoclips) should be available and ready to be used by skilled personnel. The assistance of an anesthesiologist is required in patients with severe hematemesis, and orotracheal intubation should be considered in such selected cases to prevent aspiration.[12]

The quality of endoscopy can be adversely affected by poor visibility in patients requiring urgent endoscopy with UGIB due to obscuring blood in the gastric lumen. In 3% to 19% of the cases, no apparent cause of UGIB can be identified.[13–15]

In fact, a bleeding lesion may not be identified because of the presence of food or blood debris hampering proper endoscopic visualization (particularly for awkwardly positioned lesions) or because of the presence of lesions that are difficult to identify if not actively bleeding, specifically, vascular lesions. Apart from the routine use of water-jet pikes for irrigation and adequate suction power applied to the endoscope, the patient may need to be rolled over to positions different from the initial left lateral decubitus position to dislocate the blood pool and make the lesion visible. In the case of a large uncleared fundal pool, consider inserting a large-bore nasogastric tube to empty the stomach and repeat the examination shortly thereafter.[12]

The systematic use of a nasogastric tube before endoscopy is not recommended,[2] but in selected patients, it may offer important prognostic information.

Pre-endoscopic administration of intravenous erythromycin or metoclopramide (20–120 minutes before endoscopy) has been shown to reduce the need for repeat endoscopy to determine the site and cause of bleeding in patients with UGIB.[16,17] This adjunct is important to treatment with regard to the ability to make a diagnosis, apply definitive treatment, and avoid unnecessary exposure of patients to repeat procedures; the use of prokinetic agents is advisable in patients with a high probability of having fresh blood or a clot in the stomach when undergoing endoscopy to increase diagnostic yield (**Fig. 1**).

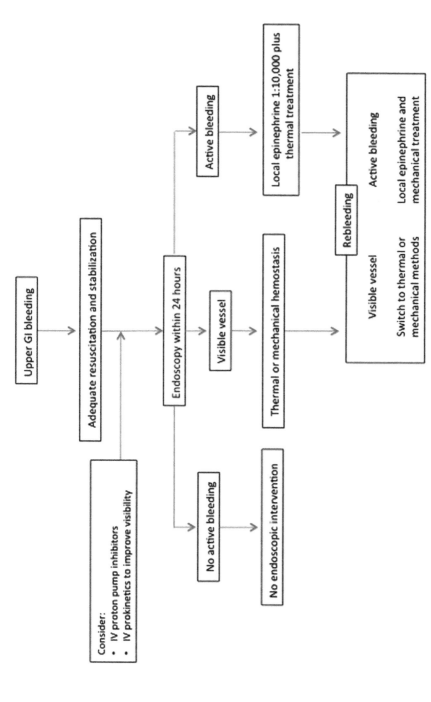

Fig. 1. Treatment algorithm for patients with NVUGIB. IV, intravenous.

Injection Methods

Endoscopic injection is widely used for the arrest of active ulcer bleeding and for the prevention of rebleeding from ulcers with visible vessels. The principle of injection therapy is to create a combination of hydrostatic pressure, tissue edema, vasoconstriction, and inflammatory changes in the region of the ulcer.[18–22]

Injection needles are single-use or autoclavable, Teflon or stainless steel, 7-Fr catheter sheaths with retractile needles varying from 19 to 25 G. The length of the needle may vary from 4 to 6 mm, although recommended needle length is 4 mm (**Fig. 2A**).[21]

The most commonly used injectates[18–23] for bleeding control are the following:

- Epinephrine
- Sclerosants
- Tissue adhesives or glues (acrylates and fibrin glue)

Epinephrine

Because of its widespread availability, low cost, and simplicity, local epinephrine is the most commonly used injective therapy. Epinephrine is usually injected as diluted 1:10,000 or 1:20,000 saline solution by a standard needle at 0.5- to 2-mL aliquots per injection. Higher doses of injected epinephrine are more likely to cause cardiovascular side effects, particularly when injected around the region of gastroesophageal junction and the distal esophagus; some endoscopists advocate the use of more diluted solution (1: 100,000) to avoid complications.[24]

Injections are placed tangentially into and around the bleeding source until the bleeding halts or slows and the surface becomes pale.

The proposed mechanisms of action of epinephrine injection involve the following[18]:

1. Local tamponade effect induced by the volume of solution injected with vessel squeezing;
2. Vasoconstriction but not vessel thrombosis;
3. Direct effect on the clotting process at the site of the arterial defect (platelet aggregation).

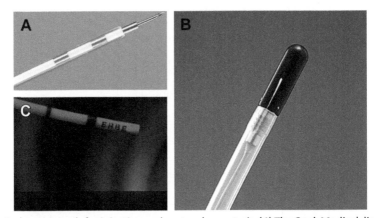

Fig. 2. Endoscopic tools for injection and cautery hemostasis. (*A*) The Cook Medical disposable injector needle (7-Fr sheath with 23-G, 4-mm-long needle extruded). (*B*) The 3.7-mm hydrothermal probe (Heater Probe, Olympus, Bloomfield, CT). (*C*) The 3.2-mm ERBE APC forward probe. (*Courtesy of* [*A*] Cook Medical, Inc, Bloomington, IL; with permission; [*B*] Olympus America, Inc; with permission; [*C*] ERBE USA Inc, Marietta, GA; with permission.)

Different studies have investigated the optimal volume needed to obtain a hemostatic effect of epinephrine. Injection of large volumes (13–20 mL) of epinephrine is superior to low volumes (5–10 mL) in reducing the rate of recurrent bleeding in high-risk patients.[25] Also, data from Korea showed that injection of 35 to 45 mL of epinephrine was more effective in preventing recurrent bleeding from ulcers in the gastric body than injection of 15 to 25 mL (0% vs 17.1%).[26] Although endoscopic injection of epinephrine is considered safe, the injected volume of epinephrine should not be unlimited, because of the risk of systemic absorption.[18,27] Even if infrequent, adverse cardiac events have been described after a high volume (30 mL) of epinephrine for treatment of a bleeding Mallory-Weiss tear.[28,29]

Sclerosants

Sclerosants agents, such as polidocanol, ethanol, and ethanolamine, induce local inflammation and subsequent fibrosis, obliterating the lumen of the vessel. The technique is similar to that used for epinephrine, but volumes are much smaller (usually a maximum of 1 mL, divided in 0.1–0.3 mL aliquots per injection at 3–4 sites around or into the visible vessel) due to the potential risk of ulceration, necrosis, and perforation described for those agents.[18] In clinical trials, when tested in combination with epinephrine, no additive effect of sclerosants was observed, either as a subsequent injection or as a mixture of the 2.[30] Moreover, polidocanol has been associated with transmural necrosis, and injections in the gastric fundus are contraindicated because of the risk of late perforations.[31] If ethanol is used, caution is recommended to avoid tissue necrosis and perforation.

The use of sclerosants for NVUGIB should be avoided in routine practice but still can be considered a valuable alternative option to treat bleeding lesions when a second method is not feasible.

Cyanoacrylate

N-butyl-2-cyanoacrylate is a tissue adhesive that on contact with water polymerizes into a firm clot. It is commonly used in Europe in the treatment of bleeding varices and has been tested also for the treatment of refractory peptic ulcer bleeding.

The glue can be used either undiluted or as a mixture of cyanoacrylate and lipiodol, an oily contrast agent to delay polymerization. The injection technique is not as user-friendly as an epinephrine injection because the glue hardens quickly and there is the potential risk of damaging the endoscope, the operator, and patient if the glue is accidentally dispersed.

Briefly, the technique of acrylate injection is as follows:

- The 21-G or 23-G metal luer-lock injector needle must be preinjected with sterile water;
- Acrylate glue is then slowly injected directly into the bleeding point (the glue is sticky with a considerable resistance to injection). To minimize the risk of embolization, not more than 1 or 2 mL glue is injected.
- Glue injection is immediately followed by 2 to 4 mL of distilled water to deliver the glue from the "dead space" of the catheter. The endoscopy assistant announces the end of this second injection, and the operator retracts the needle.

At the end of the injection procedure, the glue spills with formation of a hard plug obliterating the bleeding point. If the bleeding persists more than 60 seconds after the first injection, a second 1 mL can be injected with the same modality.[32] If the glue sticks to the lens, the endoscope should be withdrawn and cleaned with ethanol or nail polish remover immediately. The endoscopy assistant should be well trained in the injection technique; the presence of a second nurse is recommended for preparing the additional injection catheters and cyanoacrylate vials. Care must be taken to protect the eyes of the patient and the clinical personnel. Goggles are required for eye protection during preparation and injection of the glue.

In a randomized trial comparing cyanoacrylate with hypertonic saline-epinephrine injection in 126 patients with high-risk bleeding peptic ulcers, there were no differences in outcomes between the 2 groups, but 2 cases (1 fatal) of arterial embolization occurred in the cyanoacrylate group.[33] This complication was also reported in other case series (as both arterial and portal venous embolization).[34,35] Cyanoacrylate has also been successfully used to treat bleeding Dieulafoy lesions and as a spray to treat difficult-to-control malignant and nonmalignant GI bleeding.[36,37]

In the endoscopy setting, acrylate glue injection should be limited to selected cases of refractory nonvariceal bleeding as rescue therapy in patients after failure of conventional endoscopic therapies.

Fibrin glue

Fibrin glue is a 2-component system in which concentrated fibrinogen and factor XIII are combined with thrombin and calcium to simulate the final stage of the clotting cascade. Components are injected either as a subsequent injection in a standard 23-G injector needle or as a mixture of the 2 trough, a special dual-channel needle, to mix and activate the clotting cascade only when injected.

In patients pretreated with epinephrine, multiple fibrin sealant injections were associated with less recurrent bleeding compared with polidocanol.[38] Other studies did not confirm any advantage in adding the fibrin glue to epinephrine injection alone.[39] The precise role for fibrin sealant remains to be defined. Moreover, because the substance is relatively expensive and its use can be associated with the potential transmission of infectious diseases today, the use of fibrin glue is discouraged as a primary treatment modality.

Sodium hyaluronate

Sodium hyaluronate is a natural polysaccharide with peculiar viscoelastic characteristics that make it an excellent candidate for endoscopic submucosal dissection because of its ability to create a persistent submucosal cushion. In 2 case reports, sodium hyaluronate has been used to successfully achieve endoscopic hemostatic in bleeding ulcers; however, clinical trials are needed.[40,41]

Outcomes of Injection Therapy

Randomized trials indicate epinephrine injection is effective at achieving initial hemostasis in patients with active bleeding.[9] However, epinephrine monotherapy provides suboptimal efficacy and is inferior to other monotherapies or to combination therapy that uses 2 or more methods in preventing further bleeding in patients with high-risk stigmata.[6,7,10,11] Compared with injection monotherapy, other monotherapies provide a significantly superior protection against the risk of recurrent bleeding (relative risk [RR] 0.58; confidence interval, [CI] 95%, 0.36 to 0.93), with clinically relevant number needed to treat (NNT) of 9.[7]

Several meta-analyses indicate that adding a second procedure, such as a second injectate (for example, alcohol, thrombin, or fibrin glue), thermal contact, or clips, is superior to epinephrine injection alone.[6,9,10] A recent systematic review confirmed that the use of a second procedure (regardless of which second procedure is applied) following epinephrine injection significantly reduces the risk of further bleeding (RR 0.53 [CI 95%, 0.35 to 0.81]) and the need for emergency surgery (RR 0.68 [CI 95%, 0.50 to 0.93]), but did not affect mortality.[11] Also, combined therapy significantly reduced the rebleeding rate for ulcers with active bleeding (either spurting or oozing) but not for nonactively bleeding ulcers (exposed vessels or adherent clots).

International consensus recommendations advocate that if epinephrine is used to treat peptic ulcer bleeding with high-risk stigmata, it should not be used alone, but a second endoscopic treatment modality should also be used.[2,3]

Injection therapy can also be used after clip placement or cautery therapy to treat residual oozing.

CAUTERY METHODS

Thermal endoscopic hemostasis is based on the principle that electrical current flowing through a tissue causes overheating of the tissue itself with edema, coagulation of tissue protein, and contraction of vessels and arteries with subsequent activation of the clotting cascade. Tissue coagulation requires a temperature of approximately 60° to 100°C. Thermal devices can be classified as either contact or noncontact devices (**Table 1**).[20]

Contact devices (hydrothermal probes, bipolar probes, monopolar probes) provide a double hemostatic effect because of the appositional pressure and tissue coagulation (called coaptation), whereas noncontact devices (namely, argon plasma coagulation [APC]) deliver high-frequency monopolar current to the tissue through an ionized gas. The use of laser, a noncontact thermal method, is rarely used today for hemostatic endoscopic purpose because of the excessive depth of coagulation resulting in high rates of perforation as well as the excessive maintenance costs.

Heater Probe

The heater probe technique uses a multiple-uses 7-Fr or 10-Fr hydrothermal contact probe (see **Fig. 2**B) connected to a heat-generating device (HPU unit; Olympus, Bloomfield, CT). The probe is positioned directly on the bleeding point, and firm tamponade is applied with the tip before foot-pedal activation. For high-risk lesions, the 10-Fr probe is recommended with power settings of 25 to 30 J, delivering 4 to 8 pulses, regardless of location in the upper GI tract.[42] As all coaptive devices, the heater probe combines pressure and coagulation applied directly on the bleeding site until the end-point of vessel cavitation and "tissue whitening" is achieved.

Heater probe coagulation has been shown to be an effective hemostatic intervention in most bleeding ulcers. When added to epinephrine injection, the heater probe was shown to decrease the need for emergency surgery and blood transfusion and reduce the length of hospital stay for patients with spurting hemorrhage, compared with injection therapy alone.[43] The heater probe was compared in randomized clinical trials with hemoclip application in patients with major stigmata of ulcer bleeding, showing comparable efficacy in terms of initial hemostasis, but proving inferior in preventing recurrent bleeding.[25,42] When compared with monopolar soft-coagulation forceps, the hydrothermal probe was less efficacious in primary hemostasis (96% vs 67%) as well as in rebleeding rate, with one perforation occurring in the heater probe group.[44]

Table 1
Thermal probes most commonly used for cautery hemostasis

Type of Coagulation	Device Name and Manufacturer	Sheath Diameter (Fr)	Pulse Duration (s)	Fire Direction	Power	Supplementary Features	Gas Flow (Lt/min)
Contact thermal devices							
Hydrothermal	Heater probe (*Olympus*)	7, 10	3–4		25–30 J	Reusable[a]	—
Bipolar	Gold Probe (*Boston*)	7, 10	5–10		15–25 W	25-G retractile injector needle	—
	Injector Gold Probe Quicksilver (*Cook*)						
	BiCoag Probe (*Olympus*)						
	Bicap (*ConMed*)						
	Bipolar probe (*US Endoscopy*)						
Noncontact thermal devices							
APC	Canady Plasma (*Canady*)	5, 7		Straight, side	30–60 W		1.5–3
	Beamer argon (*ConMed*)	5, 7, 10		Straight	30–60 W		1.5–3
	APC (*ERBE*)	5, 7, 10		Straight, side, circumferential	30–60 W		1.5–3

Note. Fr, French (7 Fr = 2.3 mm; 10 Fr = 3.2 mm).
[a] According to local protocols.

Bipolar Probes

In bipolar devices, alternating arrays of positive and negative electrodes are located at the tip of the probe, where the electrical circuit is completed. No grounding pad is therefore required. Different types of probes are available on the market, but all of them share the same modality of coaptive coagulation and the same parameters for safe use (see **Table 1**).

Bipolar and heat probe coagulation have been shown to be equivalent in the treatment of patients with high-risk bleeding ulcers and to be more effective than injection therapy alone.[45–50]

The Gold Probe (Boston Scientific Corp, Natick, MA, USA) is a combination catheter that includes an integrated 25-G retractile injection needle and a bipolar electrocoagulation device (see **Fig. 2**C). Similarly to other contact thermal devices (Bicap, Quicksilver, BiCoag Probe), this injector-bipolar combination probe works with a combination of pressure and coagulation applied directly on the bleeding site, but with the supplementary possibility to inject. Another difference that the endoscopist should keep in mind when choosing a device is that the heater probe must be applied in a perpendicular manner, whereas the bicap may be applied perpendicularly or tangentially.

In patients with high-risk peptic ulcer bleeding, the combined treatment modality of the injector-bipolar combination probe was better than epinephrine injection alone in reducing the rate of recurrent bleeding and superior to bipolar coagulation alone in achieving initial hemostasis in patients with active bleeding.[50,51] In this subgroup of patients, indeed, the clinical advantage of the injector-Gold Probe treatment was particularly evident, with an absolute risk reduction of 31.6% (CI 95%, 5.4 to 57.7) and an NNT of 3 (CI 95%, 2 to 18).

Argon Plasma Coagulation

Argon is a gas that becomes electrically conductive when ionized by electrical current. A high-voltage spark, delivered at the tip of the probe, ionizes the argon gas as it is sprayed out from the probe tip in the direction of the target tissue, delivering the thermal energy both linearly and tangentially with a maximum depth of penetration of 3 mm, for applications up to 5 seconds. APC can be performed using either a 7-Fr or a 10-Fr probe, with straight or side fire direction. Generator setting, gas flow, and duration of application are reported in **Table 1**. The operative distance from the probe tip to the target tissue should be around 2 mm.

In this form of noncontact electrocoagulation, the electric field is proportional to the electric voltage and inversely proportional to the distance between the electrode and the tissue surface. During APC, the generated spark desiccates tissue and an electrically insulated steam layer develops as soon as fluids in the tissue being treated reach the boiling point; this increases the electrical resistance, which gradually suppresses further conduction of current. As the coagulum forms on the surface, in fact, continued application of the APC to the same area would result in a shift of the electrical energy to an adjacent nondesiccated segment as current seeks a return pathway to the external return electrode on the skin. Coagulation is virtually smokeless (tissue is desiccated and not carbonized) and multidirectional (see **Fig. 2**D). The direction of the current is determined by the electric field generated between the ionized gas and the tissue. Therefore, the probe can be used adjacent to tissue that requires coagulation, which is not dependent on the direction of the argon flow or positioning of the probe.

APC is easy to perform, allowing treatment of lesions in awkward positions with a reduced depth of penetration. APC has been proven to be effective in treating extended superficial vascular lesions, such as vascular ecstasies and watermelon stomach, but also in controlling NVUGIB. However, because of the superficial coagulation provided by this noncontact device, APC may miss deeper vessels with insufficient hemostasis and thus its use should be limited to nonactively bleeding lesions, preferably within protocols of combined therapy.

In comparative studies, rebleeding rate after APC in ulcers was comparable to injective therapy, to hemoclips, and also to other contact thermal devices such as the heater probe.[52–55]

APC is considered a safe procedure even if the occurrence of colonic and gastric explosions due to the presence of combustible gases such as methane has been described.

Monopolar Probes

Clinical experience and data for endoscopic hemostasis with monopolar cautery devices are limited. The hemostatic grasper is a novel monopolar electrosurgical hemostatic forceps with a rotatable tip that has been used for GI lower bleeding. The jaws are closed around the target vessel, and then monopolar electrocautery is used to coagulate the tissue. In nonvariceal upper GI bleeding, the clinical experience with this device is very limited, so further studies are required.[56,57]

OUTCOMES OF THERMAL THERAPY

Overall, contact cautery methods were shown to be significantly more effective than no endoscopic therapy in achieving initial hemostasis (RR 11.70 [CI 95%, 5.15 to 26.56]), reducing recurrent bleeding (RR 0.44 [CI 95%, 0.36 to 0.54]; NNT 4), and mortality (RR 0.58 [CI 95%, 0.34 to 0.98]; NNT 33) in a meta-analysis of 15 randomized trials.[7] Also APC was significantly more effective than injection therapy in preventing recurrent bleeding.[19]

Any method of contact thermal coagulation can be used in patients with high-risk lesions, alone or in combination with epinephrine injection. No single cautery method is superior to another and the choice depends essentially on the confidence that the operator has with the different devices.[6,7]

COMPLICATIONS AND MANAGEMENT

As in all medical procedures, there are potential adverse events related to the use of injection and cautery methods of endoscopic hemostasis.[18,19,23,46,58] These potential adverse events may be the following:

- Perforation (0.8%–1.6%): this complication is more frequent for duodenal ulcers and in the case of a second thermal treatment. Perforation of the ulcer bed usually requires surgical repair, although in recent years endoscopic clipping, such as over-the-scope-clip system, was successfully used to treat iatrogenic perforations[59,60];
- Induced bleeding in a nonbleeding lesion (13%–45%): indeed, it can be considered a sort of "expected" occurrence rather than a true adverse event when the exposed vessel is treated. This reason is the most practical to preinject epinephrine before removal of adherent clots or for treatment of visible vessels. Induced bleeding is usually controllable with on-going hemostasis in most cases and exceptionally requires radiologic or surgical treatment;
- Parietal wall necrosis can mainly be related to the use of sclerosing agents.

Apart from operator's expertise, some practical tricks to avoid adverse events may include the follows:

- Use 1:10,000 to 1:20,000 diluted epinephrine (maximum, 30 mL);
- Avoid sclerosants;
- Avoid too deep an injection (maximum length of needles, 4 mm);
- Avoid intravascular injection;
- Stick to coagulation parameters automatically set by the cautery unit or recommended by the manufacturer;
- Avoid re-treatment with contact thermal probes.

SUMMARY

Endoscopic methods to control nonvariceal upper GI bleeding are injection, thermal, or mechanical. Endoscopic hemostasis should be performed by skilled operators in adequately equipped settings, always within a multidisciplinary team approach after an appropriate resuscitation and stabilization of hemodynamic parameters. Injection of epinephrine is the most commonly used hemostatic method, but it should always be combined with a second endoscopic modality (both thermal and mechanical). Other injectates are sclerosants and acrylate glue, which might be used as rescue therapy in selected cases.

Cautery methods include contact and noncontact electrocoagulation probes. All of them are equally effective in achieving hemostasis, their choice depending essentially on the preference of the operator according to the type and the site of the bleeding lesion.

REFERENCES

1. Gralnek IM, Barkun AN, Bardou M. Management of acute bleeding from a peptic ulcer. N Engl J Med 2008;359:928–37.
2. Barkun AN, Bardou M, Kuipers EJ, et al. International consensus recommendations on the management of patients with nonvariceal upper gastrointestinal bleeding. Ann Intern Med 2010;152:101–13.
3. Laine L, Jensen DM. Management of patients with ulcer bleeding. Am J Gastroenterol 2012;107:345–60 [quiz: 361].
4. Hwang JH, Fisher DA, Ben-Menachem T, et al. The role of endoscopy in the management of acute non-variceal upper GI bleeding. Gastrointest Endosc 2012;75: 1132–8.
5. Lu Y, Loffroy R, Lau JY, et al. Multidisciplinary management strategies for acute non-variceal upper gastrointestinal bleeding. Br J Surg 2014;101:e34–50.
6. Barkun AN, Martel M, Toubouti Y, et al. Endoscopic hemostasis in peptic ulcer bleeding for patients with high-risk lesions: a series of meta-analyses. Gastrointest Endosc 2009;69:786–99.
7. Laine L, McQuaid KR. Endoscopic therapy for bleeding ulcers: an evidence-based approach based on meta-analyses of randomized controlled trials. Clin Gastroenterol Hepatol 2009;7:33–47 [quiz: 1–2].
8. Sung JJ, Tsoi KK, Lai LH, et al. Endoscopic clipping versus injection and thermocoagulation in the treatment of non-variceal upper gastrointestinal bleeding: a meta-analysis. Gut 2007;56:1364–73.
9. Calvet X, Vergara M, Brullet E, et al. Addition of a second endoscopic treatment following epinephrine injection improves outcome in high-risk bleeding ulcers. Gastroenterology 2004;126:441–50.

10. Marmo R, Rotondano G, Piscopo R, et al. Dual therapy versus monotherapy in the endoscopic treatment of high-risk bleeding ulcers: a meta-analysis of controlled trials. Am J Gastroenterol 2007;102:279–89 [quiz: 469].
11. Vergara M, Bennett C, Calvet X, et al. Epinephrine injection versus epinephrine injection and a second endoscopic method in high-risk bleeding ulcers. Cochrane Database Syst Rev 2014;10:CD005584.
12. Rotondano G. Epidemiology and diagnosis of acute nonvariceal upper gastrointestinal bleeding. Gastroenterol Clin North Am 2014;43:643–63.
13. Marmo R, Koch M, Cipolletta L, et al. Predicting mortality in non-variceal upper gastrointestinal bleeders: validation of the Italian PNED score and prospective comparison with the Rockall score. Am J Gastroenterol 2010;105:1284–91.
14. Marmo R, Koch M, Cipolletta L, et al. Predictive factors of mortality from nonvariceal upper gastrointestinal hemorrhage: a multicenter study. Am J Gastroenterol 2008;103:1639–47 [quiz: 1648].
15. Enestvedt BK, Gralnek IM, Mattek N, et al. An evaluation of endoscopic indications and findings related to nonvariceal upper-GI hemorrhage in a large multicenter consortium. Gastrointest Endosc 2008;67:422–9.
16. Barkun AN, Bardou M, Martel M, et al. Prokinetics in acute upper GI bleeding: a meta-analysis. Gastrointest Endosc 2010;72:1138–45.
17. Altraif I, Handoo FA, Aljumah A, et al. Effect of erythromycin before endoscopy in patients presenting with variceal bleeding: a prospective, randomized, double-blind, placebo-controlled trial. Gastrointest Endosc 2011;73:245–50.
18. Church NI, Palmer KR. Injection therapy for endoscopic haemostasis. Baillieres Best Pract Res Clin Gastroenterol 2000;14:427–41.
19. Kovacs TO. Management of upper gastrointestinal bleeding. Curr Gastroenterol Rep 2008;10:535–42.
20. Cappell MS. Therapeutic endoscopy for acute upper gastrointestinal bleeding. Nat Rev Gastroenterol Hepatol 2010;7:214–29.
21. Conway JD, Adler DG, Diehl DL, et al. Endoscopic hemostatic devices. Gastrointest Endosc 2009;69:987–96.
22. Lau JY, Leung JW. Injection therapy for bleeding peptic ulcers. Gastrointest Endosc Clin N Am 1997;7:575–91.
23. Savides TJ, Jensen DM. Therapeutic endoscopy for nonvariceal gastrointestinal bleeding. Gastroenterol Clin North Am 2000;29:465–87, vii.
24. Liu JJ, Saltzman JR. Endoscopic hemostasis treatment: how should you perform it? Can J Gastroenterol 2009;23:481–3.
25. Lin HJ, Hsieh YH, Tseng GY, et al. A prospective, randomized trial of endoscopic hemoclip versus heater probe thermocoagulation for peptic ulcer bleeding. Am J Gastroenterol 2002;97:2250–4.
26. Park CH, Lee SJ, Park JH, et al. Optimal injection volume of epinephrine for endoscopic prevention of recurrent peptic ulcer bleeding. Gastrointest Endosc 2004; 60:875–80.
27. Choudari CP, Palmer KR. Endoscopic injection therapy for bleeding peptic ulcer; a comparison of adrenaline alone with adrenaline plus ethanolamine oleate. Gut 1994;35:608–10.
28. von Delius S, Thies P, Umgelter A, et al. Hemodynamics after endoscopic submucosal injection of epinephrine in patients with nonvariceal upper gastrointestinal bleeding: a matter of concern. Endoscopy 2006;38:1284–8.
29. Schlag C, Karagianni A, Grimm M, et al. Hemodynamics after endoscopic submucosal injection of epinephrine in a porcine model. Endoscopy 2012;44: 154–60.

30. Lin HJ, Perng CL, Lee FY, et al. Endoscopic injection for the arrest of peptic ulcer hemorrhage: final results of a prospective, randomized comparative trial. Gastrointest Endosc 1993;39:15–9.
31. Dorta G, Michetti P, Burckhardt P, et al. Acute ischemia followed by hemorrhagic gastric necrosis after injection sclerotherapy for ulcer. Endoscopy 1996;28:532.
32. Cipolletta L, Zambelli A, Bianco MA, et al. Acrylate glue injection for acutely bleeding oesophageal varices: a prospective cohort study. Dig Liver Dis 2009; 41:729–34.
33. Lee KJ, Kim JH, Hahm KB, et al. Randomized trial of N-butyl-2-cyanoacrylate compared with injection of hypertonic saline-epinephrine in the endoscopic treatment of bleeding peptic ulcers. Endoscopy 2000;32:505–11.
34. Kobilica N, Flis V, Sojar V. Major complication after Histoacryl injection for endoscopic treatment of bleeding peptic ulcer. Endoscopy 2012;44(Suppl 2 UCTN): E204–5.
35. Peixoto P, Ministro P, Sadio A, et al. Embolic complications associated with endoscopic injection of cyanoacrylate for bleeding duodenal ulcer. Endoscopy 2008; 40(Suppl 2):E126.
36. Walia SS, Sachdeva A, Kim JJ, et al. Cyanoacrylate spray for treatment of difficult-to-control GI bleeding. Gastrointest Endosc 2013;78:536–9.
37. D'Imperio N, Papadia C, Baroncini D, et al. N-butyl-2-cyanoacrylate in the endoscopic treatment of Dieulafoy ulcer. Endoscopy 1995;27:216.
38. Rutgeerts P, Rauws E, Wara P, et al. Randomised trial of single and repeated fibrin glue compared with injection of polidocanol in treatment of bleeding peptic ulcer. Lancet 1997;350:692–6.
39. Pescatore P, Jornod P, Borovicka J, et al. Epinephrine versus epinephrine plus fibrin glue injection in peptic ulcer bleeding: a prospective randomized trial. Gastrointest Endosc 2002;55:348–53.
40. Kim HH, Park SJ, Park MI, et al. Hyaluronic acid injection for sustained control of bleeding from a sclerotic ulcer base. Endoscopy 2012;44(Suppl 2 UCTN): E169–70.
41. Cho YK, Kim CS, Kim SY, et al. The hemostatic effect of endoscopic sodium hyaluronate injection in peptic ulcer bleeding. Hepatogastroenterology 2007;54: 1276–9.
42. Cipolletta L, Bianco MA, Marmo R, et al. Endoclips versus heater probe in preventing early recurrent bleeding from peptic ulcer: a prospective and randomized trial. Gastrointest Endosc 2001;53:147–51.
43. Chung SS, Lau JY, Sung JJ, et al. Randomised comparison between adrenaline injection alone and adrenaline injection plus heat probe treatment for actively bleeding ulcers. BMJ 1997;314:1307–11.
44. Nunoue T, Takenaka R, Hori K, et al. A randomized trial of monopolar soft-mode coagulation versus heater probe thermocoagulation for peptic ulcer bleeding. J Clin Gastroenterol 2014. [Epub ahead of print].
45. Chau CH, Siu WT, Law BK, et al. Randomized controlled trial comparing epinephrine injection plus heat probe coagulation versus epinephrine injection plus argon plasma coagulation for bleeding peptic ulcers. Gastrointest Endosc 2003;57: 455–61.
46. Kumar P, Fleischer DE. Thermal therapy for gastrointestinal bleeding. Gastrointest Endosc Clin N Am 1997;7:593–609.
47. Chung SC, Lau JY, Rutgeerts P, et al. Thermal coagulation for nonvariceal bleeding. Endoscopy 2002;34:89–92.

48. Cook DJ, Guyatt GH, Salena BJ, et al. Endoscopic therapy for acute nonvariceal upper gastrointestinal hemorrhage: a meta-analysis. Gastroenterology 1992;102: 139–48.

49. Sacks HS, Chalmers TC, Blum AL, et al. Endoscopic hemostasis. An effective therapy for bleeding peptic ulcers. JAMA 1990;264:494–9.

50. Lin HJ, Tseng GY, Perng CL, et al. Comparison of adrenaline injection and bipolar electrocoagulation for the arrest of peptic ulcer bleeding. Gut 1999;44:715–9.

51. Bianco MA, Rotondano G, Marmo R, et al. Combined epinephrine and bipolar probe coagulation vs. bipolar probe coagulation alone for bleeding peptic ulcer: a randomized, controlled trial. Gastrointest Endosc 2004;60:910–5.

52. Wang HM, Hsu PI, Lo GH, et al. Comparison of hemostatic efficacy for argon plasma coagulation and distilled water injection in treating high-risk bleeding ulcers. J Clin Gastroenterol 2009;43:941–5.

53. Peng YC, Chen SW, Tung CF, et al. Comparison the efficacy of intermediate dose argon plasma coagulation versus hemoclip for upper gastrointestinal nonvariceal bleeding. Hepatogastroenterology 2013;60:2004–10.

54. Skok P, Krizman I, Skok M. Argon plasma coagulation versus injection sclerotherapy in peptic ulcer hemorrhage–a prospective, controlled study. Hepatogastroenterology 2004;51:165–70.

55. Cipolletta L, Bianco MA, Rotondano G, et al. Prospective comparison of argon plasma coagulator and heater probe in the endoscopic treatment of major peptic ulcer bleeding. Gastrointest Endosc 1998;48:191–5.

56. Coumaros D, Tsesmeli N. Active gastrointestinal bleeding: use of hemostatic forceps beyond endoscopic submucosal dissection. World J Gastroenterol 2010; 16:2061–4.

57. Yamasaki Y, Takenaka R, Nunoue T, et al. Monopolar soft-mode coagulation using hemostatic forceps for peptic ulcer bleeding. Hepatogastroenterology 2014;61: 2272–6.

58. Laine L, Estrada R. Randomized trial of normal saline solution injection versus bipolar electrocoagulation for treatment of patients with high-risk bleeding ulcers: is local tamponade enough? Gastrointest Endosc 2002;55:6–10.

59. Weiland T, Fehlker M, Gottwald T, et al. Performance of the OTSC System in the endoscopic closure of iatrogenic gastrointestinal perforations: a systematic review. Surg Endosc 2013;27:2258–74.

60. Mangiavillano B, Viaggi P, Masci E. Endoscopic closure of acute iatrogenic perforations during diagnostic and therapeutic endoscopy in the gastrointestinal tract using metallic clips: a literature review. J Dig Dis 2010;11:12–8.

Mechanical Hemostasis Techniques in Nonvariceal Upper Gastrointestinal Bleeding

CrossMark

Andrew S. Brock, MD*, Don C. Rockey, MD*

KEYWORDS

• Hemorrhage • High risk • Stigmata • Hemoclip • Band • Ligation • Endoloop

KEY POINTS

- Mechanical hemostasis is safe and effective for the treatment of nonvariceal upper gastrointestinal (GI) bleeding associated with high-risk stigmata.
- Hemoclips remain the most commonly used modality, owing to the weight of evidence supporting their use, ease of application, widespread availability, and familiarity among endoscopists.
- Although other mechanical techniques are less evidence based, their use is conceptually logical and they may be applied at the discretion of the endoscopist.

INTRODUCTION

Mechanical hemostatic techniques have gained popularity over time owing to their safety, efficacy, ease of application, and widespread availability. The mainstay of mechanical hemostasis involves placement of through-the-scope hemoclips, but newer modalities (eg, over-the-scope clips [OTSCs]) and methods borrowed from other endoscopic therapies (eg, band ligation) have emerged as alternatives. These therapies can be applied to a variety of lesions with much overlap in terms of which device is chosen. This review highlights mechanical techniques used to control bleeding specifically in patients with nonvariceal upper GI bleeding, typically ulcer bleeding.

MECHANICAL HEMOSTATIC TECHNIQUES
Hemoclips

Endoscopic clipping devices were first described in 1975[1] but were initially abandoned because of their complexity. They were reintroduced for use in hemostasis in 1988.[2] Further modifications to clip design resulted in improved ease of use and higher

Department of Internal Medicine, Medical University of South Carolina, Charleston, SC, USA
* Corresponding authors. Department of Internal Medicine, Medical University of South Carolina, 96 Jonathan Lucas Street, Suite 803, MSC 623, Charleston, SC 29425.
E-mail addresses: brockas@musc.edu; rockey@musc.edu

Gastrointest Endoscopy Clin N Am 25 (2015) 523–533
http://dx.doi.org/10.1016/j.giec.2015.03.003
1052-5157/15/$ – see front matter © 2015 Elsevier Inc. All rights reserved.

giendo.theclinics.com

levels of clinical efficacy. In the early 1990s, endoclips were reported to have a 100% success rate in 88 patients with ulcer bleeding.[3]

Initial devices required preloading onto the applicator and subsequent sheathing, making the delivery slow and cumbersome, which was problematic in the setting of acute bleeding.[4] However, multiple advances in endoclip design have taken place, resulting in clips that come preloaded and are easier to position and deploy. Furthermore, currently available endoclips have longer-lasting retention rates. In aggregate, these advances and the ever-increasing familiarity of endoclips have made them one of the most commonly used and effective endoscopic therapeutic techniques.

Mechanism

Hemoclips are metallic devices that can be applied directly to a blood vessel or by apposition of tissue on either side of a vessel or bleeding lesion, resulting in direct vessel occlusion or tamponade. Initial hemostasis of nonvariceal lesions is achieved in 85% to 98% of patients,[5] with rebleeding rates in the 10% to 20% range.

When hemoclips fail, the reasons are often technical or due to operator error, although patient factors may on occasion be responsible. For example, advanced patient age may play a role in the failure to control bleeding.[6] The most common technical reason for hemoclip failure is because the lesion is found in a position that makes en-face application technically difficult (eg, a lesion on the posterior wall of the antrum, lesser curve side of the duodenal bulb, or posterior wall of duodenal bulb). Additional causes of failure include operator error, often with tangential approaches and placing hemoclips improperly or in a fibrotic ulcer base where they are likely to fall off and thus fail to provide optimal vessel compression. It is the authors' practice to visualize the target lesion with aggressive water lavage so as to map out clip deployment, because blood may obscure the lesion. The clip is then positioned as close to the lesion as possible and firmly abut the clip to the mucosa with each prong on either side of the vessel before deploying; if the scope is too far from the target lesion, one loses mechanical advantage and may miss the target. It is important not to scrape the vessel or to deploy around it rather than directly on it. Finally, more than 1 clip may be necessary to fully ligate a vessel, particularly if of large caliber.

Difficulty in applying hemoclips may be overcome by repositioning the lesion with the use of a distal attachment[7] or by using an endoscope with a therapeutic channel at the 5-o'clock position. Distal attachments are clear caps that extend off the end of the scope. Use of a clear cap can be particularly helpful if the lesion is tangential; in this situation, the clear cap can push the mucosa so as to put the target area in a more en-face position for the clip to grasp. Because clips reach only the mucosa and submucosa, there is minimal risk of deep or surrounding tissue injury,[2] although rare reports of causing delayed hemorrhage when applied to normal tissue exist.[8] In addition, they can assist with ulcer healing if normal tissue on either side can be approximated.[9]

Although hemoclips are generally thought to fall off after approximately 2 weeks, there are reports of clip retention for up to 2 years.[10–12] Whether there is a relationship between hemoclips retention and control of bleeding is unknown.

Types of hemoclips

The first generation of hemoclips had a reusable loading device, but reloading was cumbersome and slow; these were largely abandoned once disposable clips were introduced in the early 2000s. Many variations of the single-use devices have been developed, with variations in opening diameter, ease of rotation, and presence of a sheath. A theme across the field is that there have been many advances in clip design. For example, the TriClip (Cook Endoscopy, Winston Salem, NC, USA), introduced in

2003, is a 3-pronged design, which attempted to obviate rotation. The Instinct hemoclip (Cook Endoscopy, Winston Salem, NC) is a sheathless, wide-opening (16 mm opening diameter), 2-pronged device that is easy to rotate and advance and can be opened and closed, a marked improvement over older devices.

The QuickClip was introduced in 2002 and the QuickClip2 in 2005 (both Olympus America, Center Valley, PA, USA). Versions of the QuickClip2 have opening diameters of 9 to 11 mm and working lengths of 165 to 270 cm, with the longer being designed to accommodate enteroscopes. The QuickClip Pro has an opening width of 11 mm and a working length of 1650 to 2300 mm. It was designed to improve ease of rotation to orient the clip to a target lesion and can be opened and closed.

The Resolution clip (Boston Scientific, Natick, MA, USA) can also be opened and closed and has an 11-mm opening diameter and a working length of 155 to 235 cm, thus also allowing accommodation of an enteroscope.

Applications

Hemoclips have been used to treat and are effective for the treatment of many lesions, including ulcers (see later discussion; **Figs. 1–4**), Dieulafoy lesions (**Fig. 5**),[13,14] Mallory-Weiss tears,[15] angioectasia,[16] diverticula,[17] endoscopic resection sites, and mucosal lesions such as tumors and polyps.[18] Hemoclips are most commonly used and were largely developed for use in patients with peptic ulcer lesions. However, they have been shown to be effective in patients with all of the lesions highlighted earlier.

Effectiveness

Several randomized controlled trials have examined hemoclips, comparing them to other single modalities such as injection or heater probe or combined approaches (ie, injection plus hemoclip).[19–24] Results from these studies have been mixed and difficult to interpret given the nuances in study design. Evidence in this area is confounded by different comparison groups. For example, there are multiple comparison groups such as hemoclip versus injection, hemoclip versus thermocoagulation, injection hemoclip versus injection plus thermocoagulation, and so on. Some studies have shown superior hemostatic control with hemoclips compared with other modalities,[22,25] whereas others have found that they are no different or even less effective

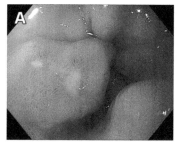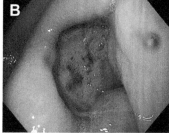

Fig. 1. Peptic ulcers for which mechanical endoscopic therapy is not indicated. In (*A*) is shown an example of a clean-based antral ulcer, with a flat ulcer base and well-demarcated margins that appear to be healing. This lesion does not have any evidence of recent bleeding and represents a lesion with essentially no risk of rebleeding (and thus should not be treated with endoscopic therapy). In (*B*) is shown a large, deep, duodenal bulb ulcer that has only flat spot stigmata of recent bleeding. Not only does this lesion not have a readily identifiable vessel but also because of its depth, large size, and fibrotic base, it would be difficult to approach with a hemoclip (or other mechanical approach).

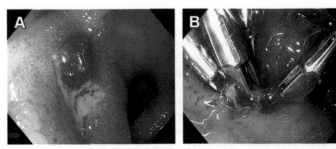

Fig. 2. Hemoclipping of a gastric ulcer with visible vessel. In (*A*) is shown a gastric ulcer, with an exudative ulcer base and a clearly visible protuberant purple punctum (representing an artery). This example represents an ideal candidate for placement of hemoclips. In (*B*) is shown the same lesion after placement of 4 hemoclips. The patient had no further bleeding.

than injection therapy or thermocoagulation therapy.[24,26] A meta-analysis suggested that hemoclips were not superior to other endoscopic modalities in terms of initial hemostasis, rebleeding rate, and the need for emergency surgery.[27] In addition, there was no difference in all-cause mortality irrespective of the modalities of endoscopic treatment. Thus, rigorous data comparing hemoclips with other modalities do not yet exist. Although the authors prefer combination therapy in certain circumstances (ie, injection plus hemoclips for actively bleeding lesions), whether this is better than hemoclip alone is somewhat controversial, and small studies have failed to demonstrate an advantage of epinephrine plus hemoclip over hemoclip alone.[19,28] The authors also inject epinephrine into large clots before removal if they are adherent after washing and to large vessels where the risk of rupture could result in substantial bleeding, as with the gastroduodenal or left gastric arteries, although data to guide this practice are limited.

Limited comparative data exist among the various types of clips, and most studies have examined older clips, which had conflicting retention and hemostasis rates.[29–31] One study that compared the hemoclip device with the TriClip device in patients with high-risk bleeding peptic ulcers found that initial hemostasis was obtained in 47 patients (94%) of the Hemoclip group and in 38 patients (76%) of the TriClip group (*P* = .011). Rebleeding episodes, volume of blood transfusion, hospital stay, numbers

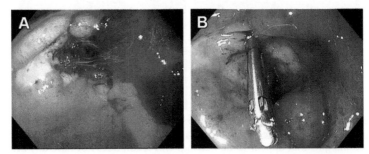

Fig. 3. Hemoclipping of a gastric ulcer with oozing visible vessel. In (*A*) is shown a complex gastric ulcer with readily visible areas of exudate in the ulcer bed along with a visible vessel that is actively oozing blood (fresh blood is seen pooling on the right side of the image). In (*B*) is shown the same lesion after washing, injection of epinephrine, and a single hemoclip was placed on the vessel. No fresh blood can be seen. The patient had no further bleeding.

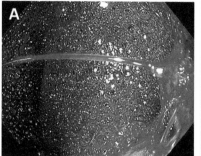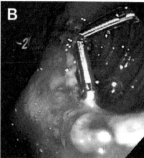

Fig. 4. Hemoclipping of an actively spurting gastrojejunal anastomotic ulcer in a patient who has undergone Roux-en-Y gastric bypass. In (A) is shown a stream of blood emanating from the artery in the ulcer bed (the ulcer is poorly visualized because of the orientation of the ulcer and the large amount of blood present). In (B) is shown the same lesion after 2 hemoclips were placed. The ulcer bed is now also more clearly seen in the retroflexed position. The patient had no further bleeding.

of patients requiring urgent operation, and mortality were not statistically different between the 2 groups.[31] It was speculated that the mechanism for the difference in initial hemostasis was that the TriClip device was more difficult to maneuver in sites where it was difficult to apply. In aggregate, no real conclusions can be drawn, and there is no clear evidence that one type of clip is better than another. **Table 1** highlights specifications of currently available through-the-scope clips.

Hemoclips may be useful in patients who are coagulopathic or who may require ongoing anticoagulation. They may produce more rapid healing than thermal methods,[9] so they may be preferred in situations in which more rapid healing is desired.

Limitations

The major drawback of hemoclips is that they may be difficult to use in hard-to-access areas, such as the lesser curvature, the posterior duodenum, or the cardia. They may not be effective in controlling bleeding in lesions that are fibrotic (such as chronic ulcers), particularly with smaller hemoclips or those that cannot be rotated. Other drawbacks to the use of clips include the inability to approach certain lesions owing to the lesion's tangential nature and the possibility that the clip may attach improperly or fall off (especially with a fibrotic ulcer base) and thus fail to

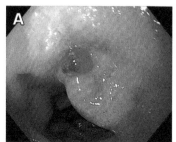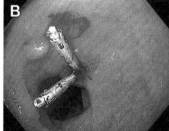

Fig. 5. Hemoclipping of a Dieulafoy lesion in the duodenal bulb. In (A) is shown a typical, nonspurting, Dieulafoy lesion in the duodenal bulb. In (B) is shown the same lesion after 2 hemoclips were placed. The patient had no further bleeding.

Table 1
Available through-the-scope endoclips

Clip	Opening Diameter (mm)	Prongs	Catheter Length (cm)	Minimum Channel Size (mm)	Manufacturer	Introduced (Year)
TriClip	12	3	205	2.8–3.2	Cook Medical	2003
Resolution	11	2	155–235	2.8	Boston Scientific	2004
QuickClip2	9–11	2	165–270	2.8	Olympus	2005
Instinct	16	2	230	2.8	Cook Medical	2013
QuickClip Pro	11	2	165–230	2.8	Olympus	2014

provide optimal vessel compression. In aggregate, although hemoclips may clearly be effective with certain vessel types, further investigation is required to understand how best to use them.

Over-the-Scope Clip

The use of a novel OTSC was first reported in 2007 (Ovesco Endoscopy GmbH, Tübingen, Germany; http://www.ovesco.com/).[32] The OTSC is mounted onto an applicator cap that is fitted to the end of the endoscope in a manner similar to a banding device (**Fig. 6**A). The firing mechanism is also akin to banding in that a wheel that pulls a thread attached to the cap is rotated, which allows release of the clip after suctioning the lesion into the cap. Two accompanying implements, the Twin Grasper and Anchor (Ovesco Endoscopy GmbH), may be used to assist with the grasping of lesions before clip placement.

Although the OTSC has since been predominantly used to close perforations and fistulae, it is also effective in treating nonvariceal GI bleeding (see **Fig. 6**B, C).[32–34] It is particularly effective in cases of bleeding refractory to conventional endoscopic therapy and lesions in locations that make en-face treatment challenging with through-the-scope clips or electrocautery.[34] The larger diameter aids in treatment of large or fibrotic ulcer bases. Although the OTSC is safe, it can be challenging (although possible) to remove once applied to a lesion.[35] The major limiting factor, however, is lack of widespread availability.

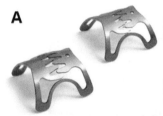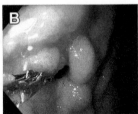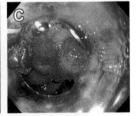

Fig. 6. Placement of a large over-the-scope clip over a bleeding mucosal defect. In (A) is shown an artists rendition of the over-the-scope clip (Ovesco Endoscopy GmbH). In (B) is shown an oozing mucosal defect of unclear cause in a patient with acute pancreatitis complicated by fluid collection; the defect is highlighted by opening with biopsy forceps. In (C) is shown the same lesion after Ovesco clip placement, resulting in cessation of bleeding and stabilization of hemoglobin.

Band Ligation

Although band ligation is not often used for nonvariceal bleeding, it is a conceptually feasible mechanical modality to treat any bleeding lesion that can be suctioned into the ligation cap (**Fig. 7**).[36] Reports of band ligation for nonvariceal bleeding date back nearly to the inception of band ligation, and this method is particularly useful in coagulopathic patients in whom mucosal injury or removal of a lesion might be avoided.[37] Despite this extensive longitudinal experience, much of the literature is still based on case series or case reports.[38]

It has been used for postpolypectomy sites[39] to treat bleeding nodular gastric antral vascular ectasia,[40] Dieulafoy lesions,[41] Mallory-Weiss tears, and even peptic ulcers.[42,43] One small randomized trial comparing epinephrine injection to band ligation demonstrated 100% primary hemostasis with no rebleeding in patients undergoing band ligation for treatment of Dieulafoy lesions.[44] Efficacy with low rebleeding rates has been demonstrated for other lesions, including high-risk stigmata peptic ulcers.[43] Similar results have been reported for Dieulafoy lesions treated by a combination of epinephrine injection and band ligation.[45] A prospective study comparing band ligation with bipolar electrocautery in patients with Dieulafoy lesions, Mallory-Weiss tears, postpolypectomy gastric ulcers, and gastric angiodysplasia showed 100% primary hemostasis in the banding group with no rebleeding compared with 84% hemostasis in the electrocautery group.[46]

Detachable Snares

Detachable snares (PolyLoop, Olympus America) are most commonly used to ligate the base of large pedunculated polyps before resection for prevention of postpolypectomy bleeding (**Fig. 8**).[47–49] These nylon loops come in a preloaded sheath, which is placed through the endoscope working channel. They are mechanistically similar to standard polypectomy snares except that once deployed they remain around the target lesion and are no longer attached to the sheath. The lesion generally sloughs off with time because of local tissue necrosis, and the loop falls off thereafter. Detachable snares have also been shown in limited reports to be useful for refractory ulcer bleeding[50,51] and bleeding due to submucosal tumors.[52] Although not studied, logic

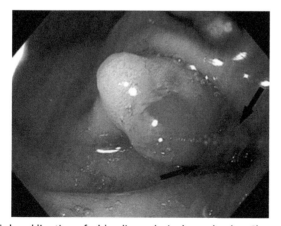

Fig. 7. Endoscopic band ligation of a bleeding pyloric channel polyp. Shown is an image of a sessile-appearing polyp with a bleeding distal tip in which a rubber band was placed around the polyp base (the band is difficult to be seen in the top part of the polyp, but its white edge can be seen at the bottom aspect of the polyp).

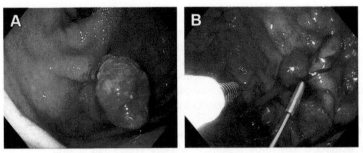

Fig. 8. Endoloop treatment of a bleeding gastric fundal polyp. In (*A*) is shown a hemorrhagic and spontaneously oozing polyp. In (*B*), a detachable snare was placed around the polyp to ensure hemostasis before snare polypectomy.

would suggest that they might be used for bleeding polyps when resection may not be safe because of coagulopathy or other extenuating circumstances. Care must be taken to avoid accidental transection during deployment.[53]

SUMMARY AND FUTURE DIRECTIONS

Mechanical hemostatic techniques are well established and commonly used for non-variceal upper GI bleeding. Hemoclips are the most commonly used devices and will likely remain the preferred modality because of their ease of use and widespread availability. Band ligation, OTSCs, and detachable snares remain alternatives in select situations depending on local expertise and availability.

Head-to-head trials comparing hemoclips and other mechanical modalities with injection and thermocoagulation techniques are needed for specific lesions. Further advancements in hemoclip design that would be beneficial include improvements in ease of clip advancement out of the working channel and ease of clip rotation to target lesions. OTSCs could benefit from improved accessory devices for tissue apposition.

REFERENCES

1. Hayashi T, Yonezawa M, Kuwabara T, et al. The study on staunch clip for the treatment by endoscopy. Gastroenterological Endoscopy 1975;17:92–101.
2. Hachisu T. Evaluation of endoscopic hemostasis using an improved clipping apparatus. Surg Endosc 1988;2(1):13–7.
3. Binmoeller KF, Thonke F, Soehendra N. Endoscopic hemoclip treatment for gastrointestinal bleeding. Endoscopy 1993;25(2):167–70.
4. Devereaux CE, Binmoeller KF. Endoclip: closing the surgical gap. Gastrointest Endosc 1999;50(3):440–2.
5. Raju GS, Gajula L. Endoclips for GI endoscopy. Gastrointest Endosc 2004;59(2):267–79.
6. Peng YC, Chen SY, Tung CF, et al. Factors associated with failure of initial endoscopic hemoclip hemostasis for upper gastrointestinal bleeding. J Clin Gastroenterol 2006;40(1):25–8.
7. Kim JI, Kim SS, Park S, et al. Endoscopic hemoclipping using a transparent cap in technically difficult cases. Endoscopy 2003;35(8):659–62.
8. van den Broek JW, Jones DP, Godino J. Hemodynamically significant upper-GI bleeding after hemoclip application. Gastrointest Endosc 2007;66(4):843–5.

9. Jensen DM, Machicado GA, Hirabayashi K. Randomized controlled study of 3 different types of hemoclips for hemostasis of bleeding canine acute gastric ulcers. Gastrointest Endosc 2006;64(5):768–73.

10. Ooi BP, Hassan MR, Kiew KK, et al. Case report of a hemostatic clip being retained for 2 years after deployment. Gastrointest Endosc 2010;72(6):1315–6.

11. Volfson A, McKinley MJ. Prolonged endoclip retention time. Gastrointest Endosc 2011;74(3):727–8.

12. Swellengrebel HA, Marijnen CA, Vincent A, et al. Evaluating long-term attachment of two different endoclips in the human gastrointestinal tract. World J Gastrointest Endosc 2010;2(10):344–8.

13. Parra-Blanco A, Takahashi H, Mendez Jerez PV, et al. Endoscopic management of Dieulafoy lesions of the stomach: a case study of 26 patients. Endoscopy 1997; 29(9):834–9.

14. Ljubicic N. Efficacy of endoscopic clipping and long-term follow-up of bleeding Dieulafoy's lesions in the upper gastrointestinal tract. Hepatogastroenterology 2006;53(68):224–7.

15. Yamaguchi Y, Yamato T, Katsumi N, et al. Endoscopic hemoclipping for upper GI bleeding due to Mallory-Weiss syndrome. Gastrointest Endosc 2001;53(4):427–30.

16. Brock AS, Cook JL, Ranney N, et al. Clinical problem-solving. A not-so-obscure cause of gastrointestinal bleeding. N Engl J Med 2015;372(6):556–61.

17. Simpson PW, Nguyen MH, Lim JK, et al. Use of endoclips in the treatment of massive colonic diverticular bleeding. Gastrointest Endosc 2004;59(3):433–7.

18. Parra-Blanco A, Kaminaga N, Kojima T, et al. Hemoclipping for postpolypectomy and postbiopsy colonic bleeding. Gastrointest Endosc 2000;51(1):37–41.

19. Chung IK, Ham JS, Kim HS, et al. Comparison of the hemostatic efficacy of the endoscopic hemoclip method with hypertonic saline-epinephrine injection and a combination of the two for the management of bleeding peptic ulcers. Gastrointest Endosc 1999;49(1):13–8.

20. Chung IK, Kim EJ, Lee MS, et al. Bleeding Dieulafoy's lesions and the choice of endoscopic method: comparing the hemostatic efficacy of mechanical and injection methods. Gastrointest Endosc 2000;52(6):721–4.

21. Nagayama K, Tazawa J, Sakai Y, et al. Efficacy of endoscopic clipping for bleeding gastroduodenal ulcer: comparison with topical ethanol injection. Am J Gastroenterol 1999;94(10):2897–901.

22. Cipolletta L, Bianco MA, Marmo R, et al. Endoclips versus heater probe in preventing early recurrent bleeding from peptic ulcer: A prospective and randomized trial. Gastrointest Endosc 2001;53(2):147–51.

23. Buffoli F, Graffeo M, Nicosia F, et al. Peptic ulcer bleeding: comparison of two hemostatic procedures. Am J Gastroenterol 2001;96(1):89–94.

24. Gevers AM, De Goede E, Simoens M, et al. A randomized trial comparing injection therapy with hemoclip and with injection combined with hemoclip for bleeding ulcers. Gastrointest Endosc 2002;55(4):466–9.

25. Chou YC, Hsu PI, Lai KH, et al. A prospective, randomized trial of endoscopic hemoclip placement and distilled water injection for treatment of high-risk bleeding ulcers. Gastrointest Endosc 2003;57(3):324–8.

26. Lin HJ, Hsieh YH, Tseng GY, et al. A prospective, randomized trial of endoscopic hemoclip versus heater probe thermocoagulation for peptic ulcer bleeding. Am J Gastroenterol 2002;97(9):2250–4.

27. Yuan Y, Wang C, Hunt RH. Endoscopic clipping for acute nonvariceal upper-GI bleeding: a meta-analysis and critical appraisal of randomized controlled trials. Gastrointest Endosc 2008;68(2):339–51.

28. Saltzman JR, Strate LL, Di Sena V, et al. Prospective trial of endoscopic clips versus combination therapy in upper GI bleeding (PROTECCT–UGI bleeding). Am J Gastroenterol 2005;100(7):1503–8.

29. Shin EJ, Ko CW, Magno P, et al. Comparative study of endoscopic clips: duration of attachment at the site of clip application. Gastrointest Endosc 2007;66(4): 757–61.

30. Jensen DM, Machicado GA. Hemoclipping of chronic canine ulcers: a randomized, prospective study of initial deployment success, clip retention rates, and ulcer healing. Gastrointest Endosc 2009;70(5):969–75.

31. Lin HJ, Lo WC, Cheng YC, et al. Endoscopic hemoclip versus TriClip placement in patients with high-risk peptic ulcer bleeding. Am J Gastroenterol 2007;102(3): 539–43.

32. Kirschniak A, Kratt T, Stuker D, et al. A new endoscopic over-the-scope clip system for treatment of lesions and bleeding in the GI tract: first clinical experiences. Gastrointest Endosc 2007;66(1):162–7.

33. Manta R, Galloro G, Mangiavillano B, et al. Over-the-scope clip (OTSC) represents an effective endoscopic treatment for acute GI bleeding after failure of conventional techniques. Surg Endosc 2013;27(9):3162–4.

34. Chan SM, Chiu PW, Teoh AY, et al. Use of the over-the-scope clip for treatment of refractory upper gastrointestinal bleeding: a case series. Endoscopy 2014;46(5): 428–31.

35. Schmidt A, Riecken B, Damm M, et al. Endoscopic removal of over-the-scope clips using a novel cutting device: a retrospective case series. Endoscopy 2014;46(9):762–6.

36. Lo CC, Hsu PI, Lo GH, et al. Endoscopic banding ligation can effectively resect hyperplastic polyps of stomach. World J Gastroenterol 2003;9(12):2805–8.

37. Tseng C, Burke S, Connors P, et al. Endoscopic band ligation for treatment of non-variceal upper gastrointestinal bleeding. Endoscopy 1991;23(5):297–8.

38. Abi-Hanna D, Williams SJ, Gillespie PE, et al. Endoscopic band ligation for non-variceal non-ulcer gastrointestinal hemorrhage. Gastrointest Endosc 1998;48(5): 510–4.

39. Slivka A, Parsons WG, Carr-Locke DL. Endoscopic band ligation for treatment of post-polypectomy hemorrhage. Gastrointest Endosc 1994;40(2 Pt 1):230–2.

40. Prachayakul V, Aswakul P, Leelakusolvong S. Massive gastric antral vascular ectasia successfully treated by endoscopic band ligation as the initial therapy. World J Gastrointest Endosc 2013;5(3):135–7.

41. Cheng CL, Liu NJ, Lee CS, et al. Endoscopic management of Dieulafoy lesions in acute nonvariceal upper gastrointestinal bleeding. Dig Dis Sci 2004;49(7–8): 1139–44.

42. Krishnan A, Velayutham V, Satyanesan J, et al. Role of endoscopic band ligation in management of non-variceal upper gastrointestinal bleeding. Trop Gastroenterol 2013;34(2):91–4.

43. Park CH, Joo YE, Kim HS, et al. A prospective, randomized trial comparing mechanical methods of hemostasis plus epinephrine injection to epinephrine injection alone for bleeding peptic ulcer. Gastrointest Endosc 2004;60(2):173–9.

44. Park CH, Joo YE, Kim HS, et al. A prospective, randomized trial of endoscopic band ligation versus endoscopic hemoclip placement for bleeding gastric Dieulafoy's lesions. Endoscopy 2004;36(8):677–81.

45. Mumtaz R, Shaukat M, Ramirez FC. Outcomes of endoscopic treatment of gastroduodenal Dieulafoy's lesion with rubber band ligation and thermal/injection therapy. J Clin Gastroenterol 2003;36(4):310–4.

46. Matsui S, Kamisako T, Kudo M, et al. Endoscopic band ligation for control of non-variceal upper GI hemorrhage: comparison with bipolar electrocoagulation. Gastrointest Endosc 2002;55(2):214–8.
47. Li L, Shen Z, Ji F, et al. Combined application of clip and endoloop for the prevention of postpolypectomy complications in large pedunculated colonic polyps: a better choice. Int J Colorectal Dis 2015;30(2):287–8.
48. Ji JS, Lee SW, Kim TH, et al. Comparison of prophylactic clip and endoloop application for the prevention of postpolypectomy bleeding in pedunculated colonic polyps: a prospective, randomized, multicenter study. Endoscopy 2014;46(7): 598–604.
49. Luigiano C, Ferrara F, Ghersi S, et al. Endoclip-assisted resection of large pedunculated colorectal polyps: technical aspects and outcome. Dig Dis Sci 2010; 55(6):1726–31.
50. Lee JH, Kim BK, Seol DC, et al. Rescue endoscopic bleeding control for nonvariceal upper gastrointestinal hemorrhage using clipping and detachable snaring. Endoscopy 2013;45(6):489–92.
51. Racz I, Karasz T, Saleh H. Endoscopic hemostasis of bleeding gastric ulcer with a combination of multiple hemoclips and endoloops. Gastrointest Endosc 2009; 69(3 Pt 1):580–3.
52. Lee SH, Park JH, Park do H, et al. Endoloop ligation of large pedunculated submucosal tumors (with videos). Gastrointest Endosc 2008;67(3):556–60.
53. Katsinelos P, Kountouras J, Paroutoglou G, et al. Endoloop-assisted polypectomy for large pedunculated colorectal polyps. Surg Endosc 2006;20(8):1257–61.

Hemostatic Powders in Gastrointestinal Bleeding
A Systematic Review

Yen-I Chen, MD[a], Alan N. Barkun, MD, MSc[a,b,*]

KEYWORDS

- Gastrointestinal bleeding • Hemostatic powders • Ankaferd Blood Stopper

KEY POINTS

- Topical hemostatic agents and powders are an emerging modality in the endoscopic management of upper and lower gastrointestinal bleeding.
- This systematic review demonstrates the effectiveness and safety of these agents with special emphasis on TC-325 and Ankaferd Blood Stopper.
- The unique noncontact/nontraumatic application, ability to cover large areas of bleed, and ease of use make these hemostatic agents an attractive option in certain clinical situations, such as massive bleeding with poor visualization, salvage therapy, and diffuse bleeding from luminal malignancies.
- Because of their temporary and short luminal residency time, the effectiveness of these topical agents may not be optimal as monotherapy in lesions at high risk of rebleeding beyond a 24-hour period, such as peptic ulcer hemorrhage.

INTRODUCTION

Gastrointestinal (GI) bleeding from both the upper and the lower GI tract is a common cause for hospitalization, resulting in significant mortality, morbidity, and resource utilization. In the United States, nonvariceal upper GI bleeding (NVUGIB) is associated with a hospitalization rate of 60.6 to 78.4 per 100,000 adults and a mortality of 2.1% to 2.45%.[1–4] Lower GI bleeding (LGIB), on the other hand, is accompanied by a

Disclosure Statement: Dr A. Barkun is a consultant for Cook Medical Inc. Dr Y-I. Chen has no relevant disclosures.
[a] Division of Gastroenterology, McGill University Health Center, McGill University, Montreal, Quebec, Canada; [b] Epidemiology and Biostatistics and Occupational Health, McGill University, Montreal, Quebec, Canada
* Corresponding author. Division of Gastroenterology, The McGill University Health Center, Montreal General Hospital site, 1650 Cedar Avenue, Room D16.125, Montréal H3G 1A4, Canada.
E-mail address: alan.barkun@muhc.mcgill.ca

hospitalization and mortality rate of 21 per 100,000 adults and 2% to 4%, respectively.[5,6] The advent of endoscopic hemostatic therapies, such as clips, injection therapy, thermocoagulation, and argon plasma coagulation, have changed the management of GI bleeding and, in the case of NVUGIB, a potential benefit in mortality, need for surgery, and transfusion requirement.[7,8] However, these devices have their limitations, such as the risk for perforation, worsening of bleeding, and possible difficulty in using with large, friable bleeding surfaces, such as hemorrhage arising from GI tumors.

Over the past few years, innovative topical hemostatic modalities have been developed for endoscopic use. Although these agents are new in digestive endoscopy, topical hemostatic agents have existed over the past 50 years with widespread medical applications.[9] They were first introduced in 1909, with the use of topical fibrin for surgical hemostasis.[10] Indeed, fibrin sealants marked the beginning of a wide spectrum of topical hemostatic agents to be used in surgery. More recently, novel hemostatic products, such as the Ankaferd Blood Stopper (ABS; Ankaferd Health Products Ltd, Istanbul, Turkey), TC-325 (Hemospray; Cook Medical, Winston-Salem, NC, USA), and EndoClot (AMP; EndoClot Plus Inc, Santa Clara, CA, USA), have been adapted to digestive endoscopy and the management of GI bleed. Uncontrolled data from both TC-325 and ABS have shown promising results in a variety of bleeding pathologic abnormalities from both the upper and the lower GI tract.[11,12] In the following, the use of endoscopic topical hemostatic agents is discussed, focusing on ABS and TC-325 in terms of their composition, mechanism of action, clinical data and application, and related complications.

METHODS

A computerized systematic literature review from January 1950 through August 2014, by using OVID MEDLINE, EMBASE, CENTRAL, and ISI Web of Knowledge 5.6, was initiated. Articles were selected by using a combination of MeSH headings and text words related to TC-325, nanopowder, hemostatic or haemostatic agent, granule or powder, TC-325, Ankaferd Blood Stopper, and microporous polysaccharides. Recursive searches and cross-referencing were also carried out by using a similar articles function; hand searches of articles were identified after an initial search. Included were all adult human studies in French or English.

STUDY SELECTION

Of an initial 3799 articles, 105 articles were identified that were related to ABS as a topical hemostatic agent; however, after excluding nonendoscopic data, review articles, in vitro studies, and animal models, 17 articles were left on the endoscopic use of ABS in GI bleeding. Also identified were 23 original articles related to TC-325 use in GI bleeding and 21 articles after the exclusion of animal studies. There is only one published article on the use of AMP; therefore, most of this brief review on AMP is based on the information provided by the manufacturer's Web site.

COMPOSITION OF HEMOSTATIC POWDERS AND TECHNICAL APPLICATION
Ankaferd Blood Stopper

The ABS is an herbal extract derived from 5 different plants approved in Turkey for topical application.[13] Each 100 mL of ABS is composed of 5 mg *Thymus vulgaris*, 9 mg *Glycyrrhiza glabra*, 8 mg *Vitis vinifera*, 7 mg *Alpinia officinarum*, 6 mg *Urtica dioica*. Although the exact mechanism for hemostasis remains unclear, it likely achieves bleeding control by promoting the formation of a protein network behaving as an anchor for erythrocyte aggregation that then integrates the classic coagulation cascade without directly acting on coagulation factors and platelets.[13–15] Interestingly, ABS may have other therapeutic effects beyond hemostasis, such as its influence on angiogenesis, cellular proliferation, and vascular dynamic,[14–17] which has led to investigations into its possible anti-infective, antineoplastic, and wound-healing potentials.[18–20] Currently, ABS experience is limited mostly to Turkey and has not been approved by the Food and Drug Agency (FDA) in the United States.

Hemospray

TC-325 is composed of a proprietary inorganic biologically inert powder that, when put in contact with moisture in the GI tract, becomes coherent, thus serving as a mechanical barrier for hemostasis.[10] In addition, it may provide a scaffold, enhancing platelet aggregation and possibly activating clotting factors.[21–23] Data from an in vitro model by Holster and colleagues[24] showed decreasing clotting time with the application of TC-325 in a dose-dependent fashion. Following hemostasis, the powder sloughs off the intestinal mucosa and is completely eliminated from the GI tract, likely within 24 hours of application.[11] It is important to note that the powder only adheres to actively bleeding lesions; therefore, its use in high-risk lesions without active spurting or oozing, such as in nonbleeding visible vessels, is likely ineffective in providing appropriate hemostasis. The endoscopic use of TC-325 is currently approved in Canada, Mexico, and several countries in the Caribbean, South America, Europe, and Asia; however, it is not FDA approved.

EndoClot

AMP is composed of proprietary hemostatic polysaccharides that are derived from plant starch.[25] It is adhesive, ultra hydrophilic, and fast degrading and induces hemostasis by rapidly absorbing water from blood and thereby concentrating red cells, platelets, and coagulation factors at the bleeding site. Similarly to TC-325, AMP is delivered through a catheter inserted into the operating channel of the endoscope and propelled by an air compressor onto the bleeding lesion. AMP is currently approved in Turkey, Europe, Malaysia, and Australia according to the company's Web site. At the time of this review, only one peer-reviewed publication on the use of AMP was found in the literature. It described the application of AMP in LGIB after endoscopic mucosal resection (EMR) showing excellent hemostasis of 90% (18/20), time to hemostasis of 1.7 min, 3 documented cases of rebleeding, and no procedural related complications.[26]

Method of Delivery

At the time of this review, there were no published articles focused on the technical application of ABS. In addition, given that ABS is only available in Turkey, the authors have no technical experience and cannot provide an expert opinion as to how the hemostatic agent should be optimally delivered. They do know that ABS comes in 3 forms: ampoules, tampons, and sprays.[27] Sprays can then be applied through a disposable catheter in the operating channel of an endoscope in 50-mL vials.

TC-325, on the other hand, is propelled from a canister under CO_2 pressure and delivered through a catheter unto the bleeding lesion. The catheter should be maintained 1 to 2 cm from the high-risk lesion and application should be noncontact. As mentioned, the endoscopic powder will aggregate immediately when it comes into contact with moisture; therefore, efforts should be made to keep the tip of the catheter dry and to avoid suctioning while it is in use or while the powder is settling. Flushing the accessory channel with a 60-mL syringe of air before TC-325 application is also recommended to ensure that the tip of the catheter does not come into contact with moisture during insertion.

CLINICAL DATA ON THE USE OF ANKAFERD BLOOD STOPPER IN GASTROINTESTINAL BLEEDING

ABS has been extensively studied and deemed systemically safe in animal models and human data in a variety of nonendoscopic settings, such as dental,[28–31] ocular,[32–34] orthopedic,[35] urologic,[36–39] liver injury,[40–44] epistaxis,[45–48] plastic surgery,[49] head and neck,[50] and cardiothoracic surgery.[51,52] Intravascular application of ABS is considered a contraindication due to the potential for vascular embolization, as demonstrated by animal data.[53] In terms of ABS use in the digestive tract, high-dose oral administration of the hemostatic agent in 8 rats and 12 rabbits proved to be safe without significant deleterious effects.[54,55] In addition, oral administration of ABS in rats with caustic esophageal injury was shown to be associated with improved mucosal healing.[56]

Kurt and colleagues[57] reported one of the first cases of endoscopically applied ABS in the human digestive tract; more specifically, it was used in a case of gastrojejunostomy anastomic bleed refractory to conventional therapy. Several other case reports and series then followed describing the successful use of ABS in NVUGIB due to peptic ulcer (PUD), anastomotic ulcer, tumor, Dieulafoy lesion, gastric antral vascular ectasia (GAVE), arteriovenous malformation (AVM), Mallory-Weiss syndrome, postprocedural bleeding, esophagitis, and diffuse bleeding due to severe coagulopathy.[12,57–65] Karaman and colleagues[60] described the first large retrospective series of variceal and NVUGIB treated with ABS with an immediate hemostasis of 86.7% (26/30) and no documented rebleeding. Gungor and colleagues[59] then demonstrated a more modest immediate hemostasis rate of 73% (19/26) in NVUGIB with PUD as the major cause.

Ankaferd Blood Stopper in the Management of Nonvariceal Upper Gastrointestinal Bleeding

Overall, there are a total of 83 cases of ABS-treated NVUGIB of various causes in the literature with an immediate hemostasis of 88.0% (73/83). **Table 1** displays the immediate hemostasis rates of NVUGIB treated with ABS stratified according to cause and

Table 1
Summary of Ankaferd Blood Stopper immediate hemostasis based on the current available literature stratified according to risk of rebleeding and cause

High-Risk Rebleed	N	Immediate Hemostasis	Low-Risk Rebleed	N	Immediate Hemostasis
PUD total	34	76.5% (26/34)	Mallory-Weiss syndrome	4	100% (4/4)
Anastomotic ulcer	3	100% (3/3)	Gastroduodenal erosion	1	100% (1/1)
Tumor bleeding	10	100% (10/10)	Postbiopsy	5	100% (5/5)
AVM	1	100% (1/1)	Postpolypectomy	12	100% (12/12)
Dieulafoy	5	100% (5/5)	Postsphincterotomy	2	100% (2/2)
Amyloidosis ulcer	1	100% (1/1)	Diffuse UGIB due to coagulopathy	1	100% (1/1)
GAVE	3	100% (3/3)	Esophagitis	1	100% (1/1)
Total	57	86.0% (49/57)	Total	26	100% (26/26)

risk of rebleeding. In terms of PUD bleeding, there are a total of 34 cases treated with ABS reported in the literature with an immediate hemostasis rate of 73.4% (25/34). Gungor and colleagues[59] showed a rebleeding rate of 15.8% in PUD treated with ABS monotherapy. These modest results suggest that the protein network and erythrocyte aggregation provided by ABS application may not be enough to attain optimal tamponade and successful hemostasis in PUD bleeding and that a second modality such as thermal or mechanical clip is needed to obliterate the bleeding vessel. There are also 10 cases of upper GI bleeding due to a luminal malignancy treated with ABS with excellent immediate hemostasis of 100% and no documented rebleeding.[59,60,62,65] As with TC-325, ABS may be ideal for malignant bleeding given its noncontact and nontraumatic delivery and ability to cover large areas of bleed. In addition, in vitro and animal data suggest that ABS may have some healing properties and antineoplastic activity, while Turhan and colleagues[65] reported decreased tumor vascularization post-ABS application in 2 patients with luminal cancer; however, these findings need to be confirmed and reproduced in larger trials.[14–17,56]

Ankaferd Blood Stopper in the Management of Variceal Bleeding

Although direct intravascular application of ABS has been shown to lead to systemic embolization in animal models,[53] the use of this novel hemostatic powder has been described in 12 cases of variceal bleed (7 gastric, 4 esophageal, 1 duodenal) without evidence of systemic embolization. Immediate hemostasis was excellent at 91.7% (11/12) with only 1 documented case of rebleeding. Although use of ABS seems to be safe in this setting, this topical agent is unlikely to become a definite therapy in variceal bleeding given its inability to eradicate vascular structures and may play a more important role in terms of rescue or bridging therapy. In addition, the pooled sample size is quite small and more data will be needed to confirm its safety in variceal hemorrhage.

Ankaferd Blood Stopper in the Management of Lower Gastrointestinal Bleeding

The use of ABS in LGIB has been reported in 19 cases with an excellent immediate hemostasis of 100% and no documented rebleeding. Causes of hemorrhage include luminal malignancy, postpolypectomy, radiation colitis, diverticular bleeding, and solitary rectal ulcer.[12,61,62,65,66] Interestingly, Ozaslan and colleagues reported a case of severe radiation colitis treated with 4 sessions of ABS on a weekly basis and demonstrated healing of the ulcerated and mildly necrotic mucosa. This finding again may highlight the potential healing characteristics of ABS; however, as aforementioned, larger, controlled data are needed to confirm this property.

Complications Related to Ankaferd Blood Stopper Use

The safety of ABS has been demonstrated in a wide variety of medical indications in animal, in vitro, and human studies. In terms of endoscopic application, there are a total of 115 cases described in the literature. Beyazit and colleagues[58] reported the only complication found at the time of this review by describing a case of duodenal perforation post-ABS application in a patient with amyloidosis involving the GI tract. However, it is unclear whether the perforation was related to the endoscope, the use of ABS, or to the amyloid deposits. Although systemic embolization has been reported with direct ABS use in intravascular structures in animals, this has not been found in human subjects even when ABS was applied in variceal bleeding. Finally, congruent with animal studies, no intestinal toxicity or intestinal obstruction has been described with the endoscopic use of ABS. Overall, the use of ABS in the GI tract appears to be safe; however, as with all novel medical devices, larger trials and continuous monitoring are needed to confirm its safety.

CLINICAL DATA ON THE USE OF TC-325 IN GASTROINTESTINAL BLEEDING

Giday and colleagues[67] were the first to demonstrate the effectiveness and safety of TC-325 in a porcine model. Ten animals with Forrest Ia bleeding, artificially induced in the stomach by dissecting the gastroepiploic vessel, were randomized to TC-325 treatment or sham. Immediate hemostasis in the treatment arm was achieved in 100% of the animals with only 1 case of rebleeding at 24 hours. Necropsy at 1 week revealed healed bleeding sites without evidence of systemic embolization. A subsequent study focused on local and systemic effect of TC-325 therapy in 6 animals with artificially induced Forrest Ia bleeding showed no macroscopic or microscopic evidence of residual powder, no resultant gross or histologic evidence of embolization or bowel obstruction, and no systemic coagulopathic effect on necropsy.[68]

Sung and colleagues[69] were the first to describe the use of TC-325 in human subjects. This initial prospective, pilot study included 20 patients with NVUGIB stemming from gastroduodenal ulcers with high-risk stigmata (mostly Forrest Ib). Immediate hemostasis was excellent at 95% with TC-325 monotherapy and a rebleeding rate of 10.5% (2/19). Second-look endoscopy at 72 hours, performed in all subjects, showed healing of the ulcers without any remnants of the hemostatic powder. Following this pilot study, several case reports and small case series demonstrated the successful use of TC-325 in a variety of bleeding pathologic abnormalities, including PUD, anastomotic ulcer, luminal malignancies, AVM, Dieulafoy, Mallory-Weiss tears, esophagitis, and postprocedural bleeding (therapeutic and diagnostic).[70-77] Smith and colleagues[78] were the first to perform a large retrospective study on the use of TC-325. This study included 63 patients with TC-325-treated NVUGIB composed of 30 subjects with PUD and 33 patients with a variety of non-PUD-related NVUGIB. The compiled initial hemostasis rate was 87.3% (55/63) with a 7-day rebleed rate of 16.4% (9/55). More recently, the authors' group performed a retrospective study involving 67 cases of TC-325 application in a variety of nonportal hypertensive bleeding pathologic abnormalities, including 21 nonmalignant NVUGIB, 19 malignant upper GI bleeding (UGIB), 11 LGIB, and 16 instances of intraprocedural bleeding (**Fig. 1**).[11] The initial hemostasis was 98.5% (66/67) with a 3-day rebleeding rate of 9.5% (6/63). Interestingly, the second-look endoscopy data showed no remnants of hemostatic powder even in patients who had a repeat endoscopy as early as 24 hours (3 patients), suggesting that TC-325 is eliminated by the GI tract within 1 day of application.[11]

Overall, there are a total of 195 cases of NVUGIB treated with TC-325 published in the literature at the time of this review.[11,71-73,75-78,69] Combining the above prospective series, retrospective studies, and case reports yielded an immediate hemostasis of 92.3% (180/195) and 7-day rebleed of 20.6% (**Table 2**). **Table 3** displays the combined immediate hemostasis, early rebleeding (≤72 hours), delayed rebleeding (>72 hours), and 7-day rebleeding rates stratified according to the specific bleeding cause and risk of rebleeding in time. In lesions that are considered high risk for rebleeding, such as Forrest Ia and Ib ulcers and tumor bleeding, the combined immediate hemostasis was 91.6% (120/131) with a 7-day rebleeding rate of 25.8% (31/120). Lesions at low risk of rebleeding were associated with an immediate hemostasis rate of 93.5% (29/31) and a 7-day rebleeding rate of 0% (0/29). It is important to note that many of the studies did not include data on cause-specific rates of immediate hemostasis and timing of rebleeding, therefore explaining the variable denominators and numerators shown in **Table 3**.

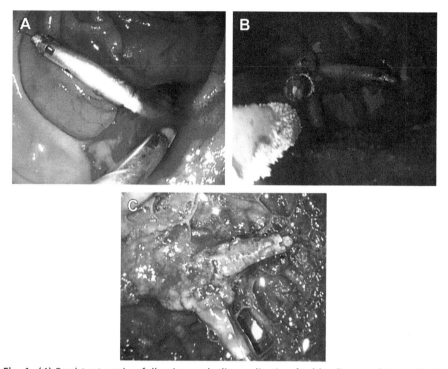

Fig. 1. (*A*) Persistent oozing following endoclip application for bleeding postbiopsy site in the duodenum. (*B*) TC-325 application. (*C*) Successful hemostasis after TC-325 application.

Table 2
Summary of TC-325 immediate hemostasis, rebleeding rates, and complications in nonvariceal upper GI bleeding, portal-hypertensive/variceal upper GI bleeding, and lower GI bleeding based on the current available published literature

	NVUGIB	Portal-Hypertensive and Variceal GIB	LGIB
N	195	20	28
Immediate hemostasis	92.3% (180/195)	100% (20/20)	100% (28/28)
Rebleed ≤72 h	20.2% (18/89)[a]	0% (0/9)	7.4% (2/27)
Rebleed >72 h	12.4% (11/89)[a]	0% (0/9)	0% (0/27)
7-d Rebleed	20.6% (37/180)[a]	0% (0/8)	7.7% (2/26)
Complications	• Pain with TC-325 delivery • Splenic infarct (unclear if related to TC-325) • Transient biliary obstruction • Hemoperitoneum (unclear if related to TC-325)	Perforated viscus (unclear if due to TC-325)	None

[a] Many of the reviewed literature did not differentiate between rebled 72 h or less and rebled greater than 72 h and only provided data on 7-day rebleed, therefore, explaining the variable denominators.

Table 3
Summary of TC-325 immediate hemostasis and rebleeding rates based on the current available literature and stratified according to cause and risk of rebleeding

High-Risk Rebleed	N	Immediate Hemostasis	Early Rebleed ≤72 h	Delayed Rebleed >72 h	7-d Rebleed*	Low-Risk Rebleed	N	Immediate Hemostasis	Early Rebleed ≤72 h	Delayed Rebleed >72 h	7-d Rebleed*
PUD total	86	89.5% (77/86)	18.9% (10/53)	7.5% (4/53)	22.1% (17/77)	Bleeding from buried PEG bumper site	1	100% (1/1)	0% (0/1)	0% (0/1)	0% (0/1)
PUD Ia	24	76.9% (10/13)	40% (4/10)	20% (2/10)	60% (6/10)	Mallory-Weiss syndrome	1	100% (1/1)	0% (0/1)	0% (0/1)	0% (0/1)
PUD Ib	59	100% (43/43)	13.0% (6/43)	4.7% (2/43)	16.3% (7/43)	Esophagitis/gastroduodenal erosion	2	100% (2/2)	0% (0/2)	0% (0/2)	0% (0/2)
Anastomotic ulcer	3	66.7% (2/3)	50% (1/2)	0% (0/2)	50% (1/2)	Postbiopsy	7	100% (7/7)	0% (0/7)	0% (0/7)	0% (0/7)
Tumor bleeding	28	100% (28/28)	4.3% (1/23)	26.1% (6/23)	25% (7/28)	Postpolypectomy	2	100% (2/2)	0% (0/2)	0% (0/2)	0% (0/2)
AVM	3	100% (3/3)	33.3% (1/3)	33.3% (1/3)	33.3% (1/3)	Post-ESD/EMR	11	100% (11/11)	0% (0/11)	0% (0/11)	0% (0/11)
Dieulafoy	5	100% (5/5)	80% (4/5)	0% (0/5)	80% (4/5)	Post-balloon dilatation	1	100% (1/1)	0% (0/1)	0% (0/1)	0% (0/1)
Postampullectomy	4	75% (3/4)	33.3% (1/3)	0% (0/3)	33.3% (1/3)	Postsphincterotomy	5	80% (4/5)	0% (0/4)	0% (0/4)	0% (0/4)
Arterial bleeding cystgastrostomy tube site	2	100% (2/2)	0% (0/2)	0% (0/2)	0% (0/2)	Duodenal diverticular bleed	1	0% (0/1)	N/A	N/A	N/A
Total	131	91.6% (120/131)	17.6% (16/91)	12.1% (11/91)	25.8% (31/120)	Total	31	93.5% (29/31)	0% (0/29)	0% (0/29)	0% (0/29)

Abbreviations: PEG, percutaneous endoscopic gastrostomy.
* Includes both early and delayed rebleeding.

TC-325 in the Management of Peptic Ulcer Bleeding

In terms of the efficacy of TC-325 specifically in the management PUD bleeding, the initial study by Sung and colleagues[69] showed very promising results (immediate hemostasis of 95% and rebleeding of 10.5%); however, the subsequent series by Smith and colleagues[78] demonstrated a much more modest rate of immediate hemostasis and 7-day rebleeding rate of 76% (19/25) and 15.8% (3/19), respectively, when TC-325 was used as monotherapy for ulcer bleeding. Overall, there are a total of 86 PUD bleeds treated with TC-325 reported in the literature with an immediate hemostasis rate of 89.5% (77/86) and a 7-day rebleeding rate of 22.1% (17/77).[11,71,75,77,78,69]

The variable reported efficacy of TC-325 might be related to the fact that the hemostatic powder was often used as a salvage modality following failure with standard endoscopic therapy. Also, it is important to remember that TC-325 has not been shown to induce tissue healing. In addition, powder residency time is most likely less than or equal to 24 hours; therefore, lesions that are at high risk of rebleeding beyond the 24-hour period, such as ulcers with high-risk stigmata, may not be adequately treated with TC-325 as monotherapy. As such, a second modality including endoclips or thermal therapy should be considered following TC-325 use either during the index endoscopy or on second look.

TC-325 in the Management of Malignant Nonvariceal Upper Gastrointestinal Bleeding

GI bleeding arising from malignant tumors is increasingly recognized as a result of oncologic advances and improved detection methods and stems from local vessel damage and tumor invasion with associated derangements in the hemostatic system.[79,80] The authors performed the first case series of 5 patients with malignant UGIB treated with TC-325 and showed promising results with an initial hemostasis of 100% and only 1 case of rebleeding.[70] Leblanc and colleagues[72] subsequently published a case series showing very similar results in 5 patients with a 100% immediate hemostasis and 2 cases of rebleeding. Most recently, the authors' center looked at the largest retrospective series of tumor bleeding from the upper GI tract treated with TC-325, which included a total of 19 patients. Immediate hemostasis was excellent at 100% (19/19), with early ($\leq$72 hours) and delayed (>72 hours) rebleeding rates of 5.3% (1/19) and 31.6% (6/19), respectively.[11] There are a total of 28 cases of malignant NVUGIB reported in the literature with a combined immediate hemostasis of 100% (28/28), early rebleeding of 4.3% (1/23), and a 7-day rebleeding of 25% (7/28).[11,71,72,75]

Conventional endoscopic hemostasis methods improve outcomes in UGIB due to PUDs and other nonvariceal benign bleeding lesions of the upper, and perhaps the lower, GI tract. In contradistinction, data on their use in hemorrhagic, upper, or lower GI neoplasms are scarce and associated with varying success in immediate hemostasis and high rebleeding rates.[81–85] Other recognized single- or multimodality treatment approaches include radiation therapy, interventional angiography, and surgery all exhibit disappointing rebleeding rates, and in the case of emergency surgery, high mortality.[82,86–89] Challenges associated with bleeding tumors include hematologic derangements such as thrombocytopenia, disseminated intravascular coagulation, and neutropenia as well as the endoscopic manipulation of friable, diffusely bleeding surfaces when attempting hemostasis.[70,80,90] TC-325 with its noncontact and nontraumatic application and its ability to cover a large irregular surface of bleeding may be the ideal modality for tumor bleeding. The excellent immediate hemostasis and early rebleeding rate highlights TC-325's possible role as a temporizing agent, which could allow for more definitive therapy such as radiation therapy and nonemergent surgery to occur. A randomized controlled trial comparing TC-325 to current standard of care for malignant GI bleeding (GIB) is currently underway at the authors' center to better characterize the role of this novel hemostatic powder in tumor bleeding (NCT02135627).

TC-325 in Portal-Hypertensive and Esophagogastric Variceal Gastrointestinal Bleeding

The use of TC-325 in variceal bleeding is currently contraindicated as per the company's labeling because of the theoretic risk of embolization into a low-pressure system. Nonetheless, a few small studies have emerged describing its efficacy and safety in the management of variceal bleeding and other portal-hypertensive bleeding pathologic abnormalities.[71,75,91–95] Holster and colleagues[91] were the first to describe the successful use of TC-325 in the management of bleeding gastric varices refractory to cyanoacrylate injection. Since this initial report, there have been 20 cases of portal-hypertensive GI bleeding published in the literature including 9 cases of esophageal varices, 4 cases of gastric varices, 4 cases portal-hypertensive gastropathies, 2 cases of postbanding ulcers, and 1 case of hypertensive colopathy.[71,75,91–95] The overall hemostasis was 100% (20/20) with no documented cases of rebleeding.

Although the preliminary results on the use of TC-325 in variceal bleeding suggest it is safe and effective, more data are needed to recommend its use. There exists no reported systemic embolization with TC-325 use in variceal bleeding, even though the sample size is quite small with only 8 cases described in the literature. In addition, given the short residency time of the powder and the inability to obliterate varices, TC-325 may not prove to be a definite therapy for variceal bleeding and will most likely serve as a salvaging or bridging therapeutic option.

TC-325 in the Management of Lower Gastrointestinal Bleeding

Soulellis and colleagues[74] were the first to report TC-325 use in LGIB in a small case series of 4 patients with postpolypectomy bleeding (2 patients), Dieulafoy lesion, and radiation proctitis showing excellent immediate hemostasis of 100% and no rebleeding. A few case reports and small case series were then described using TC-325 in a variety of LGIB pathologic abnormalities, such as AVM, Dieulafoy, radiation proctitis, diverticulum, anastomotic ulcer, colonic ulcer, nonsteroidal anti-inflammatory drug colitis, tumor bleeding, postpolypectomy, postrectal endoscopic submucosal dissection (ESD), and postbiopsy.[74,75,96–99] Overall, there are a total of 28 cases of LGIB treated with TC-325 reported in the literature. Immediate hemostasis is excellent at 100% with only 2 cases of rebleeding (see **Table 1**).

Complications Related to TC-325 Use

Although there is a theoretic risk of vascular embolization, bowel perforation, and bowel obstruction with TC-325 use, animal studies have not demonstrated any of these complications.[68,100] There are a total of 243 cases of TC-325 use in the GI tract published in the literature with only 5 reported complications at the time of this review. Pain on the delivery of TC-325 was only documented in 1 patient[11]; however, anecdotally, the authors think that this is an underestimation of a relatively common transient side effect associated with the delivery of the powder under CO_2 pressure. Interestingly, Moosavi and colleagues[73] recently described a case of transient biliary obstruction with TC-325 use in a case of postsphincterotomy UGIB highlighting the need for cautious hemostatic powder application in this region. Smith and colleagues[94] reported 1 case of viscus perforation following TC-325 application in UGIB from portal-hypertensive gastropathy; however, according to the authors, the patient was extremely ill and it was unclear whether it was the instrumentation of the stomach with the gastroscope or the application of TC-325 that resulted in the perforation.

Finally, Yau and colleagues[77] reported 1 case of hemoperitoneum on day 0 and 1 case of splenic embolization on day 29 after TC-325 application; however, once again the authors could not conclude whether this came as a direct result of TC-325 use.

Overall, TC-325 use in NVUGIB and LGIB appears to be extremely safe; however, caution should be taken when using it in pathologic abnormalities involving thin intestinal wall at high risk of perforation, such as diverticula bleeding, near the ampulla and biliary tree to avoid biliary obstruction, and variceal bleeding due to fear of embolization, although not yet reported in the literature. As with ABS and other medical devices with limited clinical experience, greater patient numbers and continuous monitoring will be required to confidently address any safety concerns.

SUGGESTED MANAGEMENT ALGORITHM

Although the exact indications for topical hemostatic agents remain inconclusive, the following describes a management approach that is based on the literature and the authors' personal experience. However, the focus is on TC-325, given that the authors have no direct experience with the other topical agents described.

Advantages associated with TC-325 include its ease of use. Unlike other endoscopic hemostatic agents, its deployment does not require en face positioning with the bleeding lesion or precise targeting due to its diffuse application from the catheter in all directions. Therefore, it could be especially helpful in bleeding lesions that are difficult to reach, or in cases of massive bleeding where the exact bleeding source

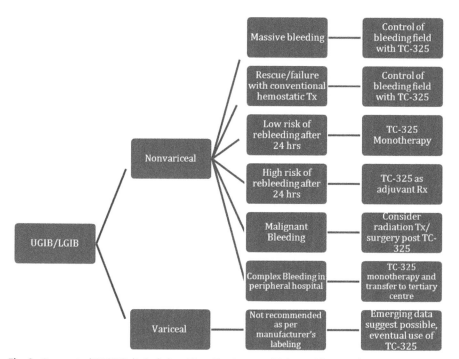

Fig. 2. Suggested TC-325 clinical algorithm. Tx, therapy. (*Adapted from* Barkun AN, Moosavi S, Martel M. Topical hemostatic agents: a systematic review with particular emphasis on endoscopic application in gastrointestinal bleeding. Gastrointest Endosc 2013;77(5):697; with permission.)

can often be hard to visualize and where immediate control of the bleeding field is crucial. In addition, TC-325 may be considered as rescue therapy following failure with standard endoscopic hemostatic modalities, which has often been the case in published reports. Retrospective data also demonstrate the luminal residency time of the hemostatic powder is probably less than 24 hours from the time of application in both the upper and the lower GI tracts. Therefore, TC-325 should probably not be used as monotherapy in lesions exhibiting a significant risk of delayed rebleeding (more than 24 hours), such as PUD lesions (that by definition are high risk since actively bleeding). In these situations, a second hemostatic agent should be considered at the time of index endoscopy or as part of a second-look endoscopy. In addition, its ability to cover large areas of bleeding and its noncontact application may make it an ideal treatment for large, friable bleeding tissues, such as those found in malignant GIB. However, given its short intestinal residency time, consideration for more definitive therapy such as radiation therapy and nonemergent surgery should be contemplated following immediate hemostasis with TC-325 in selected cases. Finally, given its ease of use and high rate of immediate hemostasis, TC-325 may emerge as a temporizing measure for complex GI bleeding in peripheral centers lacking the technical expertise for other endoscopic therapy. In other words, it may allow clinicians to attain initial hemostasis and hemodynamic stability followed by safer patient transfer to a tertiary center where more definitive endoscopic or nonendoscopic treatment may be performed. A decisional algorithm for the use of TC-325 is included in **Fig. 2**.

SUMMARY

Topical endoscopic hemostatic agents represent a novel and promising therapeutic modality for the management of GI bleeding in both the upper and lower GI tracts. This systematic review highlights the published efficacy and safety of both TC-325 and ABS, while briefly describing AMP, which has not been as extensively studied. Potential advantages with these topical agents include their ease of use, noncontact and nontraumatic application, and the ability to cover large surface areas. Immediate hemostasis rates in almost all GI bleeding pathologic abnormalities have been shown to be excellent; however, given the temporary residency time of these agents on damaged mucosa (<24 hours with TC-325), these novel products may not be adequate as monotherapy for lesions at high risk of rebleeding beyond a 24-hour period. Both TC-325 and ABS may be especially well adapted for malignant bleeding, for massive hemorrhage with poor visualization (with proximity access to the bleeding source), and as salvage therapy. Prospective controlled data and continuous safety monitoring are now needed to better characterize optimal indications for use of these hemostatic agents.

REFERENCES

1. Longstreth GF. Epidemiology of hospitalization for acute upper gastrointestinal hemorrhage: a population-based study. Am J Gastroenterol 1995;90(2):206–10.
2. van Leerdam ME, Vreeburg EM, Rauws EA, et al. Acute upper GI bleeding: did anything change? Time trend analysis of incidence and outcome of acute upper GI bleeding between 1993/1994 and 2000. Am J Gastroenterol 2003;98(7): 1494–9.
3. Laine L, Yang H, Chang SC, et al. Trends for incidence of hospitalization and death due to GI complications in the United States from 2001 to 2009. Am J Gastroenterol 2012;107(8):1190–5 [quiz: 6].

4. Abougergi MS, Travis AC, Saltzman JR. The in-hospital mortality rate for upper GI hemorrhage has decreased over 2 decades in the United States: a nation-wide analysis. Gastrointest Endosc 2014. [Epub ahead of print].
5. Longstreth GF. Epidemiology and outcome of patients hospitalized with acute lower gastrointestinal hemorrhage: a population-based study. Am J Gastroenterol 1997;92(3):419–24.
6. Farrell JJ, Friedman LS. Gastrointestinal bleeding in the elderly. Gastroenterol Clin North Am 2001;30(2):377–407, viii.
7. Sacks HS, Chalmers TC, Blum AL, et al. Endoscopic hemostasis. An effective therapy for bleeding peptic ulcers. JAMA 1990;264(4):494–9.
8. Cook DJ, Guyatt GH, Salena BJ, et al. Endoscopic therapy for acute nonvariceal upper gastrointestinal hemorrhage: a meta-analysis. Gastroenterology 1992; 102(1):139–48.
9. Sundaram CP, Keenan AC. Evolution of hemostatic agents in surgical practice. Indian J Urol 2010;26(3):374–8.
10. Barkun AN, Moosavi S, Martel M. Topical hemostatic agents: a systematic review with particular emphasis on endoscopic application in GI bleeding. Gastrointest Endosc 2013;77(5):692–700.
11. Chen YI, Barkun A, Nolan S. Hemostatic powder TC-325 in the management of upper and lower gastrointestinal bleeding: a two-year experience at a single institution. Endoscopy 2014;47:167–71.
12. Kurt M, Onal I, Akdogan M, et al. Ankaferd Blood Stopper for controlling gastrointestinal bleeding due to distinct benign lesions refractory to conventional antihemorrhagic measures. Can J Gastroenterol 2010;24(6):380–4.
13. Aydin S. Haemostatic actions of the folkloric medicinal plant extract Ankaferd Blood Stopper. J Int Med Res 2009;37(1):279.
14. Haznedaroglu BZ, Haznedaroglu IC, Walker SL, et al. Ultrastructural and morphological analyses of the in vitro and in vivo hemostatic effects of Ankaferd Blood Stopper. Clin Appl Thromb Hemost 2010;16(4):446–53.
15. Karabiyik A, Yilmaz E, Gulec S, et al. The dual diverse dynamic reversible effects of Ankaferd Blood Stopper on EPCR and PAI-1 inside vascular endothelial cells with and without LPS challenge. Turk J Haematol 2012;29(4):361–6.
16. Kandemir O, Buyukates M, Kandemir NO, et al. Demonstration of the histopathological and immunohistochemical effects of a novel hemostatic agent, Ankaferd Blood Stopper, on vascular tissue in a rat aortic bleeding model. J Cardiothorac Surg 2010;5:110.
17. Sheela ML, Ramakrishna MK, Salimath BP. Angiogenic and proliferative effects of the cytokine VEGF in Ehrlich ascites tumor cells is inhibited by Glycyrrhiza glabra. Int Immunopharmacol 2006;6(3):494–8.
18. Tasdelen Fisgin N, Tanriverdi Cayci Y, Coban AY, et al. Antimicrobial activity of plant extract Ankaferd Blood Stopper. Fitoterapia 2009;80(1):48–50.
19. Ciftci S, Keskin F, Keceli Ozcan S, et al. vitro antifungal activity of Ankaferd Blood Stopper against Candida albicans. Curr Ther Res Clin Exp 2011;72(3):120–6.
20. Demiralp Dö, Haznedaroğlu İC, Akar N. Functional proteomic analysis of Ankaferd blood stopper. Turk J Haematol 2008;27:71–7.
21. Carraway JW, Kent D, Young K, et al. Comparison of a new mineral based hemostatic agent to a commercially available granular zeolite agent for hemostasis in a swine model of lethal extremity arterial hemorrhage. Resuscitation 2008; 78(2):230–5.
22. Kheirabadi BS, Edens JW, Terrazas IB, et al. Comparison of new hemostatic granules/powders with currently deployed hemostatic products in a lethal model

of extremity arterial hemorrhage in swine. J Trauma 2009;66(2):316–26 [discussion: 327–8].

23. Ward KR, Tiba MH, Holbert WH, et al. Comparison of a new hemostatic agent to current combat hemostatic agents in a Swine model of lethal extremity arterial hemorrhage. J Trauma 2007;63(2):276–83 [discussion: 283–4].

24. Holster IL, De Maat MP, Ducharme R, et al. In vitro examination of the effects of the hemostatic powder (Hemospray) on coagulation and thrombus formation in humans. Gastrointest Endosc 2012;AB240.

25. EndoClot Plus I. Available at: http://endoclot.com/products.html. Accessed December, 2014.

26. Huang R, Pan Y, Hui N, et al. Polysaccharide hemostatic system for hemostasis management in colorectal endoscopic mucosal resection. Dig Endosc 2014; 26(1):63–8.

27. Goker H, Haznedaroglu IC, Ercetin S, et al. Haemostatic actions of the folkloric medicinal plant extract Ankaferd Blood Stopper. J Int Med Res 2008;36(1): 163–70.

28. Baykul T, Alanoglu EG, Kocer G. Use of Ankaferd Blood Stopper as a hemostatic agent: a clinical experience. J Contemp Dent Pract 2010;11(1):E088–94.

29. Beyazit Y, Kart T, Kuscu A, et al. Successful management of bleeding after dental procedures with application of blood stopper: a single center prospective trial. J Contemp Dent Pract 2011;12(5):379–84.

30. Leblebisatan G, Bay A, Karakus SC, et al. Topical Ankaferd hemostat application for the management of oral cavity bleedings in children with hemorrhagic diathesis. Blood Coagul Fibrinolysis 2012;23(6):494–7.

31. Odabas ME, Erturk M, Cinar C, et al. Cytotoxicity of a new hemostatic agent on human pulp fibroblasts in vitro. Med Oral Patol Oral Cir Bucal 2011;16(4):e584–7.

32. Alpay A, Evren C, Bektas S, et al. Effects of the folk medicinal plant extract Ankaferd Blood Stopper(R) on the ocular surface. Cutan Ocul Toxicol 2011;30(4): 280–5.

33. Alpay A, Ugurbas SC, Evren C, et al. Use of a novel haemostatic agent: ankaferd blood stopper in conjunctival incisions. Clin Exp Ophthalmol 2011;39(8): 793–8.

34. Alpay A, Bektas S, Alpay A, et al. Effects of a new hemostatic agent Ankaferd Blood Stopper((R)) on the intraocular tissues in rat model. Cutan Ocul Toxicol 2012;31(2):128–31.

35. Isler SC, Demircan S, Cakarer S, et al. Effects of folk medicinal plant extract Ankaferd Blood Stopper on early bone healing. J Appl Oral Sci 2010;18(4):409–14.

36. Yalcinkaya FR, Kerem M, Guven EO, et al. The effect of Ankaferd to stop bleeding in experimental partial nephrectomy. Bratisl Lek Listy 2011;112(12):676–8.

37. Huri E, Akgul T, Ayyildiz A, et al. First clinical experience of Ankaferd BloodStopper as a hemostatic agent in partial nephrectomy. Kaohsiung J Med Sci 2010; 26(9):493–5.

38. Kilic O, Gonen M, Acar K, et al. Haemostatic role and histopathological effects of a new haemostatic agent in a rat bladder haemorrhage model: an experimental trial. BJU Int 2010;105(12):1722–5.

39. Huri E, Akgul T, Ayyildiz A, et al. Hemostasis in retropubic radical prostatectomy with Ankaferd BloodStopper: a case report. Kaohsiung J Med Sci 2009;25(8): 445–7.

40. Aysan E, Bektas H, Ersoz F, et al. Ability of the ankaferd blood stopper(R) to prevent parenchymal bleeding in an experimental hepatic trauma model. Int J Clin Exp Med 2010;3(3):186–91.

41. Karakaya K, Ucan HB, Tascilar O, et al. Evaluation of a new hemostatic agent Ankaferd Blood Stopper in experimental liver laceration. J Invest Surg 2009; 22(3):201–6.
42. Bilgili H, Kosar A, Kurt M, et al. Hemostatic efficacy of Ankaferd Blood Stopper in a swine bleeding model. Med Princ Pract 2009;18(3):165–9.
43. Kalayci MU, Soylu A, Eroglu HE, et al. Effect of ankaferd blood stopper on hemostasis and histopathological score in experimental liver injury. Bratisl Lek Listy 2010;111(4):183–8.
44. Akarsu C, Kalayci MU, Yavuz E, et al. Comparison of the hemostatic efficiency of Ankaferd Blood Stopper and fibrin glue on a liver laceration model in rats. Ulus Travma Acil Cerrahi Derg 2011;17(4):308–12 [in Turkish].
45. Iynen I, Sogut O, Kose R. The efficacy of Ankaferd Blood Stopper in heparin-induced hemostatic abnormality in a rat epistaxis model. Otolaryngol Head Neck Surg 2011;145(5):840–4.
46. Kelles M, Kalcioglu MT, Samdanci E, et al. Ankaferd blood stopper is more effective than adrenaline plus lidocaine and gelatin foam in the treatment of epistaxis in rabbits. Curr Ther Res Clin Exp 2011;72(5):185–94.
47. Kurtaran H, Ark N, Serife Ugur K, et al. Effects of a topical hemostatic agent on an epistaxis model in rabbits. Curr Ther Res Clin Exp 2010;71(2):105–10.
48. Kurt M, Oztas E, Kuran S, et al. Tandem oral, rectal, and nasal administrations of Ankaferd Blood Stopper to control profuse bleeding leading to hemodynamic instability. Am J Emerg Med 2009;27(5):631.e1–2.
49. Al B, Yildirim C, Cavdar M, et al. Effectiveness of Ankaferd blood stopper in the topical control of active bleeding due to cutaneous-subcutaneous incisions. Saudi Med J 2009;30(12):1520–5.
50. Teker AM, Korkut AY, Gedikli O, et al. Prospective, controlled clinical trial of Ankaferd Blood Stopper in children undergoing tonsillectomy. Int J Pediatr Otorhinolaryngol 2009;73(12):1742–5.
51. Ergenoglu MU, Yerebakan H, Kucukaksu DS. A new practical alternative for the control of sternal bleeding during cardiac surgery: Ankaferd Blood Stopper. Heart Surg Forum 2010;13(6):E379–80.
52. Kilicgun A, Sarikas NG, Korkmaz T, et al. Effect of Ankaferd Blood Stopper on air leakage in the lung and prevention of bleeding: an experimental study. J Cardiothorac Surg 2011;6:20.
53. Turhan N, Bilgili H, Captug O, et al. Evaluation of a haemostatic agent in rabbits. Afr J Tradit Complement Altern Med 2011;8(1):61–5.
54. Akbal E, Koklu S, Astarci HM, et al. Oral high-dose ankaferd administration effects on gastrointestinal system. Int J Med Sci 2013;10(4):451–6.
55. Bilgili H, Captug O, Kosar A, et al. Oral systemic administration of Ankaferd blood stopper has no short-term toxicity in an in vivo rabbit experimental model. Clin Appl Thromb Hemost 2010;16(5):533–6.
56. Akbal E, Koklu S, Karaca G, et al. Beneficial effects of Ankaferd Blood Stopper on caustic esophageal injuries: an experimental model. Dis Esophagus 2012; 25(3):188–94.
57. Kurt M, Disibeyaz S, Akdogan M, et al. Endoscopic application of ankaferd blood stopper as a novel experimental treatment modality for upper gastrointestinal bleeding: a case report. Am J Gastroenterol 2008;103(8): 2156–8.
58. Beyazit Y, Onder FO, Torun S, et al. Topical application of ankaferd hemostat in a patient with gastroduodenal amyloidosis complicated with gastrointestinal bleeding. Blood Coagul Fibrinolysis 2013;24(7):762–5.

59. Gungor G, Goktepe MH, Biyik M, et al. Efficacy of ankaferd blood stopper application on non-variceal upper gastrointestinal bleeding. World J Gastrointest Endosc 2012;4(12):556–60.

60. Karaman A, Baskol M, Gursoy S, et al. Endoscopic topical application of Ankaferd Blood Stopper(R) in gastrointestinal bleeding. J Altern Complement Med 2012;18(1):65–8.

61. Karaman A, Torun E, Gursoy S, et al. Efficacy of Ankaferd Blood Stopper in post-polypectomy bleeding. J Altern Complement Med 2010;16(10):1027–8.

62. Kurt M, Akdogan M, Onal IK, et al. Endoscopic topical application of Ankaferd Blood Stopper for neoplastic gastrointestinal bleeding: a retrospective analysis. Dig Liver Dis 2010;42(3):196–9.

63. Kurt M, Kacar S, Onal IK, et al. Ankaferd Blood Stopper as an effective adjunctive hemostatic agent for the management of life-threatening arterial bleeding of the digestive tract. Endoscopy 2008;40(Suppl 2):E262.

64. Purnak T, Ozaslan E, Beyazit Y, et al. Upper gastrointestinal bleeding in a patient with defective hemostasis successfully treated with ankaferd blood stopper. Phytother Res 2011;25(2):312–3.

65. Turhan N, Kurt M, Shorbagi A, et al. Topical Ankaferd Blood Stopper administration to bleeding gastrointestinal carcinomas decreases tumor vascularization. Am J Gastroenterol 2009;104(11):2874–7.

66. Ozaslan E, Purnak T, Yildiz A, et al. The effect of Ankaferd blood stopper on severe radiation colitis. Endoscopy 2009;41(Suppl 2):E321–2.

67. Giday SA, Kim Y, Krishnamurty DM, et al. Long-term randomized controlled trial of a novel nanopowder hemostatic agent (TC-325) for control of severe arterial upper gastrointestinal bleeding in a porcine model. Endoscopy 2011;43(4):296–9.

68. Giday S, Van Alstine W, Van Vleet J, et al. Safety analysis of a hemostatic powder in a porcine model of acute severe gastric bleeding. Dig Dis Sci 2013; 58(12):3422–8.

69. Sung JJ, Luo D, Wu JC, et al. Early clinical experience of the safety and effectiveness of Hemospray in achieving hemostasis in patients with acute peptic ulcer bleeding. Endoscopy 2011;43(4):291–5.

70. Chen YI, Barkun AN, Soulellis C, et al. Use of the endoscopically applied hemostatic powder TC-325 in cancer-related upper GI hemorrhage: preliminary experience (with video). Gastrointest Endosc 2012;75(6):1278–81.

71. Holster IL, Kuipers EJ, Tjwa ET. Hemospray in the treatment of upper gastrointestinal hemorrhage in patients on antithrombotic therapy. Endoscopy 2013; 45(1):63–6.

72. Leblanc S, Vienne A, Dhooge M, et al. Early experience with a novel hemostatic powder used to treat upper GI bleeding related to malignancies or after therapeutic interventions (with videos). Gastrointest Endosc 2013;78(1):169–75.

73. Moosavi S, Chen YI, Barkun AN. TC-325 application leading to transient obstruction of a post-sphincterotomy biliary orifice. Endoscopy 2013;45(Suppl 2 UCTN):E130.

74. Soulellis CA, Carpentier S, Chen YI, et al. Lower GI hemorrhage controlled with endoscopically applied TC-325 (with videos). Gastrointest Endosc 2013;77:504–7.

75. Sulz MC, Frei R, Meyenberger C, et al. Routine use of Hemospray for gastrointestinal bleeding: prospective two-center experience in Switzerland. Endoscopy 2014;46(7):619–24.

76. Tarantino I, Barresi L, Granata A, et al. Hemospray for arterial hemorrhage following endoscopic ultrasound-guided pseudocyst drainage. Endoscopy 2014;46(Suppl 1 UCTN):E71.

77. Yau AH, Ou G, Galorport C, et al. Safety and efficacy of Hemospray(R) in upper gastrointestinal bleeding. Can J Gastroenterol Hepatol 2014;28(2):72–6.
78. Smith LA, Stanley AJ, Bergman JJ, et al. Hemospray application in nonvariceal upper gastrointestinal bleeding: results of the survey to evaluate the application of hemospray in the luminal tract. J Clin Gastroenterol 2013;48:e89–92.
79. Pereira J, Phan T. Management of bleeding in patients with advanced cancer. Oncologist 2004;9(5):561–70.
80. Dutcher JP. Hematologic abnormalities in patients with nonhematologic malignancies. Hematol Oncol Clin North Am 1987;1(2):281–99.
81. Akhtar K, Byrne JP, Bancewicz J, et al. Argon beam plasma coagulation in the management of cancers of the esophagus and stomach. Surg Endosc 2000; 14(12):1127–30.
82. Heller SJ, Tokar JL, Nguyen MT, et al. Management of bleeding GI tumors. Gastrointest Endosc 2010;72(4):817–24.
83. Laukka MA, Wang KK. Endoscopic Nd:YAG laser palliation of malignant duodenal tumors. Gastrointest Endosc 1995;41(3):225–9.
84. Loftus EV, Alexander GL, Ahlquist DA, et al. Endoscopic treatment of major bleeding from advanced gastroduodenal malignant lesions. Mayo Clin Proc 1994;69(8):736–40.
85. Savides TJ, Jensen DM, Cohen J, et al. Severe upper gastrointestinal tumor bleeding: endoscopic findings, treatment, and outcome. Endoscopy 1996; 28(2):244–8.
86. Blackshaw GR, Stephens MR, Lewis WG, et al. Prognostic significance of acute presentation with emergency complications of gastric cancer. Gastric Cancer 2004;7(2):91–6.
87. Poultsides GA, Kim CJ, Orlando R 3rd, et al. Angiographic embolization for gastroduodenal hemorrhage: safety, efficacy, and predictors of outcome. Arch Surg 2008;143(5):457–61.
88. Ripoll C, Banares R, Beceiro I, et al. Comparison of transcatheter arterial embolization and surgery for treatment of bleeding peptic ulcer after endoscopic treatment failure. J Vasc Interv Radiol 2004;15(5):447–50.
89. Sudheendra D, Venbrux AC, Noor A, et al. Radiologic techniques and effectiveness of angiography to diagnose and treat acute upper gastrointestinal bleeding. Gastrointest Endosc Clin N Am 2011;21(4):697–705.
90. Cheng AW, Chiu PW, Chan PC, et al. Endoscopic hemostasis for bleeding gastric stromal tumors by application of hemoclip. J Laparoendosc Adv Surg Tech A 2004;14(3):169–71.
91. Holster IL, Poley JW, Kuipers EJ, et al. Controlling gastric variceal bleeding with endoscopically applied hemostatic powder (Hemospray(TM)). J Hepatol 2012; 57(6):1397–8.
92. Ibrahim M, El-Mikkawy A, Mostafa I, et al. Endoscopic treatment of acute variceal hemorrhage by using hemostatic powder TC-325: a prospective pilot study. Gastrointest Endosc 2013;78(5):769–73.
93. Ibrahim M, Lemmers A, Deviere J. Novel application of Hemospray to achieve hemostasis in post-variceal banding esophageal ulcers that are actively bleeding. Endoscopy 2014;46(Suppl 1 UCTN):E263.
94. Smith LA, Morris AJ, Stanley AJ. The use of hemospray in portal hypertensive bleeding; a case series. J Hepatol 2014;60(2):457–60.
95. Stanley AJ, Smith LA, Morris AJ. Use of hemostatic powder (Hemospray) in the management of refractory gastric variceal hemorrhage. Endoscopy 2013; 45(Suppl 2 UCTN):E86–7.

96. Curcio G, Granata A, Traina M. Hemospray for multifocal bleeding following ultra-low rectal endoscopic submucosal dissection. Dig Endosc 2014;26(4): 606–7.

97. Granata A, Curcio G, Azzopardi N, et al. Hemostatic powder as rescue therapy in a patient with H1N1 influenza with uncontrolled colon bleeding. Gastrointest Endosc 2013;78(3):451.

98. Holster IL, Brullet E, Kuipers EJ, et al. Hemospray treatment is effective for lower gastrointestinal bleeding. Endoscopy 2014;46(1):75–8.

99. Kratt T, Lange J, Konigsrainer A, et al. Successful Hemospray treatment for recurrent diclofenac-induced severe diffuse lower gastrointestinal bleeding avoiding the need for colectomy. Endoscopy 2014;46(Suppl 1 UCTN):E173–4.

100. Giday SA. Preliminary data on the nanopowder hemostatic agent TC-325 to control gastrointestinal bleeding. Gastroenterol Hepatol (N Y) 2011;7(9):620–2.

New Technologies and Approaches to Endoscopic Control of Gastrointestinal Bleeding

 CrossMark

Larissa L. Fujii-Lau, MD[a], Louis M. Wong Kee Song, MD[b],
Michael J. Levy, MD[b],*

KEYWORDS

- Over-the-scope clip • Endoscopic suturing • Radiofrequency ablation • Cryotherapy
- Endoscopic ultrasound • Gastrointestinal bleeding • Hemostasis

KEY POINTS

- Emerging approaches for endoscopic hemostasis include over-the-scope clips, endoscopic suturing, mucosal ablation devices, fibrin glue injection, hemostatic spray, and endoscopic ultrasound-guided angiotherapy.
- These novel techniques may be applied as initial treatment or as rescue therapy for refractory bleeding.
- Given the experimental nature of some of these new devices for hemostasis, adequate informed consent is essential.
- The successful application of these technologies depends on proper lesion selection and operator experience in the use of these devices.

INTRODUCTION

Gastrointestinal (GI) bleeding is a common problem encountered by all gastroenterologists. Established endoscopic techniques to assist in the treatment of GI bleeding include epinephrine injection, through-the-scope clips, monopolar or bipolar coagulation, and band ligation. Because refractory GI bleeding may occur despite these therapies, new technologies are emerging to assist in the treatment algorithm. These include endoscopic methods (ie, over-the-scope clips [OTSC; Ovesco Endoscopy AG, Tubingen, Germany], endoscopic suturing, hemostatic sprays, mucosal ablation

Disclosures: None.
[a] Division of Gastroenterology and Hepatology, Washington University, 660 S. Euclid Ave Campus, Box 8124, St Louis, MO 63110, USA; [b] Division of Gastroenterology and Hepatology, Mayo Clinic, 200 1st Street Southwest, Rochester, MN 55905, USA
* Corresponding author. Mayo Clinic, 200 1st Street Southwest, Rochester, MN 55905.
E-mail address: levy.michael@mayo.edu

Gastrointest Endoscopy Clin N Am 25 (2015) 553–567
http://dx.doi.org/10.1016/j.giec.2015.02.005
1052-5157/15/$ – see front matter © 2015 Elsevier Inc. All rights reserved.

devices, stent placement, fibrin glue injection) and endoscopic ultrasound (EUS)-guided angiotherapy (ie, coil and/or glue injection). This article highlights the technique and clinical application of these new technologies. Hemostatic sprays, stent placement for hemostasis, and injection therapy are discussed elsewhere in this issue.

EMERGING ENDOSCOPIC THERAPIES FOR GASTROINTESTINAL BLEEDING
Endoscopic Over-the-Scope Clip

Technique

An OTSC has been approved in the United States since 2011 for endoscopic therapy of GI defects.[1] The caps are available in three diameters (11, 12, and 14 mm) and two working depths (3 and 6 mm), whereas the clip itself has three types of teeth (atraumatic or blunt-toothed, traumatic or sharp-toothed, and gastrostomy closure). Typically the atraumatic or traumatic clip is used for hemostasis (**Fig. 1**). The setup and deployment of the OTSC system is similar to a band ligator. The OTSC cap is affixed at the tip of the endoscope, with a string wire that runs through the scope channel connected to the deployment system that sits at the entrance port of the suction channel. Once the targeted lesion is identified, suction is applied to bring the entire lesion into the cap, followed by clip release by rotating the hand wheel of the deployment system. For fibrotic or indurated lesions, such as chronic ulcers, a dedicated tripronged anchoring device can be used to help retract the targeted lesion into the cap.

A Padlock clip (Aponos Medical Corp, Kingston, NH) is another OTSC. With this clip, the wire runs alongside the shaft of the endoscope, leaving the suction channel free to allow for better suction capability and passage of other accessories. Deployment is achieved by squeezing a handheld device. The clip has six circumferential prongs that provide radial compression on all sides and has been shown to be effective for closure of defects made in porcine stomachs and colons.[2,3] However, there are no clinical publications to date regarding its application for GI hemostasis.

Clinical applications

A randomized trial compared the OTSC with two standard hemoclips (Resolution Clip, Boston Scientific, Natick, MA; and QuickClip2, Olympus, Tokyo, Japan) on spurting vessels created at several different locations in an ex vivo porcine stomach.[1] All 45 sites (15 for each clip) were successfully treated with the assigned clip. The OTSC required significantly less time and number of clips to achieve hemostasis compared with the other clips. In the fundus, the OTSC was also thought to be more effective in

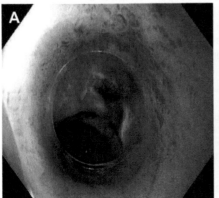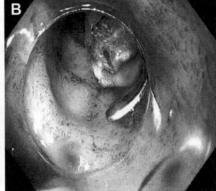

Fig. 1. (*A*) Duodenal ulcer with pigmented protuberance. (*B*) Over-the-scope clip placement.

changing the pressure measured within the vessel before and after clip placement. Similarly, a study measuring the pressure difference among clips found a significant increase in mean pressure favoring OTSC and resulting in a significant decrease in mean vessel diameter compared with the Resolution clip, QuickClip, and TriClip (Cook Medical, Limerick, Ireland).[4] The ability of the OTSC to grasp more tissue and provide greater compressive force likely translated to the observed study findings.

Chan and colleagues[5] recently described a case series on the use of the OTSC in patients with refractory (N = 6) or major bleeding caused by gastric ulcers (N = 2), duodenal ulcers (N = 5), gastric GI stromal tumor (GIST; N = 1), and ulcerative pancreatic adenocarcinoma (N = 1). The ulcers all had visible vessels and were a median of 2.5 cm (range, 1–4) in size. The technical success of achieving hemostasis during the procedure was 100%, whereas the efficacy of preventing rebleeding was achieved in seven patients (78%). The two patients who rebled had duodenal ulcers.

In a larger multicenter case series, 30 patients with refractory GI bleeding who failed conventional endoscopic therapies underwent OTSC placement.[6] Bleeding was attributed to duodenal ulcers (N = 12), gastric ulcers (N = 6), colonic endoscopic mucosal resection (N = 5), Mallory-Weiss tear (N = 2), Dieulafoy lesions (N = 2), surgical anastomosis (N = 1), colonic endoscopic submucosal dissection (ESD; N = 1), and colonic diverticulum (N = 1). Primary hemostasis immediately following OTSC placement occurred in 29 patients (97%); one patient with a posterior duodenal bulb ulcer required interventional radiology (IR) embolization for failed hemostasis. Two patients (one gastric and one duodenal bulb ulcer) rebled at 12 and 24 hours after the procedure, and they were successfully retreated with epinephrine injection to the surrounding mucosa.

The disadvantages of the OTSC are that it requires the scope to be withdrawn to load the device, the OTSC cap may make traversing the cricopharyngeus or luminal stenoses difficult, the challenge in accessing lesions in the posterior-inferior duodenal wall or the proximal lesser curvature of the stomach, and its cost. Prospective randomized trials comparing the OTSC with standard through-the-scope clips are awaited to determine its clinical role in the treatment algorithm of GI bleeding.

Endoscopic Suturing

Technique

Only one endoscopic suturing device (OverStitch; Apollo Endosurgery, Austin, TX) is currently available for clinical use. This device is mounted on a double-channel endoscope (GIF-2T160 or GIF-2T180; Olympus Corporation) and consists of a suture anchor with a detachable needle tip carrying an absorbable (2-0 or 3-0 polydioxanone) or nonabsorbable (2-0 or 3-0 polypropylene) suture that is passed through one accessory channel and coupled to the curved suturing arm of the device. The device is attached by a wire that runs alongside the scope shaft to the handle portion of the system, which is affixed to the entrance port of the working channel. Squeezing the handle component activates transfer of the needle tip, movement of the suture arm, and enables passage and exit of the suture through tissue. A dedicated corkscrew retracting device (Helix; Apollo Endosurgery) or grasping forceps can be advanced through the other working channel to facilitate tissue access to the needle. A dedicated suture-cinching tool is used to tighten, secure, and cut the suture, which can be placed in an interrupted or running fashion.

Clinical applications

Currently the use of the OverStitch device in the setting of GI bleeding is limited because of the lack of widespread availability of the device and accessories, technical complexity of the suturing system requiring specific training, impaired visibility during active hemorrhage, and restricted maneuverability of the device to access all areas of the GI tract. A bench study using porcine stomachs with submucosal splenic arteries connected to a pulsatile pump containing red ink evaluated the use of a prior generation of the endoscopic suturing device (Eagle Claw II; Apollo Endosurgery and Olympus Medical Systems Corp).[7] Of the 25 total sutures placed, 17 (68%) were successful in achieving hemostasis. The reasons behind the remaining eight that failed to treat the bleeding artery included penetration through the vessel wall (N = 4), knots that were too loose to provide hemostasis (N = 2), incorrect positioning of the suture (N = 1), and failure to penetrate an edematous gastric wall (N = 1).

One potential application of endoscopic suturing for GI bleeding may be in the setting of marginal ulcerations at an anastomosis. Three patients with chronic marginal ulcers (two presented with recurrent transfusion-dependent hemorrhage) were treated with endoscopic suturing to close the ulcer bed, followed by fibrin glue (Fibrin Sealant; Baxter, Deerfield, IL) application to the sutured area.[8] Technical success with complete ulcer closure was achieved in all patients by placing one to three 2-0 nonabsorbable stitches in an interrupted fashion. During the second case, bleeding occurred during the initial suture placement, which was successfully treated with epinephrine injection. Thereafter, the authors prophylactically injected epinephrine to the area before suturing. In the two patients with recurrent GI bleeding, repeat endoscopy at 6 weeks revealed complete ulcer resolution and they remained symptom free at 6 weeks and 1 year after the procedure.

Another possible use of endoscopic suturing is to prevent GI bleeding after ESD (**Fig. 2**). At one center, 12 patients who underwent ESD (four gastric and eight colonic lesions) had their post-ESD defects completely closed with the OverStitch device.[9] The mean size of the lesion was 42.5 mm (standard deviation [SD], 14.8) and a mean of 1.6 (SD, 1) suture was required for closure. There were no immediate or delayed adverse events, including bleeding. At surveillance endoscopy 3 months later, there was complete healing of the ESD sites.

Radiofrequency Ablation

Technique
Focal radiofrequency ablation (RFA) catheters (Barrx; Covidien, Mansfield, MA) have been used to treat GI bleeding in the setting of gastric antral vascular ectasia (GAVE) (**Fig. 3**) and radiation proctitis. The focal RFA catheters have a tilting platform that contains an array of electrodes that either is mounted at the tip or passed through the working channel of the endoscope. The active electrodes range from 15 to 40 mm in length and 7.5 to 13 mm in width. The catheters are placed in direct contact with the target tissue and the penetration of thermal energy is superficial but uniform. The typical treatment protocol is two to four applications per site using an energy density of 12 J/cm^2 and power density of 40 W/cm^2. After one site is treated, the catheter is repositioned so the probe lies at the next targeted site and the process is continued until all areas have been treated.

Clinical application
Four studies have evaluated the use of RFA in the treatment of refractory GAVE and are summarized in **Table 1**.[10–13] In the lower GI tract, RFA has been used in the treatment algorithm for radiation proctopathy following pelvic radiotherapy. Four case series reporting on a total of 27 patients who underwent RFA using the HALO^{90} (Barrx, Covidien, Mansfield) (all four studies), HALO^{90} ULTRA (one study), and the HALO^{60} (one study) device for radiation proctopathy have been described.[14–17] A total of nine (33%) patients failed prior argon plasma coagulation (APC) therapy and one (7%) failed prior bipolar coagulation. Combining the results of the four studies, a

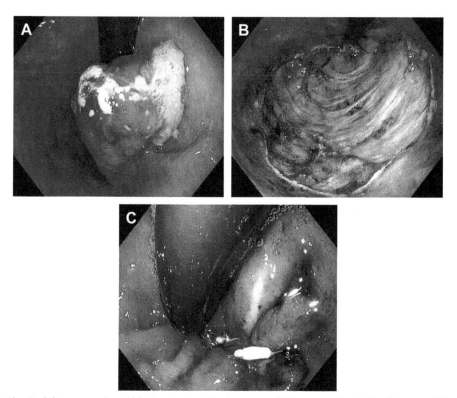

Fig. 2. (A) Large polypoid lesion in the distal rectum. (B) Large defect following ESD. (C) Complete closure of the ESD defect using an endoscopic suturing device.

mean of 1.9 (SD, 0.9) RFA sessions were performed per patient following either a full colonoscopy (N = 18) or enema-only preparation (N = 6). Clinical success with a decrease in symptoms occurred in 25 patients (93%). One patient had recurrent bleeding while on warfarin that was treated successfully with another RFA session and one patient had no change in symptoms.[15,16] Mild adverse events with the development of rectal or perianal ulcers occurred in four patients (15%); only one patient with an ulcer presented with bleeding that did not require further therapy, whereas the remaining three patients with ulcers were asymptomatic.

The limitations of RFA for GAVE using the focal catheter attached to the tip of the endoscope include the requirement to remove the scope to load the device, bulkiness of the probe making it difficult to traverse the cricopharyngeus or other areas of luminal narrowing, and need for repeated intubations to clean the probe. The disadvantages of any RFA device are its cost, limited number of pulses per probe (may require more than one probe to adequately treat the entire involved surface), and the inability to adequately contact certain areas (eg, incisura) that may require therapy.

Cryotherapy

Technique
Cryotherapy freezes the targeted tissue, resulting in cessation of blood flow in vessels less than 2 mm in size causing superficial necrosis and ulceration.[18] This results in sloughing of mucosa and re-epithelialization over several weeks.[19] The currently available endoscopic cryotherapy devices use either liquid nitrogen (CryoSpray; CSA

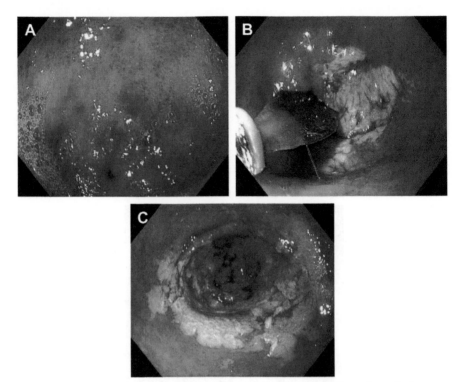

Fig. 3. (*A*) Gastric antral vascular ectasia, diffuse variant. (*B*) RFA using a through-the-scope RFA catheter. (*C*) Mucosal appearance following RFA.

Medical Inc, Lutherville, MD) or compressed carbon dioxide (CO_2) gas (Polar Wand; GI Supply, Camp Hill, PA). Because a high volume of gas is introduced with each therapy, a gastric overtube or a dedicated decompression tube is required to vent the stomach during cryotherapy application. A dedicated spray catheter is advanced through the working channel of the endoscope until it extends 1 to 2 cm distal to the tip of the endoscope. The spray is applied to the targeted mucosal surface for up to 20 seconds. A whitening of the mucosa is seen at the treated areas, signaling ice formation on the mucosa (**Fig. 4**). After each application, thawing is required while the gas is vented. The freeze-thaw cycle is repeated three to five times with each treatment session.

Clinical application

An initial pilot study using cryotherapy for the treatment of bleeding vascular lesions evaluated 26 patients (seven gastric or duodenal arteriovenous malformations, seven GAVE, five radiation-induced gastritis, and seven radiation proctopathy).[19] All had recurrent bleeding despite prior endoscopic therapy and underwent a mean of 3.4 (SD, 1.6) cryotherapy sessions using liquid nitrogen. Cryotherapy was successful in 20 patients (77%) with the formation of normal-appearing mucosa at surveillance endoscopy 6 months after therapy. Those with radiation proctopathy (100%) had the best response to cryotherapy with cessation of bleeding, followed by arteriovenous malformations (86%), GAVE (71%), and finally radiation gastritis or duodenitis (40%). Only one patient (4%) developed transient abdominal pain for which an abdominal computed tomography (CT) scan was unremarkable.

Table 1
Summary of studies on radiofrequency ablation for treatment of GAVE

Author, Year	Study Type	Definition of Refractory	Total Number of Patients	Device Used; Average[a] # Sessions	Clinical Success N (%), Definition	Average[a] Hgb (g/dL) Before/After Treatment	Adverse Events
Gross et al,[10] 2008	Prospective case series	All transfusion dependent	6	HALO[90] 1.5 (1–3)	5 (83%) no longer transfusion dependent	8.9 (12–15.5)/10.1 (9.4–11.5)	Ulcer[b] (N = 1)
McGorisk et al,[11] 2013	Prospective cohort	All failed APC and transfusion dependent	21	HALO[90] ULTRA 2 (1–3)	18 (86%) no longer transfusion dependent	7.8 (1)/10.2 (1.4)	Ulcer[b] (N = 2; 1 superficial, 1 bleeding)
Dray et al,[12] 2014	Retrospective case series	21 failed prior therapy; 23 transfusion dependent	24	HALO[90], HALO[90] ULTRA 1.8 (0.8)	15 (65%) no longer transfusion dependent	6.8 (1.4)/9.8 (1.8)	None
Raza & Diehl,[13] 2015	Retrospective case series	All failed APC and transfusion dependent	9	HALO[90] 3 (2–6)	7 (78%) no longer transfusion dependent	7.3 (1.7)/10.5 (1)	Mild abdominal pain (N = 1)

Abbreviation: APC, argon plasma coagulation.

[a] Average is reported as either mean (SD) or median (range) depending on how it was reported in the article.

[b] Found on follow-up endoscopy, resolved without intervention.

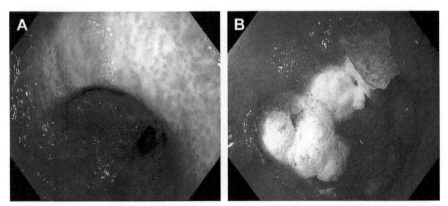

Fig. 4. (*A*) Gastric antral vascular ectasia, diffuse variant. (*B*) Application of CO_2-based cryotherapy.

Cho and colleagues[20] focused on 12 patients with GAVE treated with three sessions of CO_2-based cryotherapy. Eight (67%) had failed APC therapy. In four sessions (11%), technical problems with overtube placement (N = 1), cryogen unit (N = 1), and learning curve of the endoscopists (N = 2) limited the amount of GAVE treated to less than 90%. Six patients (50%) had a complete response (significant improvement in endoscopic appearance associated with increasing hemoglobin level and no transfusion requirements) and six patients had a partial response (incomplete ablation on endoscopy with a stable hemoglobin level and reduced transfusion requirements). Minor adverse events occurred in three patients (25%) with asymptomatic scarring or ulceration seen on surveillance endoscopy and one patient required epinephrine injection for bleeding caused by a tear of a Schatzki ring during overtube placement. Another potential application of cryotherapy in the upper GI tract includes treatment of bleeding esophageal cancer.[21]

In the lower GI tract, a prospective case series was reported on patients with radiation proctitis (N = 10) who underwent a median of one (range, 1–4) cryotherapy session with liquid nitrogen.[22] A dedicated dual-lumen venting/decompression tube was inserted to the distal sigmoid using a Savary wire and was used to vent the gas required for the procedure. Six of the seven patients (86%) who underwent cryotherapy for GI bleeding had improvement in their symptoms. One patient (10%) had rectal bleeding, requiring overnight observation 2 days following treatment, but did not require transfusions or endoscopic therapy.

ENDOSCOPIC ULTRASOUND-GUIDED ANGIOTHERAPY FOR GASTROINTESTINAL BLEEDING

With the lack of randomized control trials comparing EUS with conventional endoscopic techniques at controlling GI bleeding, EUS-guided angiotherapy has been mostly limited to experts at tertiary referral centers. EUS provides several potential advantages and disadvantages over endoscopic-guided angiotherapy, as highlighted in **Table 2**. Most reports on EUS-guided angiotherapy pertain to refractory variceal bleeding.

Endoscopic Ultrasound-Guided Coil Injection

Technique
After EUS identification of the target vessel, a fine-needle aspiration (FNA) needle is loaded with a coil. We prefer the use of 22-gauge FNA needles that allow 0.018-in coils

Table 2 Potential advantages and disadvantages of EUS over conventional endoscopic-guided angiotherapy	
Advantages	**Disadvantages**
Ability to image deep to the mucosa, visualizing submucosal vessels, and enhancing diagnosis of the source of GI bleeding	Requires fluoroscopic guidance to monitor for immediate embolization
May visualize the entire vascular network, including feeding and perforating vessels, allowing targeting of different sites	Echoendoscope has a smaller suction channel than the therapeutic endoscope, decreasing the ability to suction during active hemorrhage
Allows monitoring of treatment success through the use of Doppler imaging	Echoendoscope has a limited range of retroflexion, which may make targeting vessel in the fundus more difficult
Injection of coils before cyanoacrylate may serve as a scaffold and decrease the risk of glue embolization.[31]	High cost of repairing echoendoscope if glue becomes lodged within the scope channel

rather than larger needles and coils because of the ease of use and potential decreased risk of bleeding at the site of needle puncture. We recommend that the coiled diameter of the coil be approximately 1.25 to 1.5 times the measured diameter of the target vessel, which typically results in a 6- to 10-mm coiled diameter. To load the coil, we remove the stylet from the FNA needle, deposit the coil from the angio-catheter into the FNA needle, and use the stylet to advance the coil until it lies just short of the tip of the needle. Some prefer to use a guidewire to load the coil, but the stiffer stylet allows better pushability while not incurring the increased cost of the guidewire. Once the coil is loaded, the FNA needle is inserted through the echoen-doscope channel and the needle tip is advanced into the vessel (**Fig. 5**). We typically puncture through the entire vessel and a short distance beyond to allow anchoring of the coil and potentially decrease its risk of migration. We then slowly advance the sty-let while minimally retracting the needle to deposit most of the coil within the vessel itself, then leave the final tip of the coil at the proximal side of the vessel to serve as an additional anchor. Throughout the procedure, endosonographic and fluoroscopic images are continuously monitored to ensure proper coil placement and assess for migration. Doppler should be performed after coil insertion to document decreased or no blood flow and to determine the need for additional therapy.

Clinical application

Romero-Castro and colleagues[23] reported on the EUS-guided coil injection in four patients with gastric varices secondary to cirrhosis-related portal hypertension. A 19-gauge needle with coils that were 0.035 inches in diameter and 8 to 15 mm in coiled diameter was used in all cases. In the first patient, 13 coils were deposited into the gastric variceal complex, whereas in the following three patients two to seven coils were inserted into only the identified perforating vein. The gastric varices were erad-icated in three (75%) patients, with no adverse events, including coil migration, encountered at a median follow-up of 5 months.

The same group described a multicenter retrospective analysis on EUS-guided coil versus cyanoacrylate injection to treat gastric varices.[24] Because of its retrospective and nonrandomized study design, the two groups need to be compared cautiously.

562

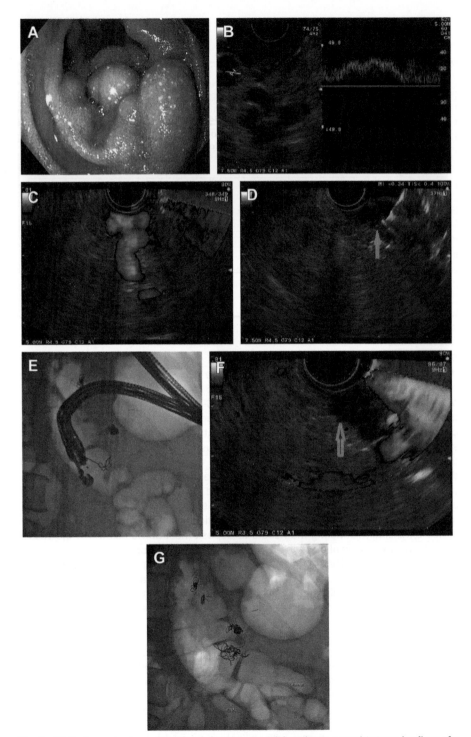

Fig. 5. (*A*) Endoscopic view of large duodenal varices. (*B*) Endosonographic Doppler flow of a duodenal varix showing a venous waveform. (*C*)Endosonographic Doppler view before coil injection. (*D*) Endosonographic view of coil injection (*arrow*). (*E*) Fluoroscopic view of the first coil being injected. (*F*) Endosonographic Doppler view after coil injection showing lack of flow (*arrow*). (*G*) Fluoroscopic view of all coils placed during the initial EUS procedure.

Of the 11 patients in the coil group, complete obliteration of the perforating vein occurred in 10 (91%). In most cases (N = 9; 82%), complete obliteration occurred after the first session. A mean of 5.8 (SD, 1.2) coils were placed per patient. Two patients (18%) required additional cyanoacrylate injection during subsequent procedures. Only one coil migrated through the gastric wall 1 month after the procedure.

At our institution, 10 patients underwent EUS-guided coil injection into esophago-gastric (N = 1), gastric only (N = 2), duodenal (N = 2), and choledochal (N = 5) varices. A mean of 4.6 (SD, 1.8) coils were placed during the index procedure into the variceal complex, whereas a mean of 7.1 (SD, 4) total coils were placed in each patient. During median follow-up of 18 months (range, 0–104 months), three patients died from their underlying disease or unrelated causes. In the remaining seven patients, four did not have any recurrent bleeding up to 8 years after their index EUS procedure. One patient with esophagogastric varices rebled from esophageal varices requiring band ligation and sclerotherapy, whereas two patients with choledochal varices rebled from their choledochal varices requiring further EUS-guided coil injection or a placement of a fully covered metal stent during endoscopic retrograde cholangiography.

Beyond treatment of varices, our institution has performed EUS-guided coil injection for an aberrant rectal artery (N = 2), intractable marginal ulcer after Roux-en-Y gastric bypass (N = 1), duodenal vascular malformation (N = 1), and descending colon arteriovenous malformation (N = 1).[25,26] After coil injection, four (80%) had no further bleeding.

Endoscopic Ultrasound-Guided Cyanoacrylate Injection

Technique
Similar to EUS-guided coil injection, the targeted vessel should be localized and thoroughly mapped during EUS before glue injection. Only after careful planning of the glue insertion do we preload the FNA needle with cyanoacrylate to minimize the risk of glue occlusion within the FNA needle. We prefer this technique over using the stylet during needle puncture and subsequent removal of the stylet before cyanoacrylate is loaded into the needle, which may potentially increase the risk of withdrawing blood into the needle and insertion of a clot or air during glue insertion. We typically use a 1:1 mixture of 2-octyl-cyanoacrylate (Dermabond; Ethicon Inc, Somerville, NJ) and lipiodol to allow fluoroscopic monitoring during glue injection. Because the risk of embolization increases with the volume of cyanoacrylate injected, we recommend to use the least amount of glue needed to achieve decreased flow through the targeted vessel.[27]

Clinical application
In a case series of five patients who underwent EUS-guided cyanoacrylate injection using a 22-gauge FNA needle into the perforating vessel, all patients had complete obliteration of the gastric varices after injecting a mean of 1.6 mL of glue.[28] During a mean follow-up of 10 months, no adverse events or recurrent bleeding were observed. Focusing on the 19 patients who underwent only EUS-guided glue embolization in the previously mentioned study, in the EUS-guided coil injection section, all 19 patients had complete obliteration of the feeding gastric vessel.[24] Only 42% of patients had successful treatment after one session of EUS-guided glue injection. A mean of 1.5 (SD, 0.1) mL of cyanoacrylate was injected per patient. Although 12 adverse events occurred in 11 patients in the cyanoacrylate group (58%), only two were symptomatic, including fever (N = 1) and chest pain (N = 1). There were nine asymptomatic pulmonary glue embolisms (47%) detected on routine chest CT scans performed in all patients, which significantly lengthened their hospital stay.

EUS-guided cyanoacrylate injection has been used at our institution to treat bleeding gastric GIST (N = 2), esophageal cancer unresponsive to APC (N = 1), duodenal ulcer refractory to IR coil embolization and surgical oversewing (N = 1), and metastatic colon cancer to the duodenum refractory to endoscopic therapy (N = 1).[26] In these patients, a median of 3.5 (range, 3–7) mL of cyanoacrylate was injected and successfully prevented recurrent bleeding during a median follow-up of 10 months (range, 0–120). Another site reported on the successful EUS-guided cyanoacrylate injection into a visceral pseudoaneurysm that failed two prior angiographic embolizations.[29] Six weeks after the procedure, CT angiogram showed almost complete resolution of the pseudoaneurysm.

Endoscopic Ultrasound-Guided Coil and Cyanoacrylate Injection

Weilert and Binmoeller[30] described an ex vivo experiment where 1 mL of cyanoacrylate was injected into heparinized blood that contained a previously placed coil. The glue clung to the fibers of the coil, allowing the glue and coil to be removed in one piece. Therefore, it was hypothesized that EUS-guided coil insertion followed by cyanoacrylate injection may decrease the risk of glue embolization.

The same group retrospectively analyzed 30 patients with acute or recent (<1 week) bleeding from gastric varices who underwent EUS-guided coil and glue embolization of a feeding vessel.[31] Technical success was reported in all 30 patients, whereas immediate hemostasis was achieved in the two patients with active bleeding. Most (93%) cases only had one coil placed and a mean of 1.4 mL of 2-octyl-cyanoacrylate injected. No immediate adverse events, including clinical evidence of pulmonary glue embolisms, occurred. Of the 24 patients with surveillance EUS, 96% had complete obliteration of the feeding vessel and no evidence of Doppler flow within the variceal complex. On endoscopic view of the area, the glue and coils were found to spontaneously extrude into the stomach and eventually form a scar. One patient had recurrent variceal bleeding 21 days after the initial procedure, which was treated with a subsequent EUS-guided coil and glue injection.

At our institution, four patients underwent combined coil and glue injection for gastric (N = 3) or duodenal (N = 1) varices that were deemed to be too large for either treatment alone. A median of seven (range, 6–8) coils and 3.25 (range, 2–3.5) mL of cyanoacrylate were injected into each patient. During subsequent follow-up of a median of 4 months (range, 1–6), all four patients had no recurrent bleeding.

Other Endoscopic Ultrasound-Guided Injectates

Standard EUS-guided injection techniques similar to those described previously have been used to inject a variety of other agents, including fibrin sealants (Tisseel Kit, Baxter Healthcare, Thetford, Norfolk, UK; or thrombin-collagen compound; D-stat, Vascular Solutions Inc, Minneapolis, MN), epinephrine, sclerosants (eg, absolute ethanol), and hyaluronate (Restylane; Medicis Anesthetics, Scottsdale, AZ). These have typically been used to treat nonvariceal GI bleeding.

There have been several case reports on EUS-guided thrombin therapy to treat pseudoaneurysms (three splenic artery and one superior mesenteric artery) secondary to pancreatitis.[32–35] These pseudoaneurysms were not able to be treated with either selective IR-guided angiotherapy or percutaneous thrombin injection because of their anatomy or location and/or presence of surrounding collateral vessels. At follow-up CT angiograms or EUS surveillance examinations, all the lesions were obliterated by the thrombin injection.

Two patients at our institution had hyaluronate injection into a bleeding gastric GIST.[26] One patient had two EUS sessions with 3 and 4 mL injected, whereas the second patient had only 1 mL of hyaluronate injected. Both patients had no subsequent bleeding 40 and 45 months, respectively, after the EUS. Four patients had absolute alcohol injected into a duodenal Dieulafoy lesion refractory to endoscopic therapy, renal cell carcinoma metastatic to the duodenum unresponsive to IR coil embolization, pancreatic pseudoaneurysm refractory to multiple IR interventions, and rectal invasion of prostate cancer. A median of 2.4 mL (range, 0.2–7.5) of alcohol was injected. Adjunctive therapy with band ligation (three bands) was performed on the duodenal Dieulafoy lesion. Three (75%) patients had no further bleeding after the EUS-guided angiotherapy, whereas the patient with rectal invasion of prostate cancer continued to bleed until he died 4 months later from unrelated causes.

SUMMARY

Several new endoscopic technologies applicable for hemostasis and EUS-guided therapies have emerged to assist in the therapy for upper and lower GI bleeding. With regard to some of these emerging techniques for endoscopic hemostasis, it is important to inform the patient and family about their experimental nature. Further studies on the long-term clinical efficacy and safety are required for all these therapies to determine their role in the treatment algorithm of GI bleeding.

REFERENCES

1. Kato M, Jung Y, Gromski MA, et al. Prospective, randomized comparison of 3 different hemoclips for the treatment of acute upper GI hemorrhage in an established experimental setting. Gastrointest Endosc 2012;75:3–10.
2. Desilets DJ, Romanelli JR, Earle DB, et al. Gastrotomy closure with the lock-it system and the Padlock-G clip: a survival study in a porcine model. J Laparoendosc Adv Surg Tech A 2010;20:671–6.
3. Guarner-Argente C, Cordova H, Martinez-Palli G, et al. Yes, we can: reliable colonic closure with the Padlock-G clip in a survival porcine study (with video). Gastrointest Endosc 2010;72:841–4.
4. Naegel A, Bolz J, Zopf Y, et al. Hemodynamic efficacy of the over-the-scope clip in an established porcine cadaveric model for spurting bleeding. Gastrointest Endosc 2012;75:152–9.
5. Chan SM, Chiu PW, Teoh AY, et al. Use of the over-the-scope clip for treatment of refractory upper gastrointestinal bleeding: a case series. Endoscopy 2014;46: 428–31.
6. Manta R, Galloro G, Mangiavillano B, et al. Over-the-scope clip (OTSC) represents an effective endoscopic treatment for acute GI bleeding after failure of conventional techniques. Surg Endosc 2013;27:3162–4.
7. Hu B, Chung SC, Sun LC, et al. Eagle Claw II: a novel endosuture device that uses a curved needle for major arterial bleeding: a bench study. Gastrointest Endosc 2005;62:266–70.
8. Jirapinyo P, Watson RR, Thompson CC. Use of a novel endoscopic suturing device to treat recalcitrant marginal ulceration (with video). Gastrointest Endosc 2012;76:435–9.
9. Kantsevoy SV, Bitner M, Mitrakov AA, et al. Endoscopic suturing closure of large mucosal defects after endoscopic submucosal dissection is technically feasible, fast, and eliminates the need for hospitalization (with videos). Gastrointest Endosc 2014;79:503–7.

10. Gross SA, Al-Haddad M, Gill KR, et al. Endoscopic mucosal ablation for the treatment of gastric antral vascular ectasia with the HALO90 system: a pilot study. Gastrointest Endosc 2008;67:324–7.
11. McGorisk T, Krishnan K, Keefer L, et al. Radiofrequency ablation for refractory gastric antral vascular ectasia (with video). Gastrointest Endosc 2013;78:584–8.
12. Dray X, Repici A, Gonzalez P, et al. Radiofrequency ablation for the treatment of gastric antral vascular ectasia. Endoscopy 2014;46:963–9.
13. Raza N, Diehl DL. Radiofrequency ablation of treatment-refractory Gastric Antral Vascular Ectasia (GAVE). Surg Laparosc Endosc Percutan Tech 2015;25(1): 79–82.
14. Zhou C, Adler DC, Becker L, et al. Effective treatment of chronic radiation proctitis using radiofrequency ablation. Therap Adv Gastroenterol 2009;2:149–56.
15. Dray X, Battaglia G, Wengrower D, et al. Radiofrequency ablation for the treatment of radiation proctitis. Endoscopy 2014;46:970–6.
16. Patel A, Pathak R, Deshpande V, et al. Radiofrequency ablation using BarRx for the endoscopic treatment of radiation proctopathy: a series of three cases. Clin Exp Gastroenterol 2014;7:453–60.
17. Pigo F, Bertani H, Manno M, et al. Radiofrequency ablation for chronic radiation proctitis: our initial experience with four cases. Tech Coloproctol 2014;18: 1089–92.
18. Pasricha PJ, Hill S, Wadwa KS, et al. Endoscopic cryotherapy: experimental results and first clinical use. Gastrointest Endosc 1999;49:627–31.
19. Kantsevoy SV, Cruz-Correa MR, Vaughn CA, et al. Endoscopic cryotherapy for the treatment of bleeding mucosal vascular lesions of the GI tract: a pilot study. Gastrointest Endosc 2003;57:403–6.
20. Cho S, Zanati S, Yong E, et al. Endoscopic cryotherapy for the management of gastric antral vascular ectasia. Gastrointest Endosc 2008;68:895–902.
21. Shah MB, Schnoll-Sussman F. Novel use of cryotherapy to control bleeding in advanced esophageal cancer. Endoscopy 2010;42(Suppl 2):E46.
22. Moawad FJ, Maydonovitch CL, Horwhat JD. Efficacy of cryospray ablation for the treatment of chronic radiation proctitis in a pilot study. Dig Endosc 2013;25: 174–9.
23. Romero-Castro R, Pellicer-Bautista F, Giovannini M, et al. Endoscopic ultrasound (EUS)-guided coil embolization therapy in gastric varices. Endoscopy 2010; 42(Suppl 2):E35–6.
24. Romero-Castro R, Ellrichmann M, Ortiz-Moyano C, et al. EUS-guided coil versus cyanoacrylate therapy for the treatment of gastric varices: a multicenter study (with videos). Gastrointest Endosc 2013;78:711–21.
25. Fujii-Lau LL, Leise MD, Kamath PS, et al. Endoscopic ultrasound-guided portal-systemic pressure gradient measurement. Endoscopy 2014;46:E654–6.
26. Law R, Fujii-Lau L, Wong Kee Song LM, et al. Efficacy of endoscopic ultrasound-guided hemostatic interventions for resistant nonvariceal bleeding. Clin Gastroenterol Hepatol 2015;13:808–12.
27. Hwang SS, Kim HH, Park SH, et al. N-butyl-2-cyanoacrylate pulmonary embolism after endoscopic injection sclerotherapy for gastric variceal bleeding. J Comput Assist Tomogr 2001;25:16–22.
28. Romero-Castro R, Pellicer-Bautista FJ, Jimenez-Saenz M, et al. EUS-guided injection of cyanoacrylate in perforating feeding veins in gastric varices: results in 5 cases. Gastrointest Endosc 2007;66:402–7.
29. Roberts KJ, Jones RG, Forde C, et al. Endoscopic ultrasound-guided treatment of visceral artery pseudoaneurysm. HPB (Oxford) 2012;14:489–90.

30. Weilert F, Binmoeller KF. EUS-guided vascular access and therapy. Gastrointest Endosc Clin N Am 2012;22:303–14, x.
31. Binmoeller KF, Weilert F, Shah JN, et al. EUS-guided transesophageal treatment of gastric fundal varices with combined coiling and cyanoacrylate glue injection (with videos). Gastrointest Endosc 2011;74:1019–25.
32. Roach H, Roberts SA, Salter R, et al. Endoscopic ultrasound-guided thrombin injection for the treatment of pancreatic pseudoaneurysm. Endoscopy 2005;37: 876–8.
33. Robinson M, Richards D, Carr N. Treatment of a splenic artery pseudoaneurysm by endoscopic ultrasound-guided thrombin injection. Cardiovasc Intervent Radiol 2007;30:515–7.
34. Lameris R, du Plessis J, Nieuwoudt M, et al. A visceral pseudoaneurysm: management by EUS-guided thrombin injection. Gastrointest Endosc 2011;73:392–5.
35. Chaves DM, Costa FF, Matuguma S, et al. Splenic artery pseudoaneurysm treated with thrombin injection guided by endoscopic ultrasound. Endoscopy 2012;44(Suppl 2 UCTN):E99–100.

Management of Patients with Rebleeding

Sunny H. Wong, MBChB, DPhil, MRCP[a,b,c], Joseph J.Y. Sung, MD, PhD, FRCP[a,b,*]

KEYWORDS

• Peptic ulcer • Rebleeding • Endoscopy • Surgery • Angiographic embolization

KEY POINTS

• Rebleeding after endoscopic hemostasis is a major risk factor for mortality.
• Risk factors for rebleeding should be recognized to identify high-risk patients.
• Newly developed devices, such as TC-325 (Hemospray; Cook Medical, Bloomington, IN) and Over-The-Scope Clip (Ovesco Endoscopy AG, Tübingen, Germany), might secure hemostasis on recurrent bleeding.
• If further rebleeding recurs after a second endoscopic attempt, transarterial angiographic embolization or surgery should be considered.
• Definitive treatment of the cause and preventive measures for peptic ulcers should always be considered to reduce disease recurrence and complications.

INTRODUCTION

Acute upper gastrointestinal bleeding is a major cause of hospitalization. Peptic ulcers accounted for 36% of all causes of acute upper gastrointestinal bleeding.[1] Despite a decreasing trend in the incidence,[2,3] peptic ulcer bleeding continues to carry a significant morbidity and mortality rate. Rebleeding may develop in up to 15% of patients after therapeutic endoscopy and is associated with a high mortality rate.[4] The mortality rate of peptic ulcer bleeding remains at about 10%.[5–7]

Medical advances over the past decades have transformed the clinical management of peptic ulcer bleeding. Endoscopic therapy has become the first-line treatment of peptic ulcer bleeding, achieving primary hemostasis in more than 90% of patients. Potent acid suppressants and eradication therapy for *Helicobacter pylori* have

Disclosure statement: The authors declare no conflict of interest.
[a] State Key Laboratory of Digestive Disease, Faculty of Medicine, Institute of Digestive Disease, The Chinese University of Hong Kong, 30-32 Ngan Shing Street, Shatin, Hong Kong, China; [b] Department of Medicine and Therapeutics, Faculty of Medicine, The Chinese University of Hong Kong, 30-32 Ngan Shing Street, Shatin, Hong Kong, China; [c] Li Ka Shing Institute of Health Sciences, Faculty of Medicine, The Chinese University of Hong Kong, 30-32 Ngan Shing Street, Shatin, Hong Kong, China
* Corresponding author. Faculty of Medicine, Institute of Digestive Disease, The Chinese University of Hong Kong, Hong Kong, China.
E-mail address: jjysung@cuhk.edu.hk

Gastrointest Endoscopy Clin N Am 25 (2015) 569–581
http://dx.doi.org/10.1016/j.giec.2015.02.007
1052-5157/15/$ – see front matter © 2015 Elsevier Inc. All rights reserved.

contributed to a decrease in hospital admissions for peptic ulcer bleeding. On the other hand, there is an increase in the number of patients taking acetylsalicylic acid and other antiplatelets for various cardiovascular diseases,[8,9] posing new challenges to disease management. These epidemiologic changes could have major implications on the disease course and outcome. Peptic ulcer bleeding is now predominantly a disease of the elderly, with more than 60% of patients older than 60 years and around 20% older than 80 years.[8] Patients with peptic ulcer bleeding now have more complex comorbidities, more diverse causes, and more elaborate lists of medications than ever before. Effective management of recurrent ulcer disease relies on the identification and modification of risk factors.

TREATMENT OF PEPTIC ULCER BLEEDING
Risk Stratification

The first step in managing patients with upper gastrointestinal bleeding is clinical evaluation and risk stratification. The aim is to determine the severity of bleeding and, hence, the priority and timing of different therapies. Patients with exsanguinating hemorrhage and unstable hemodynamics require immediate resuscitation and intensive monitoring. Prompt fluid and red cell replacement can be life saving in this situation. Nevertheless, overzealous transfusion in otherwise stable patients should be avoided, as it can be associated with higher rates of rebleeding and death.[10–13] In a randomized controlled trial involving 921 patients with severe acute upper gastrointestinal bleeding, patients receiving liberal transfusion at a hemoglobin threshold of 9 g/dL had an increased risk of further bleeding and death, compared with patients receiving transfusion only at a hemoglobin threshold of 7 g/dL.[12] Blood product transfusion also carries a risk of pulmonary edema, transfusion reaction, and blood-borne infection. Apart from the hemodynamic assessment, several risk stratification systems have been developed to predict disease outcomes. These systems include the Rockall score, which combines clinical and endoscopic parameters,[14] and the Glasgow-Blatchford score, which combines clinical and laboratory parameters to predict disease outcomes.[15] Furthermore, a risk stratification score combining albumin, International Normalized Ratio (INR), mental status assessment, systolic blood pressure and age (AIMS65) has been derived and validated in more than 60,000 patients to predict in-hospital mortality, length of stay, and costs.[16] These scores may help to risk stratify patients to different therapeutic strategies and allow some of the patients with lower risk for outpatient management.[17,18]

Pre-endoscopic Management

The role of preemptive acid suppressive therapy before endoscopy was addressed in several studies. In a randomized study involving 638 patients with upper gastrointestinal bleeding, high-dose proton-pump inhibitor was found to reduce the endoscopic grade of peptic ulcer and, hence, the need for endoscopic therapy.[19] This result was confirmed in a subsequent meta-analysis that showed an almost one-third reduction in the need for endoscopic therapy (odds ration [OR] = 0.68, 95% confidence interval [CI] = 0.50–0.93)[20]; yet there was no significant difference in blood transfusion, rebleeding, surgery, or death. The use of proton-pump inhibitors should not replace endoscopy in actively bleeding patients. In situations whereby endoscopy may be delayed or contraindicated, proton-pump inhibitor therapy improves clinical outcomes.[21]

Endoscopic Treatment

Endoscopy is now the first-line treatment of upper gastrointestinal bleeding. It has been shown to reduce further bleeding (OR = 0.38, 95% CI = 0.32–0.45), the need for surgery (OR = 0.36, 95% CI = 0.28–0.45), and mortality (OR = 0.55, 95% CI = 0.40–0.76).[22] The benefits of endoscopic therapy seem to be most significant in actively bleeding ulcers and in ulcers with a visible vessel.[23] The endoscopic grade of bleeding ulcers can be classified by the Forrest classification,[24] which predicts the risk of rebleeding and death. This classification can be used to stratify patients and guide management decisions. Peptic ulcers with high-risk features (ie, those with active spurting [IA], active oozing [IB], or nonbleeding visible bleeding vessel [IIA]) have a high risk of further bleeding and warrant endoscopic therapy to control the bleeding.[23,25] For ulcers with an adherent clot (IIB), endoscopic therapy may be performed by targeting the underlying lesion after clot removal. This strategy has been shown to reduce rebleeding as compared with medical therapy alone,[26–28] although significant heterogeneity exists among the studies.[29] Endoscopic therapy is generally not recommended for ulcers with a flat pigmented spot (IIC) or a clean base (III). Although a recent study suggested that the Forrest classification may not be accurate in predicting mortality, it remained useful to identify patients at high risk of rebleeding, especially those with Forrest IA peptic ulcers.[30]

Conventional methods of endoscopic hemostasis can be divided into injection, thermal, and mechanical methods. Although endoscopic injection of epinephrine was shown to be effective in achieving initial hemostasis,[31] injection monotherapy is insufficient for definitive hemostasis and should be coupled with a second therapy to reduce rebleeding (OR = 0.59, 95% CI = 0.44–0.80) and surgery (OR = 0.66, 95% CI = 0.49–0.89).[23,32–34] Both thermal coagulation and endoscopic clipping were effective in achieving hemostasis (81.2% vs 81.5%, P = .99) with no significant difference in rebleeding, need for surgery, and all-cause mortality.[35] These methods have become the mainstay of endoscopic therapies to treat bleeding peptic ulcers.

Apart from these conventional methods, novel endoscopic tools have been developed for hemostasis in gastrointestinal bleeding. TC-325 (Hemospray; Cook Medical, Bloomington, IN) is a hemostatic inorganic particle that becomes adhesive on contact with moisture, forming a mechanical barrier to achieve hemostasis. The absorbent power also concentrates the clotting factors to enhance clot formation.[34] Early clinical experience in 20 patients with active peptic ulcer bleeding showed that TC-325 is safe and effective, achieving a rate of acute hemostasis in 95% of patients.[36] Out of the 19 patients with successful acute hemostasis, 2 patients (10.5%) developed rebleeding by blood counts but not confirmed by endoscopy. Similar rates of efficacy were reported in several subsequent cohorts.[37,38] A higher rebleeding rate (38.9%) was observed in one study in which its main use was as a rescue therapy.[37] Although TC-325 seems to be safe and effective, prospective trials are required to determine its efficacy against other hemostatic devices.

The Over-The-Scope Clip (OTSC; Ovesco Endoscopy, Tübingen, Germany) is another novel endoscopic device for hemostasis. It is a large endoscopic clip with a greater jaw width, designed to provide a robust tissue apposition to achieve mechanical hemostasis. It has the advantages of being applicable for large ulcers with deep vessels or for closure of fistulas and perforations.[39] Early experiences in patients with gastrointestinal bleeding showed favorable rates of initial hemostasis, with rebleeding rates ranging from 7.4% to 22.2%.[40,41] Like TC-325, further studies are needed to determine its role as a primary or rescue hemostatic device in peptic ulcer bleeding.

Postendoscopy Management

Proton-pump inhibitor is effective in reducing rebleeding after endoscopy. In a randomized study of 240 patients with actively bleeding ulcers, high dose intravenous omeprazole after endoscopy treatment reduced early rebleeding within 3 days (relative risk = 4.80).[42] These results were supported by other studies showing a consistent reduction in rebleeding and the need for surgery.[43,44] Despite some studies showing benefits with a high-dose intravenous regimen,[45,46] there is now increasing evidence that standard dose or even an oral regimen may be as effective in reducing rebleeding.[47–50] A larger randomized study will be necessary to determine the equivalency or noninferiority of the two treatments in a heterogeneous patient population.

RECURRENT PEPTIC ULCER BLEEDING

Rebleeding after initial endoscopic control occurs in up to 15% of cases. It is a major risk factor for peptic ulcer–related mortality. A cohort study based on 3000 patients with peptic ulcer bleeding showed that rebleeding was an important factor contributing to mortality,[4] along with other clinical prognostic factors, including age older than 70 years, medical comorbidity, hypotension, and need for surgery.

Risk Factors for Rebleeding

Multiple prospective studies have evaluated the risk factors for rebleeding after initial endoscopic hemostasis. One of the earliest descriptions is the Forrest classification of stigmata of recent hemorrhage, which correlated the endoscopic appearance of the ulcer with the rebleeding rate.[51] Given that this classification system only comprises the endoscopic description, Rockall and colleagues[52] undertook a large prospective audit in 1995 to integrate clinical parameters with endoscopic score to predict disease outcomes, including rebleeding and mortality.[53–55] Nevertheless, with changing epidemiology and the advent of endoscopic techniques, larger cohorts have been conducted to evaluate the risk factors. A cohort study involving 1144 patients with peptic ulcer bleeding identified several clinical and endoscopic parameters as independent factors predicting rebleeding.[56] These findings were supported by 2 subsequent meta-analyses involving more than 3000 individuals, showing hemodynamic instability, active bleeding at endoscopy, large ulcer size, and ulcer location (posterior duodenal wall or lesser gastric curve) as the most important predictors for rebleeding.[57,58] These factors may be used to identify patients who are most likely to benefit from intensive monitoring and treatment.

Acute Management of Rebleeding

Repeat endoscopy can be performed in patients with clinical evidence of rebleeding after initial hemostasis (**Fig. 1**). A randomized trial comparing repeated endoscopic therapy versus surgery revealed that 73% of patients with rebleeding can be treated with a second endoscopy to achieve durable hemostasis with a lower complication rate.[59] It is, therefore, recommended to repeat endoscopy after the first episode of rebleeding. Nevertheless, it remains unknown whether the novel endoscopic devices may provide more secure hemostasis in cases of rebleeding, although initial experiences on their use as a salvage therapy were encouraging with high success rates of hemostasis.[38,60]

If further bleeding recurs after a second endoscopic attempt, transarterial angiographic embolization (TAE) or surgery may be attempted (see **Fig. 1**). A review of 15 case series with 819 intractable bleeding patients undergoing TAE showed a technical success rate of 93%.[61] In a retrospective study comparing TAE with surgery after failed endoscopic hemostasis, TAE was associated with a higher rate of rebleeding (34.4% vs 12.5%, $P = .01$) but less complications (40.6% vs 67.9%, $P = .01$). There was no difference in 30-day mortality between the two groups

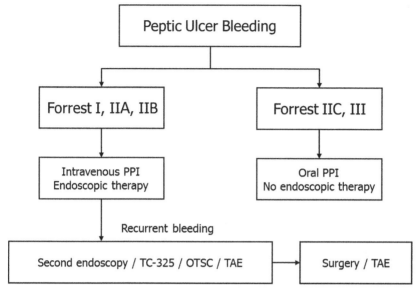

Fig. 1. A proposed algorithm for the management of acute peptic ulcer bleeding. PPI, proton pump inhibitor; TAE, transarterial angiographic embolization.

(25.0% vs 30.4%, $P = .77$),[62] a result consistent with several other retrospective studies.[63–65] The preliminary results of a randomized study in patients with massive bleeding uncontrolled by endoscopy showed an insignificantly higher failure rate with TAE than surgery (52.9% vs 21.4%, $P = .052$), despite similar outcomes in terms of hospitalization and mortality between the two groups.[66]

Preemptive Endoscopy or Angiographic Embolization

Second-look endoscopy was one of the strategies to prevent rebleeding. It is generally defined as a routine repeat endoscopy within 24 hours after initial endoscopy, with an aim to identify persistent high-grade stigmata of recent hemorrhage amendable to further therapy. Although a meta-analysis of randomized trials showed a small but significant reduction in rebleeding with second-look endoscopy,[67] most of these early studies did not use proton-pump inhibitors, which subsequently became the standard of care. This benefit, thus, becomes questionable with the addition of intensive proton-pump inhibitor therapy after endoscopy.[68] Besides, further endoscopic treatment can result in perforation, especially when thermal coagulation is repeatedly applied.[69] Two cost-effectiveness analyses suggested that selective instead of routine second-look endoscopy is more cost-effective.[70,71] Routine second-look endoscopy is not recommended in most international guidelines.

An alternative approach is to provide preemptive treatment to patients with a high risk of rebleeding. In a preliminary study of 222 patients with high-risk ulcers, early postendoscopy TAE to patients with large peptic ulcers ($\geq$1.5 cm in size) reduced rebleeding (OR = 0.18, 95% CI = 0.02–0.92) compared with patients who did not receive TAE.[72] There was no mortality at 30 days in the TAE group (0% vs 4.5%, $P = .065$).[72] A preemptive approach in selected cases of high-risk ulcer bleeding using TAE should be considered in preventing rebleeding.

Therapeutic Management of Recurrent Ulcer Disease

Peptic ulcer has a high rate of recurrence, especially if the causative agent or cause is not eliminated. Early studies before the discovery of *H pylori* and proton-pump inhibitor reported relapse rates of up to 74% during a 12-month follow-up period.[73,74] Approximately 25% to 40% of the ulcer recurrences were asymptomatic,[75,76] whereas others may present with rebleeding.[77,78] Definitive treatment and preventive measures are required to reduce ulcer recurrence and its complications.

Helicobacter Pylori Ulcers

Untreated *H pylori*–associated peptic ulcers tend to recur.[73–76] It is, therefore, important to ensure complete eradication of the bacterium. An early study comparing eradication therapy (bismuth, metronidazole, and tetracycline) with acid-suppression therapy (omeprazole) showed similar rates of gastric ulcer healing but a significantly lower rate of ulcer recurrence in the eradication group (4.5% vs 53.2%, *P*<.01).[79] This study establishes the efficacy of eradication therapy in healing *H pylori* ulcers and preventing their recurrence. A subsequent review confirmed the efficacy and revealed a recurrence rate of 0.75% per patient-year after *H pylori* eradication.[80]

Despite the importance of eradication, persistent *H pylori* may occur because of poor drug compliance or emergency of resistant organisms.[81] The importance of the eradication therapy, as well as its common side effects, should be explained to patients to enhance compliance. The local resistance pattern should be recognized in choosing an eradication regimen, and confirmation of successful eradication should be performed no sooner than 4 weeks after therapy.[82,83]

Nonsteroidal Antiinflammatory Drug–Induced Peptic Ulcers

Nonsteroidal antiinflammatory drugs (NSAIDs) have emerged as a major cause of recurrent peptic ulcer disease as the incidence of *H pylori*–associated ulcers decline. It is estimated that up to 25% of long-term NSAID users will develop peptic ulcer, of which 2% to 4% will have complications, such as bleeding or perforation.[84,85] Several studies have been performed to prevent ulcer bleeding in patients starting NSAIDs. Two studies have showed that test and eradication of *H pylori* infection can substantially reduce peptic ulcers (12.1% vs 34.4% at 6 months, *P*<.01) and the complications,[86,87] suggesting that there may be synergistic effects between *H pylori* and NSAIDs in ulcerogenesis. As for a protective strategy, a systematic review showed that proton-pump inhibitor, high-dose histamine-2 receptor antagonist, and misoprostol were all effective in the prevention of long-term NSAID-related peptic ulcers.[88] For high-risk patients with a history of ulcer bleeding, long-term prophylactic use of a proton-pump inhibitor could significantly lower the risk of recurrent ulcer bleeding (4.4% vs 18.8% at 6 months, *P*<.01).[89]

Selective cyclooxygenase-2 (COX-2) inhibitors were originally developed to be a less toxic alternative of NSAIDs. Despite early studies showing fewer gastroduodenal ulcers and complications compared with nonselective NSAIDs,[90] COX-2 inhibitors have not adequately reduced the risk of ulcer recurrence in very-high-risk patients.[91] In a randomized study of 287 patients, celecoxib usage in patients with an ulcer bleeding history had a risk of rebleeding of 4.9% over 6 months, compared with 6.4% in patients receiving diclofenac plus omeprazole.[91] Nevertheless, the risk can be lowered by adding a proton-pump inhibitor to a COX-2 inhibitor, which was found to have significantly fewer rebleeding episodes than a COX-2 inhibitor alone (0% vs 8.9% at 13 months, *P*<.01).[92] However, the increased cardiovascular risk associated with COX-2 inhibitors should be considered and balanced against the gastrointestinal risk.[93–95]

Antiplatelet-Induced Peptic Ulcers

Acetylsalicylic acid is an independent risk factor for ulcer bleeding, with an estimated OR of 2.07.[96] Because of the cardiovascular diseases pandemic, acetylsalicylic acid and other antiplatelet agents are being increasingly consumed worldwide and have, thus, become an important cause of peptic ulcers.

The strategies for reducing rebleeding in acetylsalicylic acid users include elimination of risk factors and administration of a gastroprotective agent. *H pylori* infection is an independent risk factor for ulcer bleeding (OR = 4.7, 95% CI = 2.0–10.9).[97] There is now good evidence that *H pylori* eradication could reduce rebleeding in high-risk acetylsalicylic acid users,[89,98] although the evidence for average-risk patients is less definite.[99,100] Despite claims of clopidogrel being less toxic to the gastrointestinal tract, a randomized study showed that the addition of a proton-pump inhibitor to acetylsalicylic acid was preferred to clopidogrel, with a 10-fold difference in ulcer bleeding risk (0.7% vs 8.6%, $P<.01$).[101] Therefore, adding a proton-pump inhibitor as a gastroprotective agent to low-dose acetylsalicylic acid should be preferred over clopidogrel in situations when either drug can be prescribed.

Another important question in managing peptic ulcer bleeding is the resumption of an antiplatelet agent after hemostasis. In a randomized controlled trial involving 156 patients with established cardiovascular disease, early resumption of acetylsalicylic acid after endoscopic hemostasis resulted in almost 10-fold reduction in all-cause mortality (1.3% vs 12.9%) despite a higher risk for rebleeding (10.3% vs 5.4%).[102] This may be accounted by the fact that the major causes of death in these patients were cardiovascular diseases related rather than gastrointestinal bleeding.[5] Early resumption of acetylsalicylic acid with proton-pump inhibitor in patients with established cardiovascular diseases, preferably within 1 to 3 days, should be considered to minimize the overall mortality and morbidity.

SUMMARY

The past few decades have witnessed revolutionary changes in the management of peptic ulcer disease. Despite major breakthroughs, there is still a small proportion (5%–10%) of patients who have recurrent peptic ulcer bleeding after endoscopic hemostasis. Identifying such patients using a risk stratification scoring system or key risk factors should be adopted as a routine practice. In high-risk patients, a more aggressive approach including second-look endoscopy and preemptive endoscopic treatment should be considered. The role of TC-325 and OTSC needs further evaluation. The use of TAE in elderly and fragile patients should be considered. When hemostasis is achieved, removing the underlying causes, namely, *H pylori* infection and the use of NSAIDs or antiplatelets, should be implemented. With these strategies, the risk of rebleeding would be further reduced to minimal in due course.

REFERENCES

1. Hearnshaw SA, Logan RF, Lowe D, et al. Acute upper gastrointestinal bleeding in the UK: patient characteristics, diagnoses and outcomes in the 2007 UK audit. Gut 2011;60(10):1327–35.
2. Hermansson M, Ekedahl A, Ranstam J, et al. Decreasing incidence of peptic ulcer complications after the introduction of the proton pump inhibitors, a study of the Swedish population from 1974–2002. BMC Gastroenterol 2009;9:25.
3. Loperfido S, Baldo V, Piovesana E, et al. Changing trends in acute upper-GI bleeding: a population-based study. Gastrointest Endosc 2009;70(2):212–24.

4. Chiu PW, Ng EK, Cheung FK, et al. Predicting mortality in patients with bleeding peptic ulcers after therapeutic endoscopy. Clin Gastroenterol Hepatol 2009; 7(3):311–6 [quiz: 253].
5. Sung JJ, Tsoi KK, Ma TK, et al. Causes of mortality in patients with peptic ulcer bleeding: a prospective cohort study of 10,428 cases. Am J Gastroenterol 2010; 105(1):84–9.
6. Wheatley KE, Snyman JH, Brearley S, et al. Mortality in patients with bleeding peptic ulcer when those aged 60 or over are operated on early. Br Med J 1990;301(6746):272.
7. Rockall TA. Management and outcome of patients undergoing surgery after acute upper gastrointestinal haemorrhage. Steering Group for the National Audit of Acute Upper Gastrointestinal Haemorrhage. J R Soc Med 1998;91(10):518–23.
8. Ohmann C, Imhof M, Ruppert C, et al. Time-trends in the epidemiology of peptic ulcer bleeding. Scand J Gastroenterol 2005;40(8):914–20.
9. Kang JY, Elders A, Majeed A, et al. Recent trends in hospital admissions and mortality rates for peptic ulcer in Scotland 1982–2002. Aliment Pharmacol Ther 2006;24(1):65–79.
10. Jairath V, Hearnshaw S, Brunskill SJ, et al. Red cell transfusion for the management of upper gastrointestinal haemorrhage. Cochrane Database Syst Rev 2010;(9):CD006613.
11. Hearnshaw SA, Logan RF, Palmer KR, et al. Outcomes following early red blood cell transfusion in acute upper gastrointestinal bleeding. Aliment Pharmacol Ther 2010;32(2):215–24.
12. Villanueva C, Colomo A, Bosch A, et al. Transfusion strategies for acute upper gastrointestinal bleeding. N Engl J Med 2013;368(1):11–21.
13. Hebert PC, Wells G, Blajchman MA, et al. A multicenter, randomized, controlled clinical trial of transfusion requirements in critical care. Transfusion requirements in critical care investigators, Canadian Critical Care Trials Group. N Engl J Med 1999;340(6):409–17.
14. Rockall TA, Logan RF, Devlin HB, et al. Risk assessment after acute upper gastrointestinal haemorrhage. Gut 1996;38(3):316–21.
15. Blatchford O, Davidson LA, Murray WR, et al. Acute upper gastrointestinal haemorrhage in west of Scotland: case ascertainment study. BMJ 1997;315(7107): 510–4.
16. Saltzman JR, Tabak YP, Hyett BH, et al. A simple risk score accurately predicts in-hospital mortality, length of stay, and cost in acute upper GI bleeding. Gastrointest Endosc 2011;74(6):1215–24.
17. Pang SH, Ching JY, Lau JY, et al. Comparing the Blatchford and pre-endoscopic Rockall score in predicting the need for endoscopic therapy in patients with upper GI hemorrhage. Gastrointest Endosc 2010;71(7):1134–40.
18. Stanley AJ, Ashley D, Dalton HR, et al. Outpatient management of patients with low-risk upper-gastrointestinal haemorrhage: multicentre validation and prospective evaluation. Lancet 2009;373(9657):42–7.
19. Lau JY, Leung WK, Wu JC, et al. Omeprazole before endoscopy in patients with gastrointestinal bleeding. N Engl J Med 2007;356(16):1631–40.
20. Sreedharan A, Martin J, Leontiadis GI, et al. Proton pump inhibitor treatment initiated prior to endoscopic diagnosis in upper gastrointestinal bleeding. Cochrane Database Syst Rev 2010;(7):CD005415.
21. Leontiadis GI, Sharma VK, Howden CW. Proton pump inhibitor therapy for peptic ulcer bleeding: cochrane collaboration meta-analysis of randomized controlled trials. Mayo Clin Proc 2007;82(3):286–96.

22. Cook DJ, Guyatt GH, Salena BJ, et al. Endoscopic therapy for acute nonvariceal upper gastrointestinal hemorrhage: a meta-analysis. Gastroenterology 1992; 102(1):139–48.
23. Laine L, McQuaid KR. Endoscopic therapy for bleeding ulcers: an evidence-based approach based on meta-analyses of randomized controlled trials. Clin Gastroenterol Hepatol 2009;7(1):33–47.
24. Enestvedt BK, Gralnek IM, Mattek N, et al. An evaluation of endoscopic indications and findings related to nonvariceal upper-GI hemorrhage in a large multi-center consortium. Gastrointest Endosc 2008;67(3):422–9.
25. Laine L, Kivitz AJ, Bello AE, et al. Double-blind randomized trials of single-tablet ibuprofen/high-dose famotidine vs. ibuprofen alone for reduction of gastric and duodenal ulcers. Am J Gastroenterol 2012;107(3):379–86.
26. Bleau BL, Gostout CJ, Sherman KE, et al. Recurrent bleeding from peptic ulcer associated with adherent clot: a randomized study comparing endoscopic treatment with medical therapy. Gastrointest Endosc 2002;56(1):1–6.
27. Jensen DM. Endoscopic screening for varices in cirrhosis: findings, implications, and outcomes. Gastroenterology 2002;122(6):1620–30.
28. Kahi CJ, Jensen DM, Sung JJ, et al. Endoscopic therapy versus medical therapy for bleeding peptic ulcer with adherent clot: a meta-analysis. Gastroenterology 2005;129(3):855–62.
29. Laine L, Jensen DM. Management of patients with ulcer bleeding. Am J Gastroenterol 2012;107(3):345–60 [quiz: 361].
30. de Groot NL, van Oijen MG, Kessels K, et al. Reassessment of the predictive value of the Forrest classification for peptic ulcer rebleeding and mortality: can classification be simplified? Endoscopy 2014;46(1):46–52.
31. Chung SC, Leung JW, Steele RJ, et al. Endoscopic injection of adrenaline for actively bleeding ulcers - a randomized trial. Br Med J 1988;296(6637): 1631–3.
32. Calvet X, Vergara M, Brullet E, et al. Addition of a second endoscopic treatment following epinephrine injection improves outcome in high-risk bleeding ulcers. Gastroenterology 2004;126(2):441–50.
33. Marmo R, Rotondano G, Piscopo R, et al. Dual therapy versus monotherapy in the endoscopic treatment of high-risk bleeding ulcers: a meta-analysis of controlled trials. Am J Gastroenterol 2007;102(2):279–89 [quiz: 469].
34. Barkun AN, Martel M, Toubouti Y, et al. Endoscopic hemostasis in peptic ulcer bleeding for patients with high-risk lesions: a series of meta-analyses. Gastrointest Endosc 2009;69(4):786–99.
35. Sung JJ, Tsoi KK, Lai LH, et al. Endoscopic clipping versus injection and thermo-coagulation in the treatment of non-variceal upper gastrointestinal bleeding: a meta-analysis. Gut 2007;56(10):1364–72.
36. Sung JJ, Luo D, Wu JC, et al. Early clinical experience of the safety and effectiveness of Hemospray in achieving hemostasis in patients with acute peptic ulcer bleeding. Endoscopy 2011;43(4):291–5.
37. Yau AH, Ou G, Galorport C, et al. Safety and efficacy of Hemospray (R) in upper gastrointestinal bleeding. Can J Gastroenterol Hepatol 2014;28(2):72–6.
38. Sulz MC, Frei R, Meyenberger C, et al. Routine use of Hemospray for gastrointestinal bleeding: prospective two-center experience in Switzerland. Endoscopy 2014;46(7):619–24.
39. Kirschniak A, Kratt T, Stuker D, et al. A new endoscopic over-the-scope clip system for treatment of lesions and bleeding in the GI tract: first clinical experiences. Gastrointest Endosc 2007;66(1):162–7.

40. Kirschniak A, Subotova N, Zieker D, et al. The Over-The-Scope Clip (OTSC) for the treatment of gastrointestinal bleeding, perforations, and fistulas. Surg Endosc 2011;25(9):2901–5.
41. Chan SM, Chiu PW, Teoh AY, et al. Use of the Over-The-Scope Clip for treatment of refractory upper gastrointestinal bleeding: a case series. Endoscopy 2014; 46(5):428–31.
42. Lau JY, Sung JJ, Lee KK, et al. Effect of intravenous omeprazole on recurrent bleeding after endoscopic treatment of bleeding peptic ulcers. N Engl J Med 2000;343(5):310–6.
43. Leontiadis GI, Sharma VK, Howden CW. Proton pump inhibitor treatment for acute peptic ulcer bleeding. Cochrane Database Syst Rev 2006;(1):CD002094.
44. Sung JJ, Barkun A, Kuipers EJ, et al. Intravenous esomeprazole for prevention of recurrent peptic ulcer bleeding a randomized trial. Ann Intern Med 2009; 150(7):455–64.
45. Chan WH, Khin LW, Chung YF, et al. Randomized controlled trial of standard versus high-dose intravenous omeprazole after endoscopic therapy in high-risk patients with acute peptic ulcer bleeding. Br J Surg 2011;98(5):640–4.
46. Liu N, Liu L, Zhang H, et al. Effect of intravenous proton pump inhibitor regimens and timing of endoscopy on clinical outcomes of peptic ulcer bleeding. J Gastroenterol Hepatol 2012;27(9):1473–9.
47. Andriulli A, Loperfido S, Focareta R, et al. High- versus low-dose proton pump inhibitors after endoscopic hemostasis in patients with peptic ulcer bleeding: a multicentre, randomized study. Am J Gastroenterol 2008;103(12):3011–8.
48. Wang CH, Ma MH, Chou HC, et al. High-dose vs non-high-dose proton pump inhibitors after endoscopic treatment in patients with bleeding peptic ulcer: a systematic review and meta-analysis of randomized controlled trials. Arch Intern Med 2010;170(9):751–8.
49. Sung JJ, Suen BY, Wu JC, et al. Effects of intravenous and oral esomeprazole in the prevention of recurrent bleeding from peptic ulcers after endoscopic therapy. Am J Gastroenterol 2014;109(7):1005–10.
50. Chen CC, Lee JY, Fang YJ, et al. Randomised clinical trial: high-dose vs. standard-dose proton pump inhibitors for the prevention of recurrent haemorrhage after combined endoscopic haemostasis of bleeding peptic ulcers. Aliment Pharmacol Ther 2012;35(8):894–903.
51. Forrest JA, Finlayson ND, Shearman DJ. Endoscopy in gastrointestinal bleeding. Lancet 1974;2(7877):394–7.
52. Rockall TA, Logan RF, Devlin HB, et al. Incidence of and mortality from acute upper gastrointestinal haemorrhage in the United Kingdom. Steering Committee and members of the National Audit of Acute Upper Gastrointestinal Haemorrhage. BMJ 1995;311(6999):222–6.
53. Vreeburg EM, Terwee CB, Snel P, et al. Validation of the Rockall risk scoring system in upper gastrointestinal bleeding. Gut 1999;44(3):331–5.
54. Sanders DS, Carter MJ, Goodchap RJ, et al. Prospective validation of the Rockall risk scoring system for upper GI hemorrhage in subgroups of patients with varices and peptic ulcers. Am J Gastroenterol 2002;97(3):630–5.
55. Soncini M, Triossi O, Leo P, et al. Management of patients with nonvariceal upper gastrointestinal hemorrhage before and after the adoption of the Rockall score, in the Italian gastroenterology units. Eur J Gastroenterol Hepatol 2007;19(7):543–7.
56. Wong SK, Yu LM, Lau JY, et al. Prediction of therapeutic failure after adrenaline injection plus heater probe treatment in patients with bleeding peptic ulcer. Gut 2002;50(3):322–5.

57. Elmunzer BJ, Young SD, Inadomi JM, et al. Systematic review of the predictors of recurrent hemorrhage after endoscopic hemostatic therapy for bleeding peptic ulcers. Am J Gastroenterol 2008;103(10):2625–32 [quiz: 2633].
58. Garcia-Iglesias P, Villoria A, Suarez D, et al. Meta-analysis: predictors of re-bleeding after endoscopic treatment for bleeding peptic ulcer. Aliment Pharmacol Ther 2011;34(8):888–900.
59. Lau JY, Sung JJ, Lam YH, et al. Endoscopic retreatment compared with surgery in patients with recurrent bleeding after initial endoscopic control of bleeding ulcers. N Engl J Med 1999;340(10):751–6.
60. Manta R, Galloro G, Mangiavillano B, et al. Over-the-scope clip (OTSC) represents an effective endoscopic treatment for acute GI bleeding after failure of conventional techniques. Surg Endosc 2013;27(9):3162–4.
61. Loffroy R, Rao P, Ota S, et al. Embolization of acute nonvariceal upper gastrointestinal hemorrhage resistant to endoscopic treatment: results and predictors of recurrent bleeding. Cardiovasc Intervent Radiol 2010;33(6):1088–100.
62. Wong TC, Wong KT, Chiu PW, et al. A comparison of angiographic embolization with surgery after failed endoscopic hemostasis to bleeding peptic ulcers. Gastrointest Endosc 2011;73(5):900–8.
63. Ang D, Teo EK, Tan A, et al. A comparison of surgery versus transcatheter angiographic embolization in the treatment of nonvariceal upper gastrointestinal bleeding uncontrolled by endoscopy. Eur J Gastroenterol Hepatol 2012;24(8):929–38.
64. Venclauskas L, Bratlie SO, Zachrisson K, et al. Is transcatheter arterial embolization a safer alternative than surgery when endoscopic therapy fails in bleeding duodenal ulcer? Scand J Gastroenterol 2010;45(3):299–304.
65. Loffroy R, Estivalet L, Cherblanc V, et al. Transcatheter embolization as the new reference standard for endoscopically unmanageable upper gastrointestinal bleeding. World J Gastrointest Surg 2012;4(10):223–7.
66. Lau JY, Wong KT, Chiu PW, et al. 158 transarterial angiographic embolization vs. surgery in patients with bleeding peptic ulcers uncontrolled at endoscopy; a multicenter randomized trial. Gastrointest Endosc 2014;79(5):AB113.
67. Marmo R, Rotondano G, Bianco MA, et al. Outcome of endoscopic treatment for peptic ulcer bleeding: is a second look necessary? A meta-analysis. Gastrointest Endosc 2003;57(1):62–7.
68. Tsoi KK, Chan HC, Chiu PW, et al. Second-look endoscopy with thermal coagulation or injections for peptic ulcer bleeding: a meta-analysis. J Gastroenterol Hepatol 2010;25(1):8–13.
69. Chiu PW, Sung JJ. High risk ulcer bleeding: when is second-look endoscopy recommended? Clin Gastroenterol Hepatol 2010;8(8):651–4 [quiz: e687].
70. Spiegel BM, Ofman JJ, Woods K, et al. Minimizing recurrent peptic ulcer hemorrhage after endoscopic hemostasis: the cost-effectiveness of competing strategies. Am J Gastroenterol 2003;98(1):86–97.
71. Imperiale TF, Kong N. Second-look endoscopy for bleeding peptic ulcer disease: a decision-effectiveness and cost-effectiveness analysis. J Clin Gastroenterol 2012;46(9):e71–5.
72. Lau JY, Wong KT, Chiu PW, et al. 157 early angiographic embolization after endoscopic hemostasis to high risk bleeding peptic ulcers improves outcomes. Gastrointest Endosc 2014;79(5 Supplement):AB113.
73. Bardhan KD, Cole DS, Hawkins BW, et al. Does treatment with cimetidine extended beyond initial healing of duodenal ulcer reduce the subsequent relapse rate? Br Med J (Clin Res Ed) 1982;284(6316):621–3.

74. Gudmand-Hoyer E, Jensen KB, Krag E, et al. Prophylactic effect of cimetidine in duodenal ulcer disease. Br Med J 1978;1(6120):1095–7.
75. Boyd EJ, Wilson JA, Wormsley KG. The fate of asymptomatic recurrences of duodenal ulcer. Scand J Gastroenterol 1984;19(6):808–12.
76. Wolosin JD, Gertler SL, Peterson WL, et al. Gastric ulcer recurrence: follow-up of a double-blind, placebo-controlled trial. J Clin Gastroenterol 1989;11(1):12–6.
77. Chan FK, Sung JJ. Helicobacter pylori eradication in long-term users of non-steroidal anti-inflammatory drugs. Lancet 1998;352(9145):2016 [author reply: 2017].
78. Chan FK, Sung JJ. Therapies for ulcers associated with nonsteroidal antiinflam-matory drugs. N Engl J Med 1998;339(5):349–50 [author reply: 350–1].
79. Sung JJ, Chung SC, Ling TK, et al. Antibacterial treatment of gastric ulcers associated with Helicobacter pylori. N Engl J Med 1995;332(3):139–42.
80. Gisbert JP, Khorrami S, Carballo F, et al. Meta-analysis: Helicobacter pylori erad-ication therapy vs. antisecretory non-eradication therapy for the prevention of recurrent bleeding from peptic ulcer. Aliment Pharmacol Ther 2004;19(6):617–29.
81. Tang RS, Chan FK. Therapeutic management of recurrent peptic ulcer disease. Drugs 2012;72(12):1605–16.
82. Malfertheiner P, Megraud F, O'Morain C, et al. Current concepts in the manage-ment of Helicobacter pylori infection: the Maastricht III Consensus Report. Gut 2007;56(6):772–81.
83. Chey WD, Wong BC. American College of Gastroenterology guideline on the man-agement of Helicobacter pylori infection. Am J Gastroenterol 2007;102(8):1808–25.
84. Silverstein FE, Faich G, Goldstein JL, et al. Gastrointestinal toxicity with cele-coxib vs nonsteroidal anti-inflammatory drugs for osteoarthritis and rheumatoid arthritis: the CLASS study: a randomized controlled trial. Celecoxib Long-term Arthritis Safety Study. JAMA 2000;284(10):1247–55.
85. Bombardier C, Laine L, Reicin A, et al. Comparison of upper gastrointestinal toxicity of rofecoxib and naproxen in patients with rheumatoid arthritis. VIGOR Study Group. N Engl J Med 2000;343(21):1520–8, 1522 p following 1528.
86. Chan FK, To KF, Wu JC, et al. Eradication of Helicobacter pylori and risk of peptic ulcers in patients starting long-term treatment with non-steroidal anti-in-flammatory drugs: a randomised trial. Lancet 2002;359(9300):9–13.
87. Chan FK, Sung JJ, Chung SC, et al. Randomised trial of eradication of Helico-bacter pylori before non-steroidal anti-inflammatory drug therapy to prevent peptic ulcers. Lancet 1997;350(9083):975–9.
88. Rostom A, Dube C, Wells G, et al. Prevention of NSAID-induced gastroduodenal ulcers. Cochrane Database Syst Rev 2002;(4):CD002296.
89. Chan FK, Chung SC, Suen BY, et al. Preventing recurrent upper gastrointestinal bleeding in patients with Helicobacter pylori infection who are taking low-dose aspirin or naproxen. N Engl J Med 2001;344(13):967–73.
90. Rostom A, Muir K, Dube C, et al. Gastrointestinal safety of cyclooxygenase-2 in-hibitors: a Cochrane collaboration systematic review. Clin Gastroenterol Hepatol 2007;5(7):818–28, 828.e1–5; [quiz: 768].
91. Chan FK, Hung LC, Suen BY, et al. Celecoxib versus diclofenac and omeprazole in reducing the risk of recurrent ulcer bleeding in patients with arthritis. N Engl J Med 2002;347(26):2104–10.
92. Chan FK, Wong VW, Suen BY, et al. Combination of a cyclo-oxygenase-2 inhib-itor and a proton-pump inhibitor for prevention of recurrent ulcer bleeding in pa-tients at very high risk: a double-blind, randomised trial. Lancet 2007;369(9573): 1621–6.

93. Sung JJ. Marshall and Warren lecture 2009: peptic ulcer bleeding: an expedition of 20 years from 1989–2009. J Gastroenterol Hepatol 2010;25(2):229–33.
94. Kearney PM, Baigent C, Godwin J, et al. Do selective cyclo-oxygenase-2 inhibitors and traditional non-steroidal anti-inflammatory drugs increase the risk of atherothrombosis? Meta-analysis of randomised trials. BMJ 2006;332(7553): 1302–8.
95. Solomon SD, Wittes J, Finn PV, et al. Cardiovascular risk of celecoxib in 6 randomized placebo-controlled trials: the cross trial safety analysis. Circulation 2008;117(16):2104–13.
96. Sostres C, Gargallo CJ, Lanas A. Interaction between Helicobacter pylori infection, nonsteroidal anti-inflammatory drugs and/or low-dose aspirin use: old question new insights. World J Gastroenterol 2014;20(28):9439–50.
97. Lanas A, Fuentes J, Benito R, et al. Helicobacter pylori increases the risk of upper gastrointestinal bleeding in patients taking low-dose aspirin. Aliment Pharmacol Ther 2002;16(4):779–86.
98. Chan FK, Ching JY, Suen BY, et al. Effects of Helicobacter pylori infection on long-term risk of peptic ulcer bleeding in low-dose aspirin users. Gastroenterology 2013;144(3):528–35.
99. Giral A, Ozdogan O, Celikel CA, et al. Effect of Helicobacter pylori eradication on anti-thrombotic dose aspirin-induced gastroduodenal mucosal injury. J Gastroenterol Hepatol 2004;19(7):773–7.
100. Hart J, Hawkey CJ, Lanas A, et al. Predictors of gastroduodenal erosions in patients taking low-dose aspirin. Aliment Pharmacol Ther 2010;31(1):143–9.
101. Chan FK, Ching JY, Hung LC, et al. Clopidogrel versus aspirin and esomeprazole to prevent recurrent ulcer bleeding. N Engl J Med 2005;352(3):238–44.
102. Sung JJ, Lau JY, Ching JY, et al. Continuation of low-dose aspirin therapy in peptic ulcer bleeding: a randomized trial. Ann Intern Med 2010;152(1):1–9.

Unusual Causes of Upper Gastrointestinal Bleeding

 CrossMark

Keyur Parikh, MD, Meer Akbar Ali, MD, Richard C.K. Wong, MD*

KEYWORDS

- Cameron lesions • Dieulafoy lesions • Gastric antral vascular ectasia
- Duodenal varices • Hemosuccus pancreaticus • Hemobilia • Ampullary carcinoma
- Aortoenteric fistula

KEY POINTS

- Upper gastrointestinal (GI) bleeding is a commonly encountered clinical condition managed by endoscopists, and appropriate diagnosis and treatment require the ability to recognize both common and uncommon causes of bleeding.
- Knowledge of unusual causes of upper GI bleeding will help increase clinical suspicion and allow for prompt diagnoses when these uncommon causes are encountered.
- Certain unusual causes of upper GI bleeding require multidisciplinary management, including endoscopists, surgeons, and interventional radiologists.

CAMERON LESIONS

Initially described by Philemon Truesdale in 1924[1] and then further expanded on in a case series published by Cameron in 1976,[2] Cameron lesions are best described as linear erosions or ulcerations found at the distal end of a hiatus hernia sac in close proximity to the diaphragmatic pinch (**Fig. 1**). The prevalence of these lesions has been estimated to be between 3% and 5% in the presence of any hiatal hernia and is directly related to the size of the hernia. In patients with large hiatal hernias (>5 cm), the prevalence has been reported to be greater than 12%.[3,4] Interestingly, a recent study from 2013 found a prevalence of 0.2% in patients hospitalized for overt upper gastrointestinal (GI) bleeding and 3.8% in patients hospitalized for obscure causes of GI bleeding (**Table 1**).[5] The mechanism for the formation of Cameron lesions is not clearly defined. Many experts thought they occur in patients with hiatal hernias as a result of mechanical trauma and local ischemia caused by repetitive movement of the hernia sac against the diaphragm. Histologically, the changes to the normal mucosa are consistent with ischemia, and biopsy of these lesions can often be

Disclosure Statement: Dr R.C.K. Wong receives research funding from Vascular Technology Inc, Nashua, NH. Drs K. Parikh and M.K. Ali have no financial affiliations to disclose.
Digestive Health Institute, Division of Gastroenterology and Liver Disease, University Hospitals Case Medical Center, 11100 Euclid Avenue, Cleveland, OH 44106-5066, USA
* Corresponding author.
E-mail address: Richard.wong@uhhospitals.org

Gastrointest Endoscopy Clin N Am 25 (2015) 583–605
http://dx.doi.org/10.1016/j.giec.2015.02.009

giendo.theclinics.com

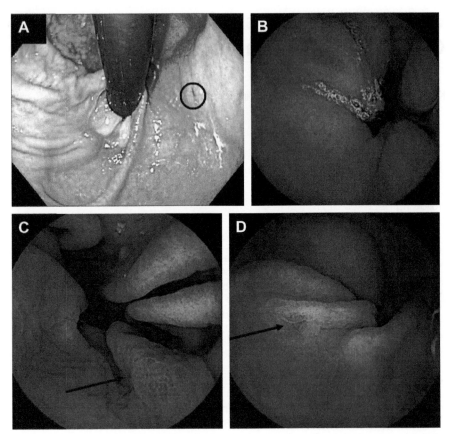

Fig. 1. Cameron lesions. (*A*) Retroflexed view during upper endoscopy showing a singular Cameron erosion with a black circle. (*B–D*) Cameron lesions as seen on capsule endoscopy denoted by the black arrows in 1C and 1D.

confused for ischemic gastritis.[6] Alternatively, there have been some reports in the literature noting that Cameron lesions can result from acid reflux, ischemia, *Helicobacter pylori* infection, gastric stasis, or vascular stasis.[7] It is likely that these lesions occur from multiple causes, including possible underlying genetic mutations, medical comorbidities, and medications.

Cameron lesions are often a source for both overt and obscure GI bleeding. They can present as frank hematemesis, melena, or iron deficiency anemia. The hernia neck and sac should be meticulously evaluated during esophagogastroduodenoscopy (EGD) and specifically in retroflexed views as small Cameron lesions can often be difficult to visualize. In addition, it is important for the endoscopist to gauge whether

Table 1	
Prevalence of Cameron lesions in various clinical scenarios	
With any hiatal hernia	3%–5%
With hiatal hernia >5 cm in size	12%
Any overt upper GI bleeding	0.2%
Obscure GI bleeding	3.8%

a patient's clinical presentation is typical for bleeding from Cameron lesions; if it is unclear, then the endoscopist should exclude other causes of GI bleeding.

Bleeding from these lesions is exacerbated by both acid exposure and nonsteroidal anti-inflammatory drug use. In a series of 95 patients with obscure GI bleeding without a clearly identified source on standard endoscopy, push enteroscopy was used to evaluate further. Of the 39 patients with an identifiable source on push enteroscopy, Cameron lesions were the second most commonly missed lesion (21%).[7] In all cases of GI bleeding, especially when an obvious source is not found, Cameron lesions should remain on the differential diagnosis. It is particularly important for Cameron lesions to remain on the differential diagnosis because Cameron lesions can come and go (that is, occur transiently) and can often be missed at the index upper endoscopy.

Treatment of Cameron lesions should be individualized to their presentation. In patients with iron deficiency anemia, acid-suppressive therapy with proton-pump inhibitors following repletion and maintenance of iron stores is generally successful.[4,8,9] Conversely, in overt GI bleeding due to Cameron lesions, endoscopic therapy with band ligation for source control has also been reported to be quite successful.[10] Alternative methods of endoscopic hemostasis, such as injection of epinephrine, thermal-contact therapy, and clipping, may be difficult to perform because of its location and movement of the hiatal hernia sac with respiration. Moreover, thermal-contact therapy, such as heat probe or multipolar electrocoagulation, can result in deep ulcers or perforations because of the thin mucosal wall in this area and the lack of underlying fibrous support. It is important to note that when patients present with recurrent or life-threatening bleeding or with persistent and severe iron deficiency anemia from Cameron lesions, surgical intervention may be necessary to repair the invariably large hiatal hernia, thus correcting a major underlying pathogenic mechanism of disease by reducing mechanical trauma caused by repetitive movement of the hernia sac against the diaphragm.[11]

DIEULAFOY LESION

This vascular lesion was originally referred to as *exulceratio simplex* in 1898 by the French surgeon Paul Georges Dieulafoy[12] because he thought that it was the first stage of a gastric ulcer. It has also been inaccurately described as an atherosclerotic aneurysm, but this is a misnomer because the caliber of the artery's walls is uniform throughout and there is no unusual degree of atherosclerosis. A Dieulafoy lesion is a vascular abnormality where persistently large-caliber arteries are present in the submucosa and occasionally the mucosa itself with a small overlying defect. Moreover, the length of the superficially located artery can be several centimeters.

Constant pressure or trauma to a singular area of mucosa ultimately leads to erosions and breakdown of tissue. Similar to the mechanism behind primary aortoenteric fistula (PAEF) formation, it is thought that persistent pressure from these large underlying arteries leads to erosion of tissue and creates a small defect with an exposed vascular wall. The most common location where a Dieulafoy lesion can be found is along the lesser curvature of the stomach, within 6 cm from the gastroesophageal junction in the gastric cardia. Other locations where these lesions have been described include the duodenum (14%), the colon (5%), surgical anastomoses (5%), the jejunum (1%), and the esophagus (1%).[13]

The clinical presentation of this lesion is usually major coffee ground emesis, hematemesis, or melena, without any preceding symptoms. This presentation is followed by recurrent intermittent bleeding that can last for several days. Before the advent of endoscopy, these lesions carried an 80% rate of mortality; however, with current endoscopic and angiographic techniques, this rate has been reduced to 13% or less.[14]

Diagnosis is made during endoscopy and requires a high index of clinical suspicion. In a patient with upper GI bleeding, finding a nonbleeding Dieulafoy lesion can be very challenging. The mucosal defect is often quite small (there is no ulcer) and can be hidden between gastric folds or the vessel itself may constrict and retract after a bleeding episode and thus be almost impossible to see. The lesion itself may also be covered in blood or underneath clot, which also contributes to its elusiveness to identification. The endoscopist should perform a meticulous endoscopic examination of the gastric cardia (where the classic Dieulafoy lesion should be located), and if nothing is seen, the authors suggest using water-jet irrigation to target wash as much of the gastric cardia as possible, particularly along the lesser curvature, with the intent of disrupting a fibrin plug and provoking active bleeding from an underlying Dieulafoy lesion (so-called technique of provocative endoscopy). Once bleeding is provoked, the diagnosis and exact location of a bleeding Dieulafoy lesion are certain and endoscopic therapy can immediately follow. Other methods that have been described to diagnose a Dieulafoy lesion include performing endoscopic ultrasound (EUS) of the stomach and mesenteric angiography.[15,16]

Dual combination endoscopic therapy is usually recommended to treat a bleeding Dieulafoy lesion (**Fig. 2**). Endoscopic hemostasis is usually achieved using thermal-contact or mechanical therapy in addition to injection of 1:10,000 diluted epinephrine. Thermal-contact therapy can be performed using heat probe or multipolar electrocoagulation, while mechanical therapy includes band ligation or endoclip placement. The latter 2 both have an equal efficacy, and trends have progressed toward favoring mechanical therapy in the management of these lesions.[17–20]

In the authors' practice, once bleeding from a Dieulafoy lesion is diagnosed, they often use a through-the-scope endoscopic Doppler ultrasound (DopUS) probe to determine the subsurface route and path of the persistently large-caliber artery (so-called technique of acoustic Doppler mapping)[21] in order that the artery can be treated by endoscopic therapy along the length of its subsurface course. Anecdotally, the authors have found the acoustic Doppler mapping technique to be useful because it permits the endoscopist to treat the entire length of the superficially located artery, which in the authors' opinion, may reduce the incidence of recurrent bleeding from this disorder. After endoscopic hemostasis is achieved, confirmation of blood flow cessation using a DopUS probe can be used to confirm successful eradication of the lesion. The Dieulafoy lesion should also be endoscopically tattooed to help locate the lesion for repeat endoscopic management if recurrent bleeding were to occur or for surgical wedge resection, if needed.[22,23]

Additional techniques to control bleeding from a Dieulafoy lesion include endoscopic band ligation or use of a large over-the-scope clip. Angiography with embolization of bleeding source should be pursued in patients who are not candidates for endoscopy or when the site of bleeding is unidentified.[14]

NONNEOPLASTIC GASTRIC POLYPS: INFLAMMATORY FIBROID POLYPS

Inflammatory fibroid polyps (IFPs) are rare submucosal lesions of the GI tract that are semipedunculated protrusions covered by normal mucosa[24] and represent an exceedingly rare cause of upper GI bleeding. In terms of all gastric polyps, which are found in 6% of all EGDs performed in the United States, IFPs represent 0.1% of them. The most common sites where IFPs occur are in the gastric antrum followed by the small bowel. Rarely, they can also occur in the gastric fundus, and very rarely in the esophagus.[25,26] They were first described by Vanek in 1949,[27] and the term "inflammatory fibroid polyps" was used by Helwig and Ranier in 1953.[28]

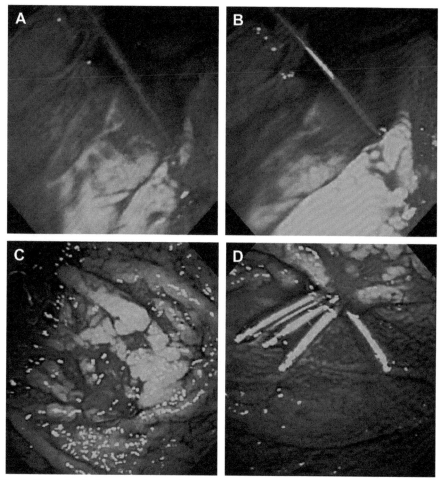

Fig. 2. Dieulafoy lesions. (*A–C*) Actively bleeding Dieulafoy lesions. (*D*) Dieulafoy lesions after dual combination endoscopic therapy with epinephrine injection and multiple endoscopic clip placement to achieve hemostasis. (*Courtesy of* [*A, B*] Drs Sapna Thomas and Saleem Chowdhry, University Hospitals Case Medical Center, Cleveland, OH.)

Clinical manifestations of IFPs are uncommon because patients are mostly asymptomatic; however, when symptoms do occur, they depend on location of the lesion and include intestinal obstruction, intussusception,[29] abdominal pain, early satiety, gastric outlet obstruction, nausea, vomiting,[25] dysphagia,[26] and rarely, GI tract hemorrhage.[30]

In cases of upper GI bleeding secondary to IFPs located in the upper GI tract, the lesion is usually identifiable on upper endoscopy; however, its endoscopic appearance may be confused with GI stromal tumor, carcinoid tumor, or lymphoma, and definitive diagnosis requires pathologic evaluation.[30] Most IFPs are less than 5 cm in size, but they have certainly been reported to be greater than 10 cm in size.[25] On endoscopy, these lesions are firm and solitary and are often ulcerated. On EUS, IFPs are characterized by an indistinct margin and homogeneous internal echopattern and are located within the second or third layer with an intact forth layer.

Histologically, IFPs consist of submucosal proliferations of spindle cells, circumferential deposition of fibroblasts around vessels, giving them an onion-skin appearance, and an inflammatory infiltrate primarily comprising of eosinophils. Classically, these lesions are not thought to carry malignant potential, but there have been published reports showing evidence of IFPs being rarely associated with gastric carcinoma.[31]

Given their size, IFPs have been historically resected surgically based on their origin, and exploratory laparotomy is often pursued based on their location. The advancement of endoscopic techniques and increasing prevalence of expertise in endoscopic mucosal resection have allowed for the resections of these lesions endoscopically.[32] Because of their rarity, limited data exist in regards to management, and therefore, each encountered case must be managed in accordance to clinical presentation and local expertise.

NONNEOPLASTIC GASTRIC POLYPS: GASTRIC HYPERPLASTIC POLYPS

Gastric hyperplastic polyps (GHPs) are a commonly encountered type of gastric polyps. They are equally common in men and women and typically occur in the sixth and seventh decades of life. Although the exact mechanism of pathogenesis is not well defined, these polyps are thought to result from a reparative or regenerative response in the setting of an underlying chronic inflammatory process. Commonly associated causes include atrophic gastritis, H pylori infection, hypergastrinemia, and autoimmune gastritis, among many others. The malignant potential of GHPs is low; however, lesions greater than 1 cm in size and pedunculated morphology are thought to carry an increased risk.[33]

Clinically, GHPs are generally asymptomatic and found incidentally on upper endoscopy performed for alternative indications. Occasionally, patients may present with symptoms including abdominal pain, gastric outlet obstruction, iron deficiency anemia from occult bleeding, and rarely, with overt upper GI bleeding,[34] which occurs more commonly in the setting of anticoagulation, antiplatelet therapy, or other causes of coagulopathy. Although it is quite rare, the exact incidence of overt bleeding from GHP is not well defined (**Fig. 3**).

Endoscopically, these lesions are classically described as smooth, dome-shaped lesions and are usually 0.5 to 1.5 cm in diameter. Larger lesions also occur, frequently become lobulated and pedunculated, and develop surface epithelium erosions, which can result in chronic occult blood loss and iron deficiency anemia. Between 1% and 20% of GHPs have been reported to harbor focal areas of dysplasia, and because of their potential cancer risk, experts have recommended that GHPs larger than 0.5 cm should be completely resected. Endoscopic resection can be performed with snare cautery polypectomy with or without saline lifting or with the assistance of endoloop ligation. If the lesion is too large or resection is unable to be performed, biopsies of the lesions should be taken, and if dysplasia is present or the biopsy is inadequate to exclude dysplasia, then the patient should be referred for surgical wedge resection, which may be able to be done laparoscopically if the endoscopist has previously tattooed the lesion or lesions.[35] According to American Society for Gastrointestinal Endoscopy guidelines, these lesions should undergo surveillance 1 year after initial resection and then at intervals of no more than every 3 to 5 years. If initial pathology is negative for dysplasia, then no further surveillance is necessary.[36] Recent reports have advocated for the use of EUS to further characterize these lesions before resection, but given limited data, no published guidelines exist, and the necessity of EUS to further characterize these lesions should be determined by the endoscopist based on local expertise and specific clinical utility. Endoscopic mucosal

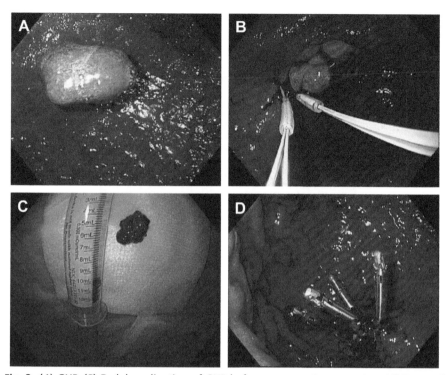

Fig. 3. (A) GHP. (B) Endoloop ligation of GHP before snare cautery resection. (C) Resected GHP. (D) Endoclipping of base of polyp after polypectomy.

resection has been used to resect these lesions to maintain its histologic integrity for pathologic evaluation,[37] but this has not been directly compared with standard snare cautery polypectomy; it is unclear whether endoscopic mucosal resection provides any advantage in clinical management.

GASTRIC ANTRAL VASCULAR ECTASIA

Gastric antral vascular ectasia (GAVE), initially described by Rider and colleagues[38] in 1953 and then further defined by Jabbari and colleagues[39] in 1984, is another uncommon cause of upper GI bleeding that can be easily confused with portal hypertensive gastropathy (PHG). In fact, it was not until 1995 that a clear distinction was made between GAVE and PHG in cirrhotic patients.[40] Overall, it is an uncommon cause of GI bleeding and is thought to be responsible for approximately 4% of nonvariceal upper GI bleeding in patients with or without portal hypertension.[41]

Classically, GAVE is described as having a "watermelon-striped" appearance in the antrum. However, 30% of patients with GAVE may also have cirrhosis, and it is in this particular group of patients that GAVE can frequently be misdiagnosed as PHG. As opposed to the usual watermelon-striped appearance, in patients with cirrhosis, GAVE can appear as multiple scattered erythematous punctuate lesions in the antrum and can have a very similar endoscopic appearance to PHG (**Fig. 4**).[42] This similarity is significant because it can lead to misdiagnosis and mismanagement, thereby resulting in continued bleeding and further unnecessary diagnostic procedures, which place the patient at increased risk for complications.

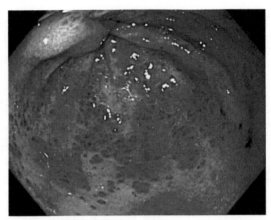

Fig. 4. Atypical appearance of GAVE initially mistaken for PHG in a patient with cirrhosis.

It is also important for the endoscopist to be aware that, despite its name, GAVE can occur in locations other than the gastic antrum. For example, GAVE can also be seen within the gastric cardia as an erythematous ring, extending just distal to the gastro-esophageal junction and described endoscopically as diminutive vascular ectasia with sparing of the stomach body.[43] GAVE can also occur in the duodenum. Another presentation of GAVE can be in a nodular pattern, known as nodular antral gastropathy, where the mucosa is often raised with visible underlying ectatic vessels.[44]

There are several steps that an endoscopist can take to help prevent confusion at the time of endoscopy and subsequently proceed with appropriate management. In patients undergoing endoscopic evaluation for bleeding or anemia and found to have lesions suspicious for PHG or GAVE, an endoscopic biopsy should be performed to help further delineate the cause. Endoscopists should also be aware that although endoscopic biopsy can be very useful in confirming a diagnosis of GAVE, a negative pathology result does not exclude that the patient has GAVE.

It is important to remember that GAVE is pathologically different from PHG and consists of vascular lesions that contain abnormally dilated and tortuous gastric mucosal capillaries (ectasia) with mural spindle cell proliferation (smooth muscle cells and myofibroblasts), fibrin thrombi, and fibrohyalinosis.[44,45] Currently, the exact pathogenesis for GAVE remains unclear; however, the microvascular ectasias are thought to be an acquired abnormality as a result of multiple biophysical factors. Mechanical stress from antropyloric dysfunction or from antroduodenal prolapse can lead to traumatic injury to the antral mucosa from inefficient, forceful peristalsis and has been postulated to contribute to the development of vascular ectasias.[46] In addition, elevated levels of several neuroendocrine hormones in cirrhotics: gastrin, vasoactive intestinal polypeptide, 5-hydroxytryptamine, prostaglandin E2, nitric oxide, and glucagon, have been implicated to play a role in the development of GAVE. It is thought that the accumulation of these vasoactive substances, which are incompletely metabolized by the cirrhotic liver, can also contribute to mucosal microvascular damage and ectasia. Hence, the mechanism for GAVE in cirrhotics is attributed to loss of liver function rather than portal hypertension and, interestingly enough, it has been reported to resolve after liver transplantation completely, whereas portal decompressive therapy seems to have no effect.[44,47–50] Almost 60% of patients with GAVE have concurrent autoimmune disease, and it has been associated with several other chronic systemic (renal, cardiac, or hematologic) diseases.[44,51,52]

Establishing a diagnosis of GAVE has important implications for patient care and its management. Initial management is the same as for any patient with GI bleeding and includes appropriate resuscitation and hemodynamic stabilization. Once this has been performed, the decision to treat lesions due to GAVE depends on the clinical scenario in which it has been discovered. Primary prophylactic treatment is not indicated if the patient is asymptomatic, if the patient does not have iron-deficiency anemia, and if GAVE was an incidental finding at endoscopy. In this scenario, it is reasonable to simply observe the patient clinically.[44] On the other hand, if these lesions are found in the setting of iron-deficiency anemia or active bleeding, first-line treatment involves thermoablative procedures that include thermal-contact and thermal noncontact methods. Examples of thermal-contact treatments include use of heat probe, multipolar electrocoagulation, and radiofrequency ablation. Examples of thermal noncontact treatments include use of argon plasma coagulation (APC) and neodymium:yttrium-aluminum garnet (Nd:YAG) laser. Although there are currently no head-to-head randomized controlled trials available and both are equally effective, the 2 techniques do differ in their safety profile. Overall, there are fewer complications associated with APC attributed to its lack of direct contact with the mucosa, thereby leading to a more superficial burn and reduced risk of perforation; however, pyloric stenosis with gastric outlet obstruction as a result of multiple APC treatments has been described in the literature.[53] Nd:YAG treatment has been associated with the development of gastric ulcers and hyperplastic gastric polyps, and one case of multifocal gastric cancer has also been reported 5 years after multiple therapy sessions.[44]

Newer techniques currently being further evaluated for the endoscopic management GAVE include a mechanically ablative procedure, endoscopic band ligation, which has been shown to result in bleeding cessation, reduced requirement for blood transfusion, and requirement of fewer treatment sessions.[54,55] A recent review of therapies for GAVE that was published in 2014 found that patients undergoing band ligation were more likely to be free from rebleeding (92%) versus those that are treated with APC (32%).[56] Other newer approaches include the use of radiofrequency ablation, which in some small published studies has shown promising results in patients who fail primary APC therapy for GAVE.[57,58] Although these results are promising, prospective randomized controlled trials are necessary to establish if one therapy is truly more successful than the other.

At the authors' institution, they use APC as primary ablative therapy for symptomatic GAVE with radiofrequency ablation being reserved for treatment failures.

DUODENAL VARICES

Variceal bleeding is a well-understood complication of portal hypertension of any cause, and the most common sites where this occurs are in the esophagus or the stomach. Occasionally, varices develop at alternative sites throughout the body, which include, but are not limited to, the small intestine, colon, rectum, and peristomal. Even more rarely, they can form around the gallbladder, bile ducts, and the pancreas and can even present as hemobilia or hemosuccus pancreaticus (HP). Overall, ectopic varices account for less than 5% of all variceal-related bleeding episodes.[59,60] Although a rare cause, bleeding from ectopic varices should be considered in all patients with known portal hypertension with overt GI bleeding without an obvious source noted in the esophagus or stomach. Duodenal varices (DV) make up 17% of cases of bleeding from ectopic varices.[59] DV most commonly occur in the bulb or in the second portion of the duodenum (**Fig. 5**).[61]

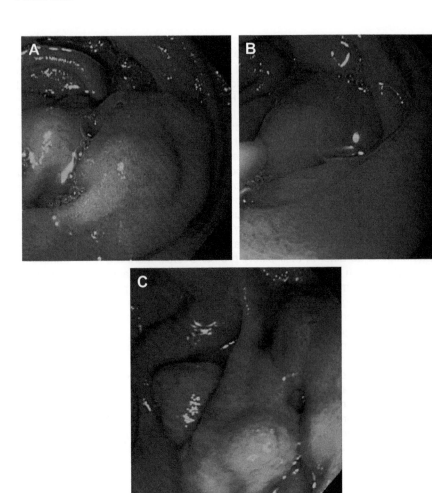

Fig. 5. (A–C) Duodenal varices. (*Courtesy of* Drs Anthony Post and Dany Raad, University Hospitals Case Medical Center, Cleveland, OH.)

Initial management of acute bleeding from DV includes hemodynamic resuscitation with intravenous fluids and blood products as needed and also the use of vasoactive agents that help reduce splanchnic blood flow such as somatostatin, its analogues such as octreotide, or vasopressin (although vasopressin has fallen out of favor because of adverse effects). Early endoscopy to assess for source and degree of bleeding should be pursued if the patient is clinically stable for the procedure.

Once a bleeding duodenal varix is identified on endoscopic evaluation, specific data regarding further management are limited to retrospective case series and case reports. In a small study published in 2009 of 14 patients, 4 patients received cyanoacrylate therapy and achieved successful hemostasis without any further evidence of recurrent bleeding.[62] Much of the authors' present management is based on data for gastric varices where initial therapy with cyanoacrylate injection has been shown to be superior to endoscopic band ligation in head to head trials. Initial hemostasis was found to be 87% with cyanoacrylate therapy versus 45% with band ligation, with rates of recurrent bleeding of 31% versus 54%, respectively.[63,64] However, an alternative study from 2006 has shown that initial hemostasis rates were similar between the 2 techniques, but that cyanoacrylate therapy had a lower incidence of recurrent bleeding, 23% versus 33.5%, for band ligation. In addition, this same study found a significantly higher recurrence rate of gastric varices with band ligation of 60%, whereas recurrence with cyanoacrylate therapy was 23%. There are reports in the literature about successful EUS-guided coil embolization for refractory bleeding from DV; however, data regarding this approach are limited and likely dependent on local expertise.[65,66] In cases where primary endoscopic management fails, it is important to remember that most DV have an afferent venous supply from either the portal vein or the superior mesenteric vein with an outflow track directly into the inferior vena cava; thus, transjugular intrahepatic portosystemic shunt (TIPS) and balloon retrograde transvenous obliteration (BRTO) procedures are possible.[63,67] A recent small case series of 5 patients found a 100% success rate with the BRTO procedure with regards to hemostasis and found no instances of recurrent bleeding for 1 year after the procedure.[68] TIPS has shown modest results. **Fig. 6** shows a flow diagram for the authors' recommended management of bleeding DV.[14]

HEMOSUCCUS PANCREATICUS

HP is an exceptionally rare and life-threatening source of upper GI bleeding that has a reported incidence of less than 1 in 1500 patients admitted for GI bleeding.[69] The clinical entity of bleeding through the ampulla of Vater from a pancreatic source was first described by Lower and Farrell[70] in a report of bleeding as a result of a splenic artery aneurysm in 1931. It was not until 1970 that Sanblom coined the term "hemosuccus pancreaticus" in a case series of patients with bleeding noted from the ampulla.[71] Other names for this condition are pseudohemobilia or *Wirsungorrhagia*. HP occurs as a consequence of numerous clinical conditions that are specifically associated with structural disorders of the pancreas or with its vascular supply. As one of the least frequently encountered sources of upper GI bleeding (**Fig. 7**), much of the data surrounding HP have been gathered mainly from retrospective studies and case reports or case series. It has been associated with many clinical conditions, which are summarized in **Box 1**. It should be noted that bleeding can also occur from the minor papilla, also known as santorinirrhage, which has been reported in cases of pancreatic divisum.

Diagnosis of HP can be quite challenging because it can present with intermittent and infrequent bleeding. Upper endoscopic evaluation has been reported to be normal in approximately half of all patients with HP in one large retrospective review.[69] Patients will typically present with abdominal pain radiating to the back with intermittent bleeding manifesting as melena, hematemesis, and rarely, hematochezia. These symptoms can be either acute or chronic over the course of months to years. Pain occurs from transient increases in intraductal pancreatic pressure by formation blood clots and improves after bleeding episodes due to the passage of clots. Other clinical features of HP include nausea, vomiting, acute pancreatitis, icterus from retrograde obstruction of bile ducts, anorexia, weight loss, and, occasionally, a palpable or pulsating epigastric mass.[72,73] Laboratory results can show various degrees of iron deficiency anemia and, occasionally, elevations in bilirubin; however, pancreatic enzyme and transaminase levels are generally normal when patients do not have abdominal pain.

Direct visualization of bleeding from the ampulla of Vater during endoscopy is uncommon because of the intermittent nature of bleeding; therefore, suspicion for HP should be increased by indirect signs of bleeding, including clots in the duodenum without an alternative explanation. Forward viewing endoscopes may not clearly visualize the papilla and, when suspicion for HP is increased, repeat endoscopy and the

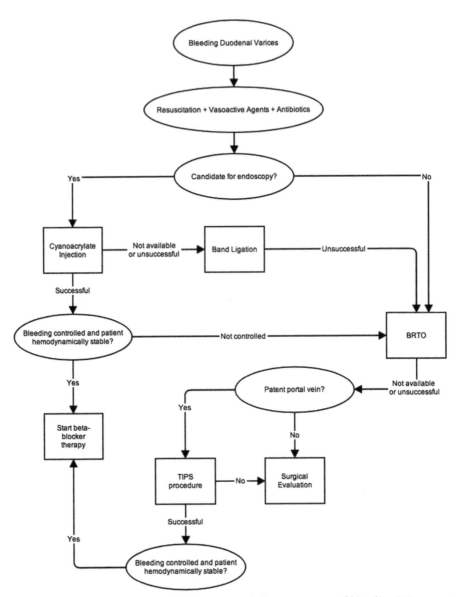

Fig. 6. Flow diagram for the authors' recommended management of bleeding DV.

adjunct of a side-viewing endoscope is almost always necessary to establish the diagnosis, but the overall sensitivity of endoscopic evaluation remains less than 50%.[69,73] Contrast-enhanced computed tomography (CT) scans with angiography and MRI can be helpful in further characterization of the local anatomy and can help lead to the diagnosis in more than 90% of cases.[69,74] Both of these imaging modalities can help distinguish pancreatic masses, aneurysms, or pseudoaneurysms of the local vasculature, or anatomic variants, including pancreatic divisum. Occasionally, CT angiography can identify active bleeding if the rate of bleeding is at least 0.4 mL/ min. On precontrast CT, the characteristic finding of clotted blood in the pancreatic

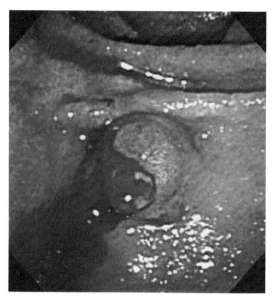

Fig. 7. HP. Blood is seen oozing out of the ampulla of Vater. (*Courtesy of* Dr Amitabh Chak, University Hospitals Case Medical Center, Cleveland, OH.)

duct, known as the sentinel clot, is seldom seen.[74] Endoscopic retrograde cholangio-pancreatography (ERCP) can be used to show extravasation of contrast, but carries increased inherent risk, including worsening of bleeding, post-ERCP pancreatitis, and disruption of the pancreatic duct. The gold standard to establish the diagnosis of HP includes selective arteriography of the celiac trunk and the superior mesenteric artery, where opacification of the pancreatic duct at angiography provides a definitive diagnosis of HP and has a reported sensitivity of 96%.[74] Pseudoaneurysms of the splanchnic arteries can present as HP in 20% of total cases.[75] These pseudoaneurysms have been reported to involve the splenic (60%–65%), gastroduodenal arteries (20%–25%), pancreaticoduodenal (10%–15%), and hepatic (5%–10%) arteries.[76] There have been recent reports of using EUS with Doppler imaging to delineate fistulous tracts originating from aneurysms.[77]

Management for HP depends on the underlying cause and, in most cases, treatment is surgical or with interventional radiology for selective arterial embolization. A definitive role of therapeutic endoscopy remains unclear at this time; however,

---

Box 1
Clinical conditions associated with Hemosuccus pancreaticus

- Acute or chronic pancreatitis
- Pancreatic malignancy
- Pancreatic pseudocysts
- Pseudoaneurysms
- Traumatic or iatrogenic damage to the pancreatic duct most commonly from ductal manipulation during ERCP
- Aneurysms of the splanchnic vasculature pancreatic divisum (bleeding from minor papilla)

there has been a recent report of successful endoscopic management of HP in a nonsurgical candidate with the use of multiple pancreatic duct stents to tamponade the hemorrhagic source.[78] This finding suggests that endoscopy may have a larger role in the future. Malignancies or other mass lesions often require surgical resection to prevent further bleeding once patients are hemodynamically stable, but in both, multiple case series have suggested reduced mortality with primary selective angiographic embolization.[69,79] The surgical management of the various causes of HP is beyond the scope of this discussion, but patients presenting with HP should be jointly evaluated by a pancreas surgeon and a therapeutic endoscopist as early as possible.

HEMOBILIA

Hemobilia, meaning bleeding from the biliary system, is a rare cause of upper GI bleeding, but should be suspected in patients with recent biliary tract or hepatic parenchymal instrumentation or trauma (**Fig. 8**). Less commonly, noniatrogenic causes can be considered. **Table 2** lists causes that can cause hemobilia. Sandblom and colleagues[80] initially described the classic triad of hemobilia consisting of obstructive jaundice, right upper quadrant abdominal pain, and either occult or overt GI bleeding in 1984; however, manifestation of all 3 signs at time of presentation is uncommon.[81] In fact, most patients have atypical presentations, which include cholestasis without jaundice, ascending cholangitis, coffee ground emesis, hematemesis, melena, pancreatitis, or even cholecystitis. The rate of bleeding may lead to clot formation in various sections of the biliary ductal system and occlusion of specific locations can lead to the aforementioned presentations.

Diagnosing hemobilia can be quite challenging and, as with HP, bleeding can be intermittent and difficult to visualize with standard forward-viewing endoscopes. Once alternative causes of upper GI bleeding are excluded by standard endoscopy, a side-viewing endoscope should be used to better visualize the ampulla of Vater for potential bleeding. Various radiological procedures have been suggested as being

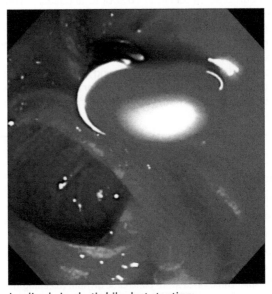

Fig. 8. Hemobilia visualized via plastic bile duct stenting.

Table 2
Pathophysiologic mechanisms and various causes of hemobilia

Mechanism	Cause of Hemobilia
Iatrogenic	• Percutaneous or transjugular liver biopsy • Percutaneous transhepatic cholangiogram • Cholecystectomy • Bile duct biopsies or stenting • TIPS placement • Angioembolization
Trauma	• Blunt abdominal trauma
Neoplastic lesions	• Hepatocellular carcinoma • Cholangiocarcinoma • Gallbladder carcinoma • Metastatic disease to liver • Gallbladder polyps
Nonneoplastic lesions	• Hepatic abscess • Hepatic cysts • Parasite infection, *Ascaris lumbricoides*
Aneurysms	• Hepatic artery aneurysm rupture (most common) • Cystic artery pseudoaneurysm
Arterial fistulization	• Arteriocholedochal fistula

helpful, including a technetium-99 tagged red blood cell scan, CT angiography[82] and mesenteric angiography, the latter of which can also be therapeutic with coil embolization.[83] There are some reports that advocate the use of EUS to help diagnose the cause of hemobilia; occasionally, endoscopic or percutaneous glue injection of an aneurysmal vessel can lead to bleeding cessation.[84,85] If minimally invasive techniques using endoscopy or angiography fail to resolve the underlying cause of bleeding, definitive management commonly involves surgical intervention specific to the cause of hemobilia.

AMPULLARY CARCINOMA

Ampullary carcinoma (AC) can also present with GI bleeding. Approximately one-third of patients present with chronic occult or overt GI bleeding. An interesting clinical sign of AC that is not often recognized is known as Thomas sign, also known as the silver stool sign, which was first described by Heneage Ogilvie in 1955. In the article, Ogilvie[86] presented 2 cases of ampullary adenocarcinoma where the pathologist, Dr A.M. Thomas, described stools as "motions having the colour of oxidized silver or aluminum paint." He noted that combination of acholic stools (white or yellow) mixed with blood from the upper GI tract (melena) led to the development of gray or silver stools.[86] These stools are reported to be a pathognomonic sign of AC.

ACs are neoplastic lesions that arise within the ampullary complex, distal to the bifurcation of the distal common bile duct and distal pancreatic duct. This type of malignancy is rare and has an incidence of 3 to 6 per million in the general population,[87] but are increased by 200- to 300-fold in the setting of hereditary polyposis syndromes.[88] A program of early screening endoscopy is an important factor in early diagnosis of ampullary lesions in patients with hereditary polyposis syndromes. On the other hand, in patients without genetic predisposition, the average age of diagnosis of sporadic AC is 60 to 70 years old. The prognosis for AC is poor and may be due to the fact that AC is often diagnosed at an advanced stage. A recent, large database study from

2008 found a 5-year survival rate for AC of 36.8%.[89] The molecular features, prognostic features, and staging of malignancy are beyond the scope of this discussion.

Up to 80% of patients with AC typically present with obstructive jaundice due to distal common bile duct compression by the ampullary mass (**Fig. 9**).[90] In addition to presenting with chronic occult or overt GI bleeding (as previously discussed), other nonspecific symptoms include abdominal pain, fever, nausea, and dyspepsia.

The standard approach for the management of primary AC is a pancreaticoduode-nectomy, also known as a Whipple operation, and permutations of the procedure as indicated in each case. As most patients present with preoperative jaundice, the role of preprocedure biliary drainage has been studied extensively with conflicting results and generally ERCP with stenting before operative management is usually performed in cases of symptomatic or asymptomatic high-grade jaundice, with a total bilirubin level greater than 15 mg/dL. Another indication for stenting before surgery is practical. Although a 2010 randomized controlled trial showed increased risk of complications with preoperative biliary drainage for cancer at the head of the pancreas, the patients in the nondrainage arm of the trial underwent surgery within 1 week of diagnosis.[91] In real-life clinical situations, surgery is often delayed for a multitude of reasons, whether it is for further preoperative evaluation or simply because of surgeon availability, and in these scenarios, the authors advocate for prior biliary tree decompression with stenting to reduce the risk of symptomatic jaundice or ascending cholangitis.

For patients who are poor surgical candidates, single-case reports and small series have been reported on the following minimally invasive nonsurgical approaches for AC:

- Endoscopic snare resection (papillectomy): a therapy option used for ampullary adenomas[92]
- Nd:YAG laser ablation has been reported to be used as palliative therapy for local control of tumor growth in patients who are poor surgical candidates[93]
- Photodynamic therapy has reported success in a small case series of 10 patients, where 3 patients underwent complete remission in those with AC confined to the ampulla and 4 others had significant reduction in tumor burden.[94]

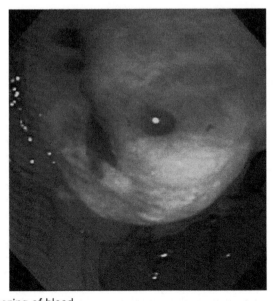

Fig. 9. AC with oozing of blood.

AORTOENTERIC FISTULAS

The formation of fistulas between the aorta and the GI tract can lead to life-threatening bleeding, which invariably has 100% mortality without intervention. Initially described in 1839,[95] a communication between the aorta and the enteric tract can occur as a result of disease processes at either site (ie, a PAEF), or as sequelae of surgical or graft intervention at the aortic aneurysmal site (ie, a secondary aortoenteric fistula [SAEF]). Overall, the reported incidence of PAEFs is 0.007 per million and SAEFs are 0.6% to 2%.[96]

The mechanism behind the development of aortoenteric fistulas (AEF) depends on whether it is a primary or secondary fistulization. In general, the rarer PAEFs develop through direct contact of the retroperitoneal duodenum with an aneurysmal aorta. The cause of the aneurysmal aorta can vary and may be from atherosclerosis, which is the most common cause in the United States, from infectious sources including tuberculosis or syphilis, or from collagen vascular disease as well as various other causes.[97–99] It is thought that persistent traumatic pulsations of an aortic aneurysm lead to local ischemia and subsequent necrosis of the intestinal wall and ultimately to direct communication of the aneurysm with the intestinal lumen. Following this, trauma from intestinal contents, pressure from peristaltic activity, or spontaneous rupture of the aneurysmal sac can lead to life-threatening upper GI bleeding.[100]

On the other hand, SAEFs form as a result of direct or indirect manipulation in and around the anatomic proximity of the abdominal aorta and the GI tract. Overall, this is the more common cause of AEF formation and can occur many years after placement of abdominal vascular grafts.[101] Fistula formation in SAEFs can occur from pressure necrosis or graft infection (**Fig. 10**). Other causes of SAEF formation include radiation therapy, foreign body perforation, trauma, tumor invasion, or ulceration.[102,103]

Classically, the presentation of AEF bleeding consists of a triad that includes massive GI bleeding, abdominal or back pain, and a pulsatile abdominal mass; however, this is only present in less than 15% of patients.[99] In most patients, bleeding may be intermittent because of clot formation and subsequent dislodgement.

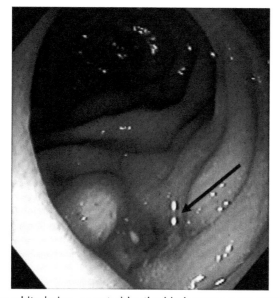

Fig. 10. SAEF. The white lesion, as noted by the black arrow, represents the aortic graft material protruding through the duodenal mucosa in this SAEF.

Paradoxically, the initial bleeding is often minor and short lived; known as a "herald bleed," it commonly presents as relatively minor GI bleeding with coffee ground emesis, hematemesis, or melena. This initial bleeding can be followed hours or days later by massive bleeding or exsanguination with or without abdominal pain, fever, or sepsis.

Diagnoses of bleeding from AEF rely on a high index of clinical suspicion and should be suspected in patients with even minor GI bleeding in addition to a history of thoracic or abdominal aortic intervention. It is imperative to recognize these bleeds as early as possible because the reported mortality nears 77% with intervention and is 100% fatal without treatment.[104] In these patients, an emergent CT angiogram with intravenous contrast may be ordered to evaluate for extravasation of contrast, to demonstrate fistula, or to evaluate for inflammation or infection around the aortic graft. The role of endoscopy in AEF depends on the degree of clinical suspicion for the entity. If a CT angiogram is diagnostic or highly suspicious for AEF, then the patient should proceed directly to emergency surgery without further endoscopic evaluation. Delays in emergent surgical management can potentially lead to fatal outcomes. On the other hand, if a CT angiogram is nondiagnostic and if the differential diagnoses include an AEF, then an urgent push enteroscopy to examine the entire duodenum should be performed to exclude other causes of GI bleeding and to evaluate for a possible AEF. During endoscopy, it is particularly important for the endoscopist to evaluate the third portion of the duodenum very carefully for the presence of an AEF and for evidence of extrinsic compression and blood. Absolutely no manipulation should be attempted if an AEF is found at endoscopy because any manipulation can result in massive bleeding and exsanguination by opening up of the AEF.

All cases of suspected GI bleeding from an AEF should be emergently and jointly evaluated by a GI endoscopist, when appropriate, and always with a vascular surgeon. Management of bleeding AEF is purely surgical. Endoscopy is only used to aid in the diagnosis and to exclude other causes of GI bleeding, when the cause is unclear and suspicion is low or moderate. There is no therapeutic role for endoscopy in this disorder. It is also important to recognize that endoscopy can diagnose an AEF, but that a negative endoscopic examination does not exclude an AEF.

REFERENCES

1. Truesdale PE. Recurring hernia of the diaphragm. Ann Surg 1924;79(5): 751–7.
2. Cameron AJ. Incidence of iron deficiency anemia in patients with large diaphragmatic hernia. A controlled study. Mayo Clin Proc 1976;51:767–9.
3. Gray DM, Kushnir V, Kalra G, et al. Cameron lesions in patients with hiatal hernias: prevalence, presentation, and treatment outcome. Dis Esophagus 2014. http://dx.doi.org/10.1111/dote.12223.
4. Weston AP. Hiatal hernia with Cameron ulcers and erosions. Gastrointest Endosc Clin N Am 1996;6(4):671–9.
5. Camus M, Jensen DM, Ohning GV, et al. Severe upper gastrointestinal hemorrhage from linear gastric ulcers in large hiatal hernias: a large prospective series of Cameron ulcers. Endoscopy 2013;45(5):397–400.
6. Katz J, Brar S, Sidhu JS. Histopathological characterization of a Cameral lesion. Int J Surg Pathol 2012;20(5):528–30.
7. Zaman A, Katon RM. Push enteroscopy for obscure gastrointestinal bleeding yields a high incidence of proximal lesions within reach of a standard endoscope. Gastrointest Endosc 1998;47:372–6.

8. Cameron AJ, Higgins JA. Linear gastric erosion. A lesion associated with large diaphragmatic hernia and chronic blood loss anemia. Gastroenterology 1986; 91:338–42.

9. Richter IA, Rabin MS. The 'riding' ulcer: a report of three cases. S Afr Med J 1979;56(15):612–4.

10. Lum DF, McQuaid K, Lee JG. Endoscopic hemostasis of non-variceal, non-peptic ulcer hemorrhage. Gastrointest Endosc Clin N Am 1997;7(4):657–70.

11. Lin C, Chen TH, How WC, et al. Endoscopic treatment of a Cameron lesion presenting as a life-threatening gastrointestinal hemorrhage. J Clin Gastroenterol 2001;33(5):423–4.

12. Dieulafoy G. Exulceratio simplex: leçons 1–3. Clinique medicale de l'Hotel Dieu de Paris. Paris: Masson et Cie; 1898. p. 1–38.

13. Lee YT, Walmsley RS, Leong RW, et al. Dieulafoy's lesion. Gastrointest Endosc 2003;58(2):236–43.

14. Feldman M, Friedman LS, Brandt LJ. Sleisenger and Fordtran's gastrointestinal and liver disease. 9th edition. Philadelphia: Saunders, Elsevier, Inc; 2010.

15. Fockens P, Meenan J, van Dullemen HM, et al. Dieulafoy's disease: endosonographic detection and endosonography-guided treatment. Gastrointest Endosc 1996;44(4):437–42.

16. Nesje LB, Skarstein A, Matre K, et al. Dieulafoy's vascular malformation: role of endoscopic ultrasonography in therapeutic decision-making. Scand J Gastroenterol 1998;33(1):104–8.

17. Park CH, Joo YE, Kim HS, et al. A prospective, randomized trial of endoscopic band ligation versus endoscopic hemoclip placement for bleeding gastric Dieulafoy's lesions. Endoscopy 2004;36(8):677–81.

18. DiMaio CJ, Stevens PD. Nonvariceal upper gastrointestinal bleeding. Gastrointest Endosc Clin N Am 2007;17(2):253–72.

19. Akhras J, Patel P, Tobi M. Dieulafoy's lesion-like bleeding: an underrecognized cause of upper gastrointestinal hemorrhage in patients with advanced liver disease. Dig Dis Sci 2007;52(3):722–6.

20. Iacoponi F, Petruzziello L, Marchese M, et al. Hemostasis of Dieulafoy's lesions by argon plasma coagulation (with video). Gastrointest Endosc 2007;66(1):20–6.

21. Wong RC. New diagnostic imaging technologies in nonvariceal upper gastrointestinal bleeding. Gastrointest Endosc Clin N Am 2011;21(4):707–20.

22. Jaspersen D. Dieulafoy's disease controlled by Doppler ultrasound endoscopic treatment. Gut 1993;34(6):857–8.

23. Acosta RD, Wong RK. Differential diagnosis of upper gastrointestinal bleeding proximal to the ligament of Treitz. Gastrointest Endosc Clin N Am 2011;21(4): 555–66.

24. Matsushita M, Uchida K, Nishio A, et al. Endoscopic and EUS features of gastric inflammatory fibroid polyps. Gastrointest Endosc 2009;69(1):188.

25. Zhang C, Cui M, Xing J, et al. Massive gastrointestinal bleeding caused by a giant gastric inflammatory fibroid polyp: a case report. Int J Surg Case Rep 2014;5(9):571–3.

26. Rawashdeh B, Meyer M, Moslemi M, et al. Unusual presentation of a giant benign inflammatory polyp in the upper esophagus. Int J Surg Case Rep 2015;6C:206–9.

27. Vanek J. Gastric submucosal granuloma with eosinophilic infiltration. Am J Pathol 1949;25(3):397–411.

28. Helwig EB, Ranier A. Inflammatory fibroid polyps of the stomach. Surg Gynecol Obstet 1953;96(3):335–67.

29. Akbulut S. Intussusception due to inflammatory fibroid polyp: a case report and comprehensive literature review. World J Gastroenterol 2012;18(40):5745–52.
30. Gutu E, Ghidirim G, Misin I, et al. Bleeding gastric inflammatory fibroid polyp (Vanek's tumor). Chirurgia (Bucur) 2010;105(1):137–40.
31. Mucientes P, Mucientes F, Klaassen R. Inflammatory fibroid polyp associated with early gastric carcinoma: a case report. Ann Diagn Pathol 2012;16(2):148–51.
32. Ergun M, Zengin N, Kayacetin E. Loop observe and snare technique for endoscopic resection of a gastric inflammatory fibroid polyp. Endoscopy 2012; 44(Suppl 2 UCTN):E86–7.
33. Jain R, Chetty R. Gastric hyperplastic polyps: a review. Dig Dis Sci 2009;54(9): 1839–46.
34. Secemsky BJ, Robinson KR, Kumar K, et al. Gastric hyperplastic polyps causing upper gastrointestinal hemorrhage in a young adult. World J Clin Cases 2013;1(1):25–7.
35. Shaib YH, Rugge M, Graham DY, et al. Management of gastric polyps: an endoscopy-based approach. Clin Gastroenterol Hepatol 2013;11(11): 1374–84.
36. Hirota WK, Zuckerman MJ, Adler DG, et al. ASGE guideline: the role of endoscopy in the surveillance of premalignant conditions of the upper GI tract. Gastrointest Endosc 2006;63(4):570.
37. Szaloki T, Toth V, Nemeth I, et al. Endoscopic mucosal resection: not only therapeutic, but a diagnostic procedure for sessile gastric polyps. J Gastroenterol Hepatol 2008;23(4):551–5.
38. Rider JA, Klotz AP, Kirsner JB. Gastritis with veno-capillary ectasia as a source of massive gastric hemorrhage. Gastroenterology 1953;24(1):118–23.
39. Jabbari M, Cherry R, Lough JO, et al. Gastric antral vascular ectasia: the watermelon stomach. Gastroenterology 1984;87(5):1165–70.
40. Payen JL, Cales P, Voight JJ, et al. Severe portal hypertensive gastropathy and antral vascular ectasia are distinct entities in patients with cirrhosis. Gastroenterology 1995;108(1):138–44.
41. Dulai GS, Jensen DM, Kovacs TO, et al. Endoscopic treatment outcomes in watermelon stomach patients with and without portal hypertension. Endoscopy 2004;36(1):68–72.
42. Ito M, Uchida Y, Kamano S, et al. Clinical comparisons between two subsets of gastric antral vascular ectasia. Gastrointest Endosc 2001;53(7):764–70.
43. Rosenfield G, Enns R. Argon photocoagulation in the treatment of gastric antral vascular ectasia and radiation proctitis. Can J Gastroenterol 2009;23(12):801–4.
44. Qureshi K, Al-Osaimi AM. Approach to the management of portal hypertensive gastropathy and gastric antral vascular ectasia. Gastroenterol Clin North Am 2014;43(4):835–47.
45. Suit PF, Petras RE, Bauer TW, et al. Gastric antral vascular ectasia. A histologic and morphometric study of "the watermelon stomach". Am J Surg Pathol 1987; 11(10):750–7.
46. Charneau J, Petit R, Cales P, et al. Antral motility in patients with cirrhosis with or without gastric antral vascular ectasia. Gut 1995;37(4):488–92.
47. Spahr L, Villeneuve JP, Dufresne MP, et al. Gastric antral vascular ectasia in cirrhotic patients: absence of relation with portal hypertension. Gut 1999; 44(5):739–42.
48. Quintero E, Pique JM, Bombi JA, et al. Gastric mucosal vascular ectasias causing bleeding in cirrhosis. A distinct entity associated with hypergastrinemia and low serum levels of pepsinogen I. Gastroenterology 1987;93(5):1054–61.

49. Saperas E, Perez Ayuso RM, Poca E, et al. Increased gastric PGE2 biosynthesis in cirrhotic patients with gastric vascular ectasia. Am J Gastroenterol 1990; 85(2):138–44.
50. Vincent C, Pomier-Layrargues G, Dagenais M, et al. Cure of gastric antral vascular ectasia by liver transplantation despite persistent portal hypertension: a clue for pathogenesis. Liver Transpl 2002;8(8):717–20.
51. Watson M, Hally RJ, McCue PA, et al. Gastric antral vascular ectasia (watermelon stomach) in patients with systemic sclerosis. Arthritis Rheum 1996; 39(2):341–6.
52. Gostout CJ, Vigiano TR, Ahlquist DA, et al. The clinical and endoscopic spectrum of the watermelon stomach. J Clin Gastroenterol 1992;15(3):256–63.
53. Farooq FT, Wong RC, Yang P, et al. Gastric outlet obstruction as a complication of argon plasma coagulation for watermelon stomach. Gastrointest Endosc 2007;65(7):1090–2.
54. Wells CD, Harrison ME, Gurudu SR, et al. Treatment of gastric antral vascular ectasia (watermelon stomach) with endoscopic band ligation. Gastrointest Endosc 2008;68(2):231–6.
55. Chong VH. Snare coagulation for gastric antral vascular ectasia ablation. Gastrointest Endosc 2009;69(6):1195.
56. Swanson E, Mahqoub A, MacDonald R, et al. Medical and endoscopic therapies for angiodysplasia and gastric antral vascular ectasia: a systematic review. Clin Gastroenterol Hepatol 2014;12(4):571–82.
57. McGorisk T, Krishnan K, Keefer L, et al. Radiofrequency ablation for refractory gastric antral vascular ectasia (with video). Gastrointest Endosc 2013;78(4): 584–8.
58. Dray X, Recpici A, Gonzalez P, et al. Radiofrequency ablation for the treatment of gastric antral vascular ectasia. Endoscopy 2014;46(11):963–9.
59. Norton ID, Andrews JC, Kamath PS. Management of ectopic varices. Hepatology 1998;28(4):1154–8.
60. Sato T, Akaike J, Toyota J, et al. Clinicopathological features and treatment of ectopic varices with portal hypertension. Int J Hepatol 2011;2011:960720.
61. Watanabe N, Toyonaga A, Kojima S, et al. Current status of ectopic varices in Japan: results of a survey by the Japan Society for portal hypertension. Hepatol Res 2010;40(8):763–76.
62. Kinzel J, Pichetshote N, Dredar S, et al. Bleeding from a duodenal varix: a unique case of variceal hemostasis achieved using EUS-guided placement of an embolization coil and cyanoacrylate. J Clin Gastroenterol 2014;48(4):362–4.
63. Hashizume M, Tanoue K, Ohta M, et al. Vascular anatomy of duodenal varices: angiographic and histopathological assessments. Am J Gastroenterol 1993; 88(11):1942–5.
64. Zamora CA, Sugimoto K, Tsurusaki M, et al. Endovascular obliteration of bleeding duodenal varices in patients with liver cirrhosis. Eur Radiol 2006; 16(1):73–9.
65. Liu Y, Yang J, Wang J, et al. Clinical characteristics and endoscopic treatment with cyanoacrylate injection in patients with duodenal varices. Scand J Gastroenterol 2009;44(8):1012–6.
66. Henry Z, Uppal D, Saad W, et al. Gastric and ectopic varices. Clin Liver Dis 2014;18(2):371–88.
67. Lo GH, Lai KH, Cheng JS, et al. A prospective, randomized trial of butyl cyanoacrylate injection versus band ligation in the management of bleeding gastric varices. Hepatology 2001;33(5):1060–4.

68. Levy MJ, Wong Kee Song LM, Kendrick ML, et al. EUS-guided coil embolization for refractory ectopic variceal bleeding (with videos). Gastrointest Endosc 2008; 67(3):572–4.
69. Rammohan A, Palaniappan R, Ramaswami S, et al. Hemosuccus pancreaticus: 15-year experience from a tertiary care GI bleed centre. ISRN Radiol 2013;2013: 191794.
70. Lower WE, Farrell JI. Aneurysm of the splenic artery: report of a case and review of literature. Arch Surg 1931;23:182–90.
71. Sandblom P. Gastrointestinal hemorrhage through the pancreatic duct. Ann Surg 1970;171(1):61–6.
72. Etienne S, Pessaux P, Tuech JJ, et al. Hemosuccus pancreaticus: a rare cause of gastrointestinal bleeding. Gastroenterol Clin Biol 2005;29(3):237–42.
73. Koren M, Kinova S, Bedeova J, et al. Hemosuccus pancreaticus. Bratisl Lek Listy 2008;109(1):37–41.
74. Koizumi J, Inoue S, Yonekawa H, et al. Hemosuccus pancreaticus: diagnosis with CT and MRI and treatment with transcatheter embolization. Abdom Imaging 2002;27(1):77–81.
75. Peroux JL, Arput JP, Saint-Paul MC, et al. Wirsungorrhagia complicating chronic pancreatitis associated with neuroendocrine tumor of the pancreas. Gastroenterol Clin Biol 1994;18(12):1142–5 [in French].
76. Gadacz TR, Trunkey D, Kieffer RF Jr. Visceral vessel erosion associated with pancreatitis. Case reports and a review of literature. Arch Surg 1978;113(12): 1438–40.
77. Pham KD, Pedersen G, Halvorsen H, et al. Usefulness of endoscopic ultrasound for the diagnosis of hemosuccus pancreaticus. Endoscopy 2014;46(Suppl 1):E528.
78. Gutkin E, Kim SH. A novel endoscopic treatment of hemosuccus pancreaticus: a stent tree tamponade. JOP 2012;13(3):312–3.
79. Akpinar H, Dicle O, Ellidokuz E, et al. Hemosuccus pancreaticus treated by transvascular selective arterial embolization. Endoscopy 1999;31(2): 213–4.
80. Sandblom P, Saegesser F, Mirkovitch V. Hepatic hemobilia: hemorrhage from the intrahepatic biliary tract, a review. World J Surg 1984;8(1):41–50.
81. Bloechele C, Izbicki JR, Rashed MY, et al. Hemobilia: presentation, diagnosis, and management. Am J Gastroenterol 1994;89(9):1537–40.
82. Delgado Millan MA, Deballon PO. Computed tomography, angiography, and endoscopic retrograde cholangiopancreatography in the nonoperative management of hepatic and splenic trauma. World J Surg 2001;25(11):1397–402.
83. Senadhi V, Arora D, Arora M, et al. Hemobilia caused by a ruptured hepatic cyst: a case report. J Med Case Rep 2011;5:26.
84. Trakarnsanga A, Sriprayoon T, Akaraviputh T, et al. Massive hemobilia from a ruptured hepatic artery aneurysm detected by endoscopic ultrasound (EUS) and successfully treated. Endoscopy 2010;42(Suppl 2):E340–1.
85. Cattan P, Cuillerier E, Cellier C, et al. Hemobilia caused by a pseudoaneurysm of the hepatic artery diagnosed by EUS. Gastrointest Endosc 1999;49(2):252–5.
86. Ogilvie H. Thomas's sign, or the silver stool in cancer of the ampulla of Vater. Br Med J 1955;1(4907):208.
87. Goodman MT, Yamamoto J. Descriptive study of gallbladder, extrahepatic bile duct, and ampullary cancers in the United States 1997–2002. Cancer Causes Control 2007;18(4):415–22.
88. Jagelman DG, DeCosse JJ, Bussey HJ. Upper gastrointestinal cancer in familial polyposis. Lancet 1988;1(8595):1149–51.

89. O'Connell JB, Maggard MA, Manunga J Jr, et al. Survival after resection of ampullary carcinoma: a national population-based study. Ann Surg Oncol 2008;15(7):1820–7.
90. Monson JR, Donohue JH, McEntee GP, et al. Radical resection for carcinoma of the ampulla of Vater. Arch Surg 1991;126(3):353–7.
91. van der Gaag NA, Rauws EA, van Eijck CH, et al. Preoperative biliary drainage for cancer of the head of the pancreas. N Engl J Med 2010;362(2):129–37.
92. Woo SM, Ryu JK, Lee WJ, et al. Feasibility of endoscopic papillectomy in early stage ampulla of Vater cancer. J Gastroenterol Hepatol 2009;24(1):120–4.
93. Fowler AL, Barham CP, Britton BJ, et al. Laser ablation of ampullary carcinoma. Endoscopy 1999;31(9):745–7.
94. Abulafi AM, Allardice JT, Williams NS, et al. Photodynamic therapy for malignant tumors of the ampulla of Vater. Gut 1995;36(6):853–6.
95. Diethrich EB, Campbell DA, Brandt RL. Gastrointestinal hemorrhage. Presenting symptom of aortoduodenal fistulization. Am J Surg 1966;112(6):903–7.
96. Vu QD, Menias CO, Bhalla S, et al. Aortoenteric fistulas: CT features and potential mimics. Radiographics 2009;29(1):197–209.
97. Voorhoeve R, Moll FL, de Letter JA, et al. Primary aortoenteric fistula: report of eight new cases and review of the literature. Ann Vasc Surg 1996;10(1):40–8.
98. Walsh AK, Gwynn BR. Atypical aorto-enteric fistula. Eur J Vasc Endovasc Surg 1995;9(3):353–4.
99. Saers SJ, Scheltinga MR. Primary aortoenteric fistula. Br J Surg 2005;92(2):143–52.
100. Champion MC, Sullivan SN, Coles JC, et al. Aortoenteric fistula: incidence, presentation, recognition, and management. Ann Surg 1982;195(3):314–7.
101. Bergqvist D, Bjorkman H, Bolin T, et al. Secondary aortoenteric fistulae— changes from 1973 to 1993. Eur J Vasc Endovasc Surg 1996;11(4):425–8.
102. Schwab CW, McMahon DJ, Phillips G, et al. Aortic balloon control of a traumatic aortoenteric fistula after damage control laparotomy: a case report. J Trauma 1996;40(6):1021–3.
103. Napoli PJ, Meade PC, Adams CW. Primary aortoenteric fistula from a posttraumatic pseudoaneurysm. J Trauma 1996;41(1):149–52.
104. Bergqvist D. Arterioenteric fistula. Review of a vascular emergency. Acta Chir Scand 1987;153(2):81–6.

Tips and Tricks on How to Optimally Manage Patients with Upper Gastrointestinal Bleeding

Michael W. Rajala, MD, PhD*, Gregory G. Ginsberg, MD

KEYWORDS

- Upper gastrointestinal bleeding • Endoscopy • Therapeutic devices
- Gastroenterology

KEY POINTS

- Make adequate resuscitation a primary goal before proceeding with endoscopy.
- Maintain knowledge of both benefits and limitations of specific therapeutic devices to best guide selection of treatment modality.
- Remain aware of evolving endoscopic devices that may influence treatment options and outcomes.
- Remain calm and composed by having knowledge and confidence in your experience, training, and preparation. If lacking, scheduled in-service training, online videos, and/or hands-on courses can boost these skills and your confidence.

Videos of hemostasis obtained following injection of epinephrine followed by bipolar diatheramy and then hemoclip placement; treatment of a variceal bleed by placement of 2 hemoclips; and the proper technique for guillotining off an adherent clot from an ulcer in the lesser curvature of the stomach accompany this article at http://www.giendo.theclinics.com/

INTRODUCTION

Presentation of a patient with acute upper GI bleeding can be a source of alarm for the consulting gastroenterologist. The consulting gastroenterologist is pivotal in key management decisions such as when to scope (ie, urgently within 24 hours vs electively)

Conflicts of interest: Neither author has any commercial or financial conflicts of interest.
Division of Gastroenterology, Department of Medicine, University of Pennsylvania Perelman School of Medicine, 3400 Spruce Street, Philadelphia, PA, USA
* Corresponding author. Perelman Center for Advanced Medicine, South Pavilion, 7th floor, 3400 Civic Center Boulevard, Philadelphia, PA 19104.
E-mail address: michael.rajala@uphs.upenn.edu

Gastrointest Endoscopy Clin N Am 25 (2015) 607–617
http://dx.doi.org/10.1016/j.giec.2015.02.004

giendo.theclinics.com

and where to scope (emergency department [ED], intensive care unit [ICU], operating room [OR], or endoscopy suite), and in performing expert endoscopic therapy while guiding adjunctive therapies to optimize the treatment plan.

This article provides tips and tricks for the successful management of acute upper GI bleeding that are complementary to the in-depth reviews that accompany it in this issue. This article offers 10 categories of tips and tricks to improve the evaluation and endoscopic management of GI bleeding.

Who Is in Charge?

One of the important first steps in the management of a patient with acute upper GI bleeding is determining who is responsible for and overseeing ongoing patient assessment and resuscitation. Although seemingly a simple task, the chain of command and delineations of responsibilities may be obscure in that patients may present with bleeding to the ED or while an inpatient on the wards. Patients with acute GI bleeding often require transfer to the ICU or specialized bleeding unit. During these times, responsibilities for assignments should be clearly dictated to avoid confusion, lapses in resuscitation, and risk for error.

Initial Management

Endoscopy for acute GI bleeding should be performed only after appropriate resuscitation. The initial evaluation of a patient with GI bleeding should focus on the presenting history, relevant comorbidities, physical examination findings, and medications that influence resuscitation and monitoring efforts.

Management of patients with severe bleeding and hemodynamic derangements must focus on the ABCs (airway, breathing, and circulation) of resuscitation. During this stage, the ability of the patient to maintain adequate ventilation should be quickly assessed. Endotracheal intubation should be considered in patients with active hematemesis, altered mentation, other risks for aspiration (eg, prior stroke), or potentially difficult airways. Peripheral or central venous access is necessary to ensure adequate administration of intravenous crystaloids, colloids, and blood products. Optimally, venous access with at least two 16-gauge to 18-gauge needles should be secured and the need for central venous access considered.

Patients with massive bleeding require blood, platelets, and clotting factors. It is imperative that blood transfusions be performed judiciously. Although it is obviously important not to under-resuscitate, a recent study showed that over-resuscitation with blood products led to increased rebleeding rates and decreased survival in patients with a liberal threshold (maintaining hemoglobin level >9 g/dL) compared with a restrictive threshold (maintaining hemoglobin level >7 g/dL).[1] The survival benefit was profoundly seen in patients with Child-Pugh class A or B cirrhosis. In a subgroup analysis, the benefit from the restrictive threshold cohort without cirrhosis only trended toward significance. Note that these thresholds were established in a patient population that excluded patients with massive GI bleeding, acute coronary syndrome, stroke, transient ischemic attack, systemic peripheral vasculopathy, or recent trauma or surgery. Although these results are applicable to most patients with GI bleeding, they therefore should not be universally generalized, and lower transfusion thresholds may not be ideal in patients with massive bleeding or ischemia. Basing transfusions on laboratory values in patients with brisk blood loss and hypotension can be misguided because hemoglobin levels may misinform.

Patients with coexisting cardiovascular, renal, or liver disease have increased overall mortality from GI bleeding. These individuals require individualized care in order to optimize resuscitation efforts. In patients with a severe bleeding and cardiovascular disease, serial enzymes and cardiac monitoring should be considered and the patient reassessed at regular intervals.

The medication review emphasizes the use of aspirin, nonsteroidal antiinflammatory agents, antiplatelet agents, and antithrombotic agents. The decision to reverse anticoagulation should be based on the severity of bleeding, the indication for anticoagulation, and the risks of reversing these agents versus the risks of further bleeding. In cases of exsanguinating GI bleeding, holding these agents and reversing their effects is recommended. However, in many other instances, a gradual reversal of anticoagulation therapy may be preferred to abrupt reversal. In cases in which the risk of a critical thromboembolic event is high, consultation of the prescribing provider or relevant specialist is advised. It is important to stay apprised of the new antithrombotic agents as they come on the market. Measures to reverse many new medications are varied and agent specific. The review of antithrombotic agents is beyond the scope of this article but these have recently been reviewed by Baron and colleagues.[2]

When to Scope?

Ideally, the triage assessment should differentiate patients who require urgent endoscopy, defined as within 24 hours, from those who can either be admitted for less urgent endoscopy or even safely evaluated as outpatients. Patients who are hemodynamically unstable on presentation or who are actively bleeding after resuscitation should undergo endoscopic evaluation as soon as they are stabilized. In such cases, early consultation with interventional radiology and surgery is recommended. Urgent endoscopy is also recommended for patients with a history concerning for variceal bleeding. An important distinction is that urgent is defined as within 12 hours for suspected variceal bleeding as opposed to within 24 hours for suspected nonvariceal bleeding. For those other patients who are hemodynamically stable but have evidence of a lesser degree of GI bleeding, considerations guiding the timing of endoscopy include the degree of GI blood loss, presence of significant comorbidities, use of anticoagulation medications, and recent medical history including instrumentation such as elective endoscopy or radiographic needle biopsy.

The main point is that the diagnostic yield of endoscopy for acute GI bleeding is related to the expediency with which endoscopy is performed. The likelihood of accurately assessing the source of bleeding is highest when endoscopy is performed sooner rather than later. This diagnostic accuracy may affect subsequent resource use, including length of stay, ICU admission, and blood products. However, only the application of endoscopic therapy has been shown to affect patient outcomes of mortality and need for operative intervention.

Upper or Lower Source?

The presenting history and physical examination are apt to help differentiate between an upper and a lower source. Given that patients are not accurate in differentiating between melena and dark stools, especially when taking medications that darken stools (iron and bismuth), a digital rectal examination, when conducted by an experienced clinician, may be an important part of the evaluation. Confirmation of melena on stool examination is fairly specific for upper GI bleeding with the caveat that it may be associated with small bowel or right colon sources in up to 5% to 10% of cases. However, it does not provide meaningful information on the severity of bleeding because melena can be observed with as little as 50 mL of acute blood loss. In contrast, although hematochezia on rectal examination is generally associated with lower GI bleeding, its presence does not exclude an upper GI source, because up to 10% of older patients with upper GI bleeding present with hematochezia.[3]

Nasogastric tube placement with lavage was once ordered on all patients presenting with suspected upper GI bleeding. Although results of a gastric lavage may be helpful in certain instances, it has a false-negative result in up to 15% of patients subsequently found to have lesions with high-risk stigmata for rebleeding.[4] Further, obtaining the lavage can delay care and often results in a considerable amount of distress for the patient. Moreover, the results of the nasogastric lavage do not typically alter clinical management or outcome.[5,6] If lavage is performed to assess for upper GI bleeding, at least a 200-mL lavage should return with bilious aspirate. A nasogastric tube can be considered when retained blood in the stomach is suspected. However, use of a prokinetic agent (discussed later) is preferred to a nasogastric lavage to clear gastric contents before endoscopy.

Where to Scope?

Few acute GI bleeding cases present during endoscopy units' normal working hours. Even when they do, endoscopy may be more appropriately performed in the ED, ICU, or even the OR. The optimal location for endoscopy has a lot to do with the timing, personnel support, and patient stability. Important considerations include the severity of bleeding, stability of the patient for transport, and ability of the different services to provide the level of care required.

In general, patients who are hemodynamically stable without severe GI bleeding or significant comorbidities are best managed in the endoscopy unit where staff are familiar with supporting endoscopic procedures and all equipment is at hand. In contrast, patients who present with signs of active bleeding, hypotension, orthostasis, hemoglobin level less than 8 g/dL, hematochezia, or major comorbidities may be best managed in locations where intensive resuscitation can occur, whether it be the ICU, ED, or OR.

While preparing to perform emergency endoscopy, the sedation plan should be considered on a case-by-case basis. Many cases can be safely and effectively performed under moderate sedation using gastroenterologist-administered narcotic and benzodiazepine. In moderate sedation, patients are expected to maintain control of their protective reflexes of cough and gag. Increasingly, monitored anesthesia care[7] sedation with propofol is administered to support endoscopic procedures. It is important to recognize that monitored anesthesia care generates deep sedation, often approaching general anesthesia. In these circumstances, patients have lost their protective reflexes and are at risk for aspiration should regurgitation of gastric contents occur during the procedure. It is important to reassess patient status frequently during the procedure and consider endotracheal intubation if an increased risk of airway compromise is perceived.

What Equipment Should Be Used when There Are so Many Options?

As the number of options for treating bleeding lesions continues to expand, it can be difficult to know which treatment modalities are best. In general, this decision should be based on the characteristics of the lesion (location and type), the benefits and limitations of the therapeutic device in treating these types of lesions, and the familiarity and experience of the endoscopist with each treatment modality.

Selection based on lesion characteristics

The location of a target can affect the utility of specific devices. In the case of lesions located on the posterior wall and lesser curvature of the stomach and the posterior wall of the duodenal bulb, a more tangential orientation of the endoscope results in more difficulty targeting the lesion enface. Multipolar cautery probes have an advantage in these locations, because they are effective for use when applied both tangentially as well as enface, compared with hemostatic clips, which are best used enface. Targets within the duodenal bulb often provide a suboptimal working distance between the scope and the lesion. Multipolar cautery probes again are often more suitable than hemostatic clips in these situations given the space required to expose, open, and deploy the clip (see supplemental Video 1). However, the use of an endoscopic cap can overcome this potential disadvantage. Endoscopic caps are transparent, hollow cylinders that can be attached to the tip of the endoscope and are used for improving visualization and access to the source of bleeding. Benefits include being able to push folds aside, improve direct engagement of the endoscope (eg, posterior wall of the stomach), and stabilize the position of the tip of the endoscope in the duodenal bulb.[8] Limitations of endoscopic caps may include decreased angle of view and extension of the scope tip that may make intubation of the esophagus more difficult.

The type of lesion being targeted should also be considered.

Gastroduodenal ulcers

Chronic ulcers with a fibrotic ulcer base or ulcers too large to approximate the margins may not be effectively treated with hemostatic clips. Iatrogenic gastric or duodenal ulcers following recent endoscopic mucosal or submucosal dissection are at greater risk of perforation caused by thermal injury and hemostatic clips are a good choice for therapy. Although the addition of epinephrine injection to either hemostatic clips or electrocoagulation therapy does not significantly increase the efficacy of either method used independently, there is a reduction in the rate of recurrent bleeding, surgery, and mortality with use of a second modality in combination with epinephrine.[9] Epinephrine injection is considered suboptimal as monotherapy and should not be used as such unless other options are not available or applicable. However, we generally opt for dual-mode therapy for active nonvariceal bleeding and for lesions with adherent clot. Initial injection with diluted epinephrine (1:10,000) into and around the base of the bleeding site provides several laudable benefits through vasoconstriction and tissue edema. First, by slowing or stopping active spurting or oozing, it typically improves visualization of the discrete bleeding site. Second, this also enables a more disciplined removal of adherent clot. In both of these cases the clinician is better able to direct definitive therapy. Third, injection can be performed strategically so as to alter the lie of the lesion by lifting the tissue, promoting a more accessible approach for definitive therapy.

Esophageal varices

For esophageal variceal bleeding, first-line treatment options include endoscopic band ligation (EBL), sclerosants, and cyanoacrylate. Although they are of equivalent efficacy, we generally use EBL rather than sclerosants, but both should be available. Cyanoacrylate is also an excellent modality if the endoscopist has sufficient training in its administration. In patients with prior therapy for esophageal varices, mucosal scarring can prevent sufficient tissue from being suctioned into the cap for effective EBL. In these cases, sclerosants are superior to EBL. If the patient has a history of recent EBL, typically within the last 1 to 2 weeks, bleeding from banding ulcers is possible. In these cases, hemostatic clips are effective in treatment of these lesions. In cases of failed hemostasis with standard methods, a recent meta-analysis detailed the potential role for fully covered self-expanding metallic stents in patients with refractory esophageal variceal bleeding, with favorable findings.[10]

Gastric varices

There is less of a role for EBL in the treatment of gastric varices greater than 2 cm beyond the gastroesophageal (GE) junction. Actively bleeding gastric varices can be treated with high-volume sclerotherapy or cyanoacrylate (if available) while coordinating referral to transjugular intrahepatic portosystemic shunt therapy. There are published descriptions of other endoscopic methods for gastric varices, including endoloop ligation and clipping. Although we have used these approaches effectively in unique circumstances, they should be considered as salvage therapies.

Tumor bleeding
In patients with bleeding related to gastric or duodenal tumors, the role of endoscopy is predominantly limited to diagnosis. Palliative treatment of bleeding tissue with argon plasma beam coagulation (APC) is of no proven value compared with transcatheter arterial embolization, surgery, or radiotherapy.[11] The new class of hemostatic powders may prove effective in this context, at least as temporizing agents.

Dieulafoy lesions
Dieulafoy lesions can be difficult to target because they are rarely visualized unless actively bleeding. They are most commonly in the proximal stomach along the lesser curvature, although they may be elsewhere in the stomach or duodenum. In cases in which these lesions are identified, hemostatic clips or contact electrocoagulation are typically used, although EBL has also been described.

Aortoenteric fistula
In patients who present with severe upper GI bleeding and have a history of aortic graft surgery, especially if there was concern for infection, an aortoduodenal fistula should be considered. Erosion typical occurs in the second or third portion of the duodenum and the graft is visible in some cases. Endoscopic intervention is not advocated. Urgent vascular surgery consultation is recommended.

Postsphincterotomy bleeding
Postsphincterotomy bleeding can be challenging. We recommend use of a duodenoscope and initial injection of epinephrine solution (1:10,000) into the apex of the sphincterotomy and then along the lateral edges. Contact thermal therapy may be applied but care must be taken to avoid thermal injury to the pancreatic duct orifice. Hemostatic clips may be used in selected cases; however, the user must have considerable experience in the use of hemostatic clips with a duodenoscope in order to expect favorable results. In cases of torrential bleeding, placement of an inflated biliary balloon for tamponade may temporize bleeding. Fully or partially covered self-expanding metal mesh biliary stents have also been described for this purpose.[12]

Selection based on expected benefits and limitations
The limitations of each treatment modality should also be considered. Neither electrocoagulation therapy nor standard clips are effective in treating visible vessels greater than 2 mm.[13] To help gauge the size of a vessel before treatment, the diameter of the lesion can be compared with that of a standard clip or probe. Newer generation hemostatic clips with longer spans and made of stronger component metal have improved opportunities for use on larger lesions, so clinicians need to stay apprised of new devices as they are approved for use. For larger lesions, use of an over-the-scope clip (Ovesco Endoscopy) that is currently approved for endoscopic closure of GI defects may be considered.[14]

Successful treatment by electrocoagulation requires that the walls of a vessel be compressed while energy is applied to allow for coaptive coagulation. If a stable position is unable to be obtained for an effective treatment cycle, there is risk of unintentionally unroofing the lesion by pulling away partially coagulated tissue adherent to the probe.

Although APC can be useful for treating vascular ectasia, its utility in acute GI bleeding is otherwise limited. Because APC is used as a noncontact means of delivering thermal energy, the absence of coaptation limits its role for lesions other than vascular ectasia and bleeding or where there is risk for bleeding vessels within a resection site base. Contact with the APC probe increases the depth of burn and risk of perforation, and risks argon injection submucosally and transmurally.

Familiarity and experience of the endoscopist

The familiarity, experience and confidence of the physician using any specific device should be taken into consideration when selecting a treatment modality. For example, the rates of successful hemostasis are comparable in the treatment of bleeding ulcers or visible vessels with either hemostatic clips or electrocoagulation. Similarly, efficacy of esophageal variceal bleeding with either banding or sclerosants is comparable, although banding is associated with fewer adverse events. In these situations, the experience of the endoscopist may have a greater impact on outcome than the modality used.

The endoscopic devices themselves are also becoming more intricate and experience in their setup and use is essential for safe and expeditious use. Although an experienced endoscopy nurse or technician is a key component of any endoscopic team, there are times when they may not be present to assist. It is therefore imperative that the endoscopist be familiar with the use and setup of all equipment and be able to instruct an assistant on its proper use before the procedure. Delays while reviewing package inserts can be frustrating, stressful, and leave clinicians more prone to error; for example, when using an inadequately setup endoscopic bander on a large varix with high-risk stigmata. Scheduled in-service training can keep all members of the endoscopic team up to date and should be conducted periodically. Attaching a list of effective and safe power settings to the generator as well as quick reference cards for setting up devices can also be helpful as a quick and easy reference.

Opportunities for providers to stay up to date on newer devices and acquire hands-on experience are readily accessible either through online videos or hands-on endoscopic technique courses offered worldwide.

Tips on the Use of Specific Devices

When using hemostatic clips, position the open clip over the lesion, apply pressure, and then apply suction to improve the compliance of the tissue. The clip should then be closed but not deployed. Air can then be insufflated and the lie of the clip examined to ensure satisfactory positioning. If the positioning is suboptimal, the clip can be opened and the process repeated. Once satisfactory positioning is ensured, the clip can be fully deployed. The deployment technique used to fire the clip differs between brands in potentially hazardous ways; for example, failure to detach the clip from the catheter effectively or advancing the deployment device into the lesion can lead to worsened bleeding by unroofing the lesion or even to perforation.

When using contact electrocautery, it is important to ensure that the catheter is compressing the lesion such that it creates a crater effect, which indicates adequate apposition of the walls of the vessel for coaptive coagulation. Once the probe is positioned properly, it is important to treat for a sufficient duration. Upwards of 8 to 10 seconds of treatment per cycle is recommended. The tendency to perform shorter duration treatment with frequent inspection can result in inadvertent withdrawal of the probe with adherent coagulum stuck to a partially treated vessel, thus unroofing the lesion and exacerbating bleeding. To facilitate less traumatic probe separation, water can be flushed onto the lesion after treatment but before withdrawing the catheter. Most commercially available electrocoagulation probes have a water channel within the probe to facilitate this.

When using EBL and suctioning a varix into the cap, it is important to ensure that there is adequate tissue within the cap to maintain a proper pseudopolyp before the rubber band is deployed. Firing the device with too little tissue in the cap may result in unroofing the varix and exacerbation of bleeding (see supplemental Video 2). If an inadequate amount of tissue is being drawn into the cap, gentle torquing of the scope while suctioning and slightly pulling back on the scope can facilitate suctioning up of sufficient tissue. In all cases, once the tissue is aspirated into the banding chamber, it is preferable to deploy a band and not reposition repeatedly. Difficulty intubating with either a cap or a band ligation kit can typically be overcome by flexing the patient's neck slightly, inserting the endoscope while insufflating air, and applying mild torque on the scope in a slight back-and-forth motion.[15] Another means to aid in the insertion of the variceal banding chamber is to first place a commercially available esophageal overtube under endoscopic guidance. The banding chamber can then easily be inserted and withdrawn via the overtube, bypassing the laryngopharynx and cervical osteophytes.

When treating esophageal varies with stigmata (eg, white clot) or in the presence of active bleeding, we generally target the discrete lesion first and then continue to band other varices in a spiral-staircase fashion over the first 5 cm above the GE junction. Although some clinicians advocate treating the distalmost aspect of the varix first to decompress the proximal aspect and thus decrease risk of massive hemorrhage should the fibrin plug become dislodged, the passage of the scope with the bander itself by a large varix can dislodge the fibrin plug and lead to brisk bleeding that compromises visualization. When using sclerotherapy, the distal aspect of the varix should be targeted, then distal and proximal to the stigmata.

Tips to Help Localize the Source of Bleeding/Improve Visualization

Whenever possible, a thorough and complete endoscopic examination should be completed before initiating therapy. If there is concern for adequate visualization of the stomach because of ongoing bleeding or old blood, intravenous (IV) erythromycin 250 mg can be used to promote gastric emptying and improve visualization. Although not shown to improve patient outcome, erythromycin reduces the need for repeat endoscopy to confidently determine and target the source of bleeding[7,16]; it also decreases the frustration of the endoscopist caused by poor visualization. If the patient has an allergy to erythromycin, or it is not available, metoclopramide 10 mg IV may be considered, although it has been shown to be less effective in reducing the need for repeat endoscopy.[17,18] Prokinetic agents should be administered once the decision to scope has been made to allow time for gastric emptying, typically while setting up the equipment. One caveat of using prokinetic agents is that increasing gastric motility increases the possibility of a clearer view of a moving target. If it is not possible to administer the prokinetic at least 30 minutes before starting, then the benefits are likely to be negligible.

Mechanical clearance of blood and debris by nasogastric lavage is as effective as erythromycin[19] in clearing the gastric contents before endoscopy; however, because of the drawbacks of patient discomfort and potential for increasing aspiration risk, as mentioned earlier, prokinetic agents are preferred. Orogastric tubes are not commonly used in our practice because of increased risk for aspiration and suboptimal results. In cases in which a large clot in the fundus is unable to be cleared and obscures the view of a suspected source, repositioning of the patient from the left lateral decubitus to a right lateral decubitus position can shift the contents from the fundus to the antrum and increase visualization. Caution should be used with this approach because repositioning may increase the risk of aspiration.

If increased motility is preventing inspection or treatment of a lesion, 0.3 mg of IV glucagon can decrease gastric and duodenal motility. The onset of effect is about 1 minute and duration of action in the range of 9 to 17 minutes. Dosing may be repeated and is generally without significant side effects in doses less than 2 mg.

Lesions with adherent clots are a conundrum for some endoscopists given concern for provoking active bleeding versus the risks of not intervening on a high-risk lesion that may be concealed under the clot. The results of a meta-analysis[20] suggest that the optimal approach is to remove the clot with subsequent treatment of any high-risk stigmata. This approach can be done by injecting epinephrine at the clot base, carefully snaring off the clot while avoiding damage to possible underlying visible vessels and treating any high-risk stigmata by standard techniques (see supplemental Video 3). The primary benefit of this approach is that it reduces recurrent hemorrhage compared with medical treatment alone. However, in this study it did not significantly alter transfusion requirement, length of stay, or mortality. We prefer the proactive approach to removing the clot.

Do Not Snatch Defeat from the Jaws of Victory

When evaluating a patient for acute GI bleeding, it is tempting to treat all lesions that are identified. Familiarity with the Forrest classification system[21] for differentiating peptic ulcers that require endoscopic therapy (spurting hemorrhage, class Ia; oozing hemorrhage, class Ib; nonbleeding visible vessel, class IIa; and adherent clot, class IIb) from those with lower risk for rebleeding that should be left alone without intervention based on low risk for rebleeding (flat pigmented spot, class IIc; clean ulcer base, class III) helps to guide endoscopists away from overtreating and risking complications. Similarly, unless actively hemorrhaging, Mallory-Weiss tears typically stop spontaneously and intervention is rarely indicated. In contrast, if there is strong suspicion for an upper GI bleed and the only significant finding on examination is esophageal varices, then varices can be presumed to be the source and eradication of the varices should be initiated, preferably with EBL.

The Zen of Endoscopy: Keep Calm and Scope on

Successful management of patients with acute upper GI bleeding is a team effort. Endoscopy is not successful in definitively treating the source of acute upper GI bleeding in up to 8% to 15% of patients, which is why gastroenterologists do not manage these patients alone. Despite this, the role of the gastroenterologist in the management of these patients is crucial and can be rewarding given that endoscopic intervention reduces the risk of rebleeding, surgery, and mortality.[22] In order to optimize opportunities for success, it is important to create an environment for endoscopy in which team members remain calm and composed, which starts with proper training and experience, a clear plan of care that is known to all members of the team, good communication, and having the proper tools and equipment on hand. In addition, it is important to discuss and share experiences, both successful and unsuccessful, with other colleagues. This practice not only improves quality of care, but also reduces the anxiety and trepidation of the endoscopist in managing patients with acute bleeding following the inevitable cases with failed hemostasis.

SUPPLEMENTARY DATA

Supplementary data related to this article can be found online at http://dx.doi.org/10.1016/j.giec.2015.02.004.

REFERENCES

1. Villanueva C, Colomo A, Bosch A, et al. Transfusion strategies for acute upper gastrointestinal bleeding. N Engl J Med 2013;368(1):11–21.
2. Baron TH, Kamath PS, McBane RD. Management of antithrombotic therapy in patients undergoing invasive procedures. N Engl J Med 2013;368(22):2113–24.
3. Jensen DM, Machicado GA. Diagnosis and treatment of severe hematochezia. The role of urgent colonoscopy after purge. Gastroenterology 1988;95(6): 1569–74.
4. Aljebreen AM, Fallone CA, Barkun AN. Nasogastric aspirate predicts high-risk endoscopic lesions in patients with acute upper-GI bleeding. Gastrointest Endosc 2004;59(2):172–8.
5. Pallin DJ, Saltzman JR. Is nasogastric tube lavage in patients with acute upper GI bleeding indicated or antiquated? Gastrointest Endosc 2011;74(5):981–4.
6. Huang ES, Karsan S, Kanwal F, et al. Impact of nasogastric lavage on outcomes in acute GI bleeding. Gastrointest Endosc 2011;74(5):971–80.
7. Bai Y, Guo JF, Li ZS. Meta-analysis: erythromycin before endoscopy for acute upper gastrointestinal bleeding. Aliment Pharmacol Ther 2011;34(2):166–71.
8. Yap CK, Ng HS. Cap-fitted gastroscopy improves visualization and targeting of lesions. Gastrointest Endosc 2001;53(1):93–5.
9. Calvet X, Vergara M, Brullet E, et al. Addition of a second endoscopic treatment following epinephrine injection improves outcome in high-risk bleeding ulcers. Gastroenterology 2004;126(2):441–50.
10. Wright G, Lewis H, Hogan B, et al. A self-expanding metal stent for complicated variceal hemorrhage: experience at a single center. Gastrointest Endosc 2010; 71(1):71–8.
11. Maluf-Filho F, Martins Bda C, de Lima MS, et al. Etiology, endoscopic management and mortality of upper gastrointestinal bleeding in patients with cancer. United European Gastroenterol J 2013;1(1):60–7.
12. Shah JN, Marson F, Binmoeller KF. Temporary self-expandable metal stent placement for treatment of post-sphincterotomy bleeding. Gastrointest Endosc 2010; 72(6):1274–8.
13. Technology Assessment C, Chuttani R, Barkun A, et al. Endoscopic clip application devices. Gastrointest Endosc 2006;63(6):746–50.
14. Kirschniak A, Subotova N, Zieker D, et al. The Over-The-Scope Clip (OTSC) for the treatment of gastrointestinal bleeding, perforations, and fistulas. Surg Endosc 2011;25(9):2901–5.
15. Baron TH, Wong Kee Song LM. Endoscopic variceal band ligation. Am J Gastroenterol 2009;104(5):1083–5.
16. Frossard JL, Spahr L, Queneau PE, et al. Erythromycin intravenous bolus infusion in acute upper gastrointestinal bleeding: a randomized, controlled, double-blind trial. Gastroenterology 2002;123(1):17–23.
17. Barkun AN, Bardou M, Martel M, et al. Prokinetics in acute upper GI bleeding: a meta-analysis. Gastrointest Endosc 2010;72(6):1138–45.
18. Daram SR, Garretson R. Erythromycin is preferable to metoclopramide as a prokinetic in acute upper GI bleeding [author reply: 5]. Gastrointest Endosc 2011; 74(1):234.

19. Pateron D, Vicaut E, Debuc E, et al. Erythromycin infusion or gastric lavage for upper gastrointestinal bleeding: a multicenter randomized controlled trial. Ann Emerg Med 2011;57(6):582–9.
20. Kahi CJ, Jensen DM, Sung JJ, et al. Endoscopic therapy versus medical therapy for bleeding peptic ulcer with adherent clot: a meta-analysis. Gastroenterology 2005;129(3):855–62.
21. Forrest JA, Finlayson ND, Shearman DJ. Endoscopy in gastrointestinal bleeding. Lancet 1974;2(7877):394–7.
22. Cook DJ, Guyatt GH, Salena BJ, et al. Endoscopic therapy for acute nonvariceal upper gastrointestinal hemorrhage: a meta-analysis. Gastroenterology 1992; 102(1):139–48.

Moving?

Make sure your subscription moves with you!

To notify us of your new address, find your **Clinics Account Number** (located on your mailing label above your name), and contact customer service at:

Email: journalscustomerservice-usa@elsevier.com

800-654-2452 (subscribers in the U.S. & Canada)
314-447-8871 (subscribers outside of the U.S. & Canada)

Fax number: 314-447-8029

Elsevier Health Sciences Division
Subscription Customer Service
3251 Riverport Lane
Maryland Heights, MO 63043

*To ensure uninterrupted delivery of your subscription, please notify us at least 4 weeks in advance of move.

Printed and bound by CPI Group (UK) Ltd, Croydon, CR0 4YY

03/10/2024

01040491-0002